TEXTBOOK OF DERMATOLOGY

VOLUME 2

INFECTIOUS, PIGMENTARY, GENETIC, AND PEDIATRIC DERMATOLOGICAL DISORDERS

Dr. Mariya Kharodawala

ALLIED HEALTH PRESS

Textbook of Dermatology

Volume 2: Infectious, Pigmentary, Genetic, and Pediatric Dermatological Disorders

Author: **Dr. Mariya Kharodawala**

Allied Health Press
4164 Lakeshore Road
Burlington ON L7L 1A4
Canada
www.alliedhealthpress.com
Email: orders@arclereducation.com

ISBN: 978-1-77956-826-7

ABOUT THE AUTHOR

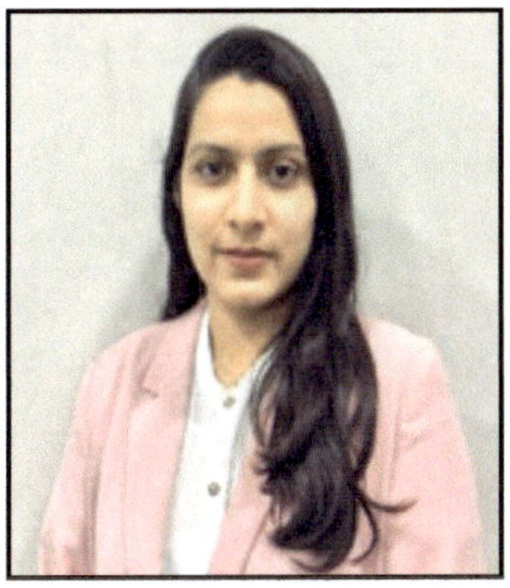

Dr. Mariya Kharodawala holds an MBBS degree with a gold medal from The Maharaja Sayajirao University of Baroda and an MD in Dermatology, Venereology, and Leprosy from B. J. Medical College, Pune, both of which are among the premier medical institutes in India. She is currently working as a Senior Resident in Dermatology. Her areas of interest include clinical dermatology, dermatopathology, and academic writing. Over the years, she has contributed to peer-reviewed journals and actively participated in national and international conferences. Her professional journey is driven by a passion for continuous learning, research, and teaching. Alongside her academic pursuits, she is committed to bridging the gap between medical knowledge and public awareness through digital platforms. Reviewing this comprehensive dermatology textbook has been an intellectually rewarding experience, and she is delighted to contribute to the academic growth of future dermatologists.

Brief Table of Contents

1. Fungal Infections	**1**
2. Parasitic Infestations	**27**
3. Cutaneous Tuberculosis and Leprosy	**47**
4. Hyperpigmentation Disorders	**73**
5. Hypopigmentation and Depigmentation Disorders	**97**
6. Vesiculobullous Diseases	**117**
7. Connective Tissue Diseases	**141**
8. Vasculitis and Purpura	**161**
9. Sarcoidosis and Granulomatous Skin Conditions	**187**
10. Genetic Skin Disorders	**213**
11. Pediatric Dermatology: Common Childhood Skin Conditions	**233**
12. Neonatal Dermatology and Birthmarks	**261**
Index	**285**

Getting Started with This Book

Chapter Openers

A list of Chapter Outline is presented providing a brief Introduction to what will be covered in the chapter.

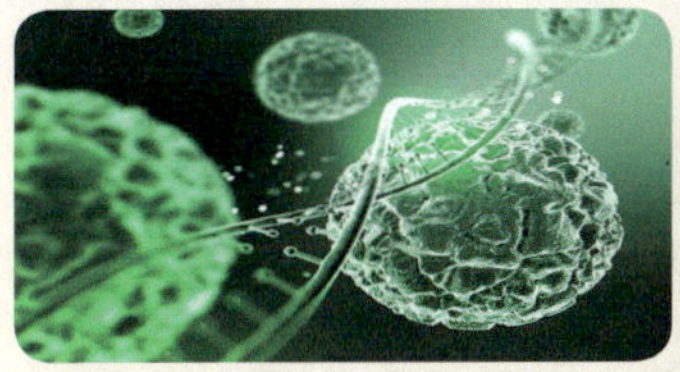

LEARNING OBJECTIVES

After studying this chapter, you will be able to:

1. Discuss the scientific method in biology;
2. Explain the cell theory;
3. Discuss the genetics and heredity;
4. Evolution and natural selection;
5. Focus on ecology and ecosystems;
6. Learn about human biology;
7. Evaluate the plant biology;
8. Explain the microbiology;
9. Focus on current trends in biology.

Introduction

Often referred to as the science of life, biology is a broad field of study aimed at comprehending the several kinds of life on Earth, from tiny creatures to sophisticated multicellular entities. Comprising several subfields, including molecular biology, ecology, and evolutionary biology, each of which advances our knowledge of living systems, this field clarifies the mechanisms controlling life events, including development, reproduction, and interaction with the surroundings, which is the central goal of biology. Moreover, biology fills in the void between the natural sciences and medicine by offering a necessary understanding of health, illness, and the interactions between organisms and their environments. Dealing with urgent global issues such as climate change, biodiversity loss, and new diseases depends on an awareness of these complex biological interactions, therefore highlighting the critical part biology plays in modern civilization. Fundamentally, biology explores and tests ideas about the living world using the scientific method. Through methodical observation and experimentation,

Learning Outcomes

1.1. The Scientific Method in Biology

Learning Outcome

1. Describe the steps of the scientific method;
2. Focus on hypothesis formation;
3. Learn about experimental design.

The beginning of each section of every chapter contains a set of Learning Outcomes that inform students of concepts they should understand. These outcomes help students understand what they should be able to do if they have mastered the material in that section.

Test Your Knowledge

Throughout each chapter, Test Your Knowledge cues you to note which topics have been covered and to self-test your understanding of the material presented.

Test Your Knowledge

1. Explain why correlation does not imply causation in scientific experiments.
2. How does the scientific method help reduce the influence of personal opinions in research?

Chapter Summary

The Summary Section appear at the end of each chapter and summarize main concepts covered throughout the chapter. These points provide key concepts in an engaging and meaningful way.

Summary

The investigation of biological principles highlights the importance of a comprehensive view of life by reflecting the intricate interactions that occur within living systems. The complexity of biology goes beyond individual species or systems, as this essay highlights; it also includes the interactions that mold ecosystems and affect biodiversity. Researchers can conduct in-depth analyses of metabolomic data using sophisticated technologies like MetaboAnalyst, which offer insights into the molecular mechanisms underlying these interactions. As demonstrated by the developments in MetaboAnalyst, for example, the integration of diverse omics data promotes a thorough understanding of metabolic pathways and helps identify important biological markers necessary for research on development and disease (Chong et al., 2018). Additionally, the phenomenon of ecological invasions is a key component of biological research and a vital field of study. The introduction of non-native species into unfamiliar habitats has significant ramifications and calls for multidisciplinary management strategies. Examining the origins and effects of these biological incursions, invasion science has become a crucial field that highlights the need to comprehend ecological dynamics and community interactions. As interest in biological invasions increases, new findings are emerging that put conventional ecological theories and practices to the test. The importance of incorporating various scientific viewpoints is shown by this developing discipline, which also highlights how invasive species shape ecosystems and advances our knowledge of ecological resilience (David et al., 2013). When taken as a whole, these discoveries from invasion science and metabolomics highlight the value of multidisciplinary biology research. Fostering cross-disciplinary collaboration and utilizing technological breakthroughs to improve our comprehension of intricate biological interactions are crucial as we look to the future of biological research. In addition to deepening our understanding of the complexities of life, this method lays the groundwork for tackling urgent environmental issues. Future studies can ensure the continued relevance of biology in a world that is constantly changing by acknowledging the interconnection of biological systems and opening the door to creative solutions that support sustainability and biodiversity conservation. We might imagine a thorough comprehension of life that serves both academia and society at large through ongoing investigation and integration of scientific knowledge.

Knowledge Assessment

The chapter includes material designed to review and reinforce each content. It includes Critical Thinking Questions to help test of your understanding of information presented in the chapter and Short answer Questions to review your understanding of the key concepts presented in the chapter.

Critical Thinking Questions

1. **Who is known as the "Father of Modern Biology"?**
   a. Aristotle
   b. Charles Darwin
   c. Gregor Mendel
   d. Louis Pasteur
2. **What is the basic unit of life?**
   a. Atom
   b. Molecule
   c. Cell
   d. Organism
3. **Which branch of biology studies the interaction of organisms with their environment?**
   a. Genetics
   b. Ecology
   c. Physiology
   d. Botany
4. **Which macromolecule is the main source of energy for living organisms?**
   a. Proteins
   b. Lipids
   c. Carbohydrates
   d. Nucleic acids
5. **DNA is primarily responsible for which function in living organisms?**
   a. Energy production
   b. Protein synthesis
   c. Storing genetic information
   d. Regulating body temperature

Short Answer Questions

1. What is biology, and why is it important to study biology?
2. What are the three main domains of life, and how are they different from one another?
3. Define homeostasis and give an example of how it works in living organisms.
4. What is the cell theory, and why is it fundamental to biology?
5. How do autotrophs and heterotrophs differ in the way they obtain energy?
6. What is the scientific method, and how is it applied in biological research?
7. Discuss how biology helps address global challenges such as climate change, disease, and food security.
8. Explain the levels of biological organization from the smallest unit to the largest. Provide examples at each level.
9. Describe the relationship between structure and function in biology, giving specific examples from cells or organs.
10. How has the discovery of genetics shaped our understanding of inheritance and variation among organisms?

Supplementary Materials

Key Terms: A list of key terms is given for quick reference

KEY TERMS FROM THIS CHAPTER

Annotation enrichment analysis	Biological structure	Cell
Cell theory	Cellular structure	Ecology
Ecosystems	Genetics	Human biology
Microbiology	Natural selection	Organism
Plant biology		

Further Resources: Recommendations for additional readings, websites, and multimedia resources.

References

1. Argelaguet, R., Velten, B., Arnol, D., Dietrich, S., Zenz, T., Marioni, J. C., Buettner, F., et al. (2018). Multi-omics factor analysis—A framework for unsupervised integration of multi-omics data sets. *Molecular Systems Biology, 14*. https://doi.org/10.15252/msb.20178124.
2. Bacher, S., Blackburn, T. M., Essl, F., & Genovesi, P. (2017). *Socio-Economic Impact Classification of Alien Taxa (SEICAT)*. https://core.ac.uk/download/286567949.pdf (accessed on 8th March 2025).
3. Barnett, R., Brace, S., Cucchi, T., & Dobney, K. (2013). *Divergent Evolutionary Processes Associated with Colonization of Offshore Islands*. https://core.ac.uk/download/20664364.pdf (accessed on 8th March 2025).

Detailed Table of Contents

List of Figures *xvii*
Preface *xxix*

CHAPTER 1

Fungal Infections 1

Introduction **1**
1.1. Superficial Mycoses **2**
1.1.1. Definition and Characteristics 2
1.1.2. Common Types of Superficial Mycoses 3
1.1.3. Causative Agents of Superficial Mycoses 3
1.1.4. Risk Factors for Superficial Infections 3
1.1.5. Symptoms and Clinical Manifestations 4
1.1.6. Diagnosis of Superficial Mycoses 4
1.1.7. Treatment Options for Superficial Infections 5
1.1.8. Prevention Strategies 5
1.2. Deep Mycoses **6**
1.2.1. Definition and Characteristics 6
1.2.2. Common Types of Deep Mycoses 6
1.2.3. Causative Agents of Deep Mycoses 7
1.2.4. Risk Factors for Deep Infections 7
1.2.5. Symptoms and Clinical Manifestations 8
1.2.6. Diagnosis of Deep Mycoses 8
1.2.7. Treatment Options for Deep Infections 8
1.2.8. Complications Associated with Deep Mycoses 9
1.3. Epidemiology of Fungal Infections **10**
1.3.1. Global Prevalence of Fungal Infections 10
1.3.2. Demographic Factors Influencing Infection Rates 11
1.3.3. Geographic Distribution of Mycoses 11
1.3.4. Trends in Fungal Infection Outbreaks 12
1.3.5. Role of Climate Change in Fungal Infections 12
1.3.6. Impact of Immunocompromised Populations 13
1.3.7. Surveillance and Reporting Systems 13
1.3.8. Public Health Initiatives 14
1.3.9. Future Directions in Epidemiological Research 14
1.4. Advances in Research and Treatment **15**
1.4.1. Recent Developments in Antifungal Therapies 15
1.4.2. Novel Drug Targets and Mechanisms 16
1.4.3. Role of Immunotherapy in Fungal Infections 16
1.4.4. Advances in Diagnostic Techniques 17
1.4.5. Research on Vaccine Development 17
1.4.6. Importance of Microbiome Studies 17
1.4.7. Challenges in Antifungal Resistance 18
1.4.8. Role of Technology in Fungal Infection Management 18
1.4.9. Future Research Priorities 19
Summary **20**
References **22**

CHAPTER 2

Parasitic Infestations 27

Introduction **27**
2.1. Scabies **28**

2.1.1. Causative Agent: Sarcoptes scabiei 28
2.1.2. Transmission and Risk Factors 29
2.1.3. Symptoms and Clinical Presentation 29
2.1.4. Diagnosis Methods 29
2.1.5. Treatment Options 30
2.1.6. Prevention Strategies 30
2.1.7. Complications Associated with Scabies 31
2.1.8. Scabies in Different Populations 31
2.1.9. Global Prevalence and Epidemiology 31
2.2. Lice 33
2.2.1. Types of Lice: Head Lice, Body Lice, and Pubic Lice 33
2.2.2. Life Cycle of Lice 33
2.2.3. Symptoms and Signs of Infestation 34
2.2.4. Diagnosis and Identification 34
2.2.5. Treatment and Management Strategies 35
2.2.6. Social Stigma and Psychological Impact 35
2.2.7. Prevention and Control Measures 35
2.2.8. Lice in Various Demographics 36
2.3. Leishmaniasis 37
2.3.1. Causative Agents: Leishmania Species 37
2.3.2. Transmission Through Sandflies 38
2.3.3. Types of Leishmaniasis: Cutaneous, Visceral, and Mucocutaneous 38
2.3.4. Symptoms and Clinical Manifestations 38
2.3.5. Diagnosis Techniques 39
2.3.6. Treatment Options and Challenges 39
2.3.7. Impact on Affected Populations 40
2.3.8. Prevention and Control Strategies 40
2.3.9. Global Distribution and Epidemiological Trends 40
Summary 42
References 44

CHAPTER 3

Cutaneous Tuberculosis and Leprosy 47

Introduction 47
3.1. Pathophysiology of Cutaneous Tuberculosis 48
3.1.1. Causative Agent: Mycobacterium tuberculosis 48
3.1.2. Mechanism of Skin Involvement 49
3.1.3. Immune Response to Infection 49
3.1.4. Types of Cutaneous Lesions 50
3.1.5. Diagnostic Methods for Cutaneous Tuberculosis 50
3.1.6. Differential Diagnosis with Other Skin Conditions 51
3.1.7. Complications Associated with Untreated Cases 51
3.1.8. Role of Genetics in Susceptibility 51
3.2. Pathophysiology of Leprosy 53
3.2.1. Causative Agent: Mycobacterium leprae 53
3.2.2. Mechanism of Skin and Nerve Involvement 54
3.2.3. Immune Response and Its Variations 54
3.2.4. Types of Leprosy and Their Clinical Features 55
3.2.5. Diagnostic Methods for Leprosy 55
3.2.6. Differential Diagnosis with Other Dermatological Diseases 56
3.2.7. Complications and Long-term Effects 56
3.2.8. Genetic Factors Influencing Disease Progression 57
3.2.9. Recent Advancements in Understanding Leprosy 57
3.3. Treatment and Management 58
3.3.1. Standard Treatment Protocols for Cutaneous Tuberculosis 58
3.3.2. Standard Treatment Protocols for Leprosy 59
3.3.3. Role of Antibiotics in Treatment 60
3.3.4. Importance of Early Diagnosis and Intervention 60
3.3.5. Management of Complications and Co-morbidities 61
3.3.6. Patient Education and Adherence to Treatment 61
3.3.7. Role of Public Health Initiatives 61
3.3.8. Challenges in Treatment Accessibility 62
3.4. Societal and Cultural Implications 63
3.4.1. Historical Stigma Associated with Both Diseases 64
3.4.2. Impact on Mental Health and Well-being 64
3.4.3. Cultural Perceptions and Misconceptions 65
3.4.4. Role of Advocacy and Awareness Campaigns 65
3.4.5. Socioeconomic Factors Influencing Disease Spread 65

3.4.6. Integration of Care into Community Health Systems 66
3.4.7. Global Health Policies Addressing These Diseases 66
3.4.8. Future Challenges in Societal Acceptance 67
Summary **68**
References **70**

CHAPTER 4

Hyperpigmentation Disorders 73

Introduction **73**
4.1. Understanding Hyperpigmentation **74**
4.1.1. Definition and Mechanisms of Hyperpigmentation 74
4.1.2. Types of Hyperpigmentation Disorders 75
4.1.3. Role of Melanin in Skin Pigmentation 75
4.1.4. Genetic Factors Influencing Hyperpigmentation 76
4.1.5. Environmental Triggers (Sun Exposure and Pollution) 76
4.1.6. Hormonal Influences (Pregnancy and Contraceptives) 76
4.1.7. Skin Types and their Susceptibility 77
4.1.8. Psychological Effects of Hyperpigmentation 77
4.1.9. Importance of Skin Care in Prevention 78
4.2. Melasma **78**
4.2.1. Definition and Characteristics of Melasma 79
4.2.2. Common Causes and Risk Factors 79
4.2.3. Diagnosis and Clinical Evaluation 79
4.2.4. Treatment Options (Topical and Procedural) 80
4.2.5. Role of Sun Protection in Management 80
4.2.6. Recurrence Rates and Long-term Management 81
4.2.7. Differences between Melasma and Other Disorders 81
4.2.8. Impact of Melasma on Self-esteem 82
4.3. Post-Inflammatory Hyperpigmentation (PIH) **83**
4.3.1. Definition and Causes of Post-Inflammatory Hyperpigmentation (PIH) 83
4.3.2. Common Conditions Leading to Post-Inflammatory Hyperpigmentation (PIH) 84
4.3.3. Mechanism of Post-Inflammatory Hyperpigmentation (PIH) Development 84
4.3.4. Diagnosis and Differentiation from Other Disorders 84
4.3.5. Treatment Strategies for Post-Inflammatory Hyperpigmentation (PIH) 85
4.3.6. Role of Skin Care in Prevention 85
4.3.7. Psychological Impact of Post-Inflammatory Hyperpigmentation (PIH) 86
4.3.8. Importance of Patient Education 86
4.3.9. Emerging Therapies and Research 87
4.4. Other Hyperpigmentation Disorders **88**
4.4.1. Overview of Less Common Hyperpigmentation Disorders 88
4.4.2. Lentigines and Their Characteristics 89
4.4.3. Nevus of Ota and Its Implications 89
4.4.4. Drug-induced Hyperpigmentation 89
4.4.5. Role of Systemic Diseases in Hyperpigmentation 90
4.4.6. Diagnosis and Management of Rare Disorders 90
4.4.7. Importance of Differential Diagnosis 91
4.4.8. Patient Support and Resources 91
Summary **92**
References **94**

CHAPTER 5

Hypopigmentation and Depigmentation Disorders 97

Introduction **97**
5.1. Vitiligo **98**
5.1.1. Definition and Classification of Vitiligo 98
5.1.2. Causes and Risk Factors 98
5.1.3. Symptoms and Clinical Presentation 99
5.1.4. Diagnosis and Differential Diagnosis 100
5.1.5. Psychological Impact on Patients 100
5.1.6. Treatment Options and Management Strategies 100
5.1.7. Role of Lifestyle and Home Remedies 101
5.2. Albinism **102**
5.2.1. Definition and Types of Albinism 102
5.2.2. Genetic Basis and Inheritance Patterns 103

5.2.3. Physical Characteristics and Symptoms 103
5.2.4. Associated Health Issues (e.g., Vision Problems) 103
5.2.5. Social and Cultural Implications 104
5.2.6. Diagnosis and Screening Methods 104
5.2.7. Treatment and Management of Symptoms 105
5.2.8. Advocacy and Support for Individuals with Albinism 105
5.3. Societal and Cultural Perspectives 106
5.3.1. Historical Views on Skin Color and Beauty 106
5.3.2. Media Representation of Hypopigmentation Disorders 107
5.3.3. Cultural Beliefs and Myths Surrounding Vitiligo and Albinism 107
5.3.4. Impact of Social Media on Awareness and Acceptance 108
5.3.5. Role of Advocacy Groups and Organizations 108
5.3.6. Education and Outreach Programs 108
5.3.7. Legal Protections and Discrimination Issues 109
5.3.8. Global Perspectives on Skin Disorders 109
5.3.9. Future Trends in Societal Attitudes 110
Summary 111
References 113

CHAPTER 6

Vesiculobullous Diseases 117

Introduction 117
6.1. Pemphigus: An Overview 118
6.1.1. Definition and Classification of Pemphigus 118
6.1.2. Types of Pemphigus (e.g., Pemphigus Vulgaris, Pemphigus Foliaceus) 119
6.1.3. Etiology and Risk Factors 119
6.1.4. Pathophysiology of Pemphigus 120
6.1.5. Clinical Manifestations and Symptoms 120
6.1.6. Diagnostic Methods and Criteria 121
6.1.7. Treatment Options and Management Strategies 121
6.1.8. Prognosis and Potential Complications 122
6.2. Bullous Pemphigoid: An Overview 122
6.2.1. Definition and Classification of Bullous Pemphigoid 123
6.2.2. Etiology and Risk Factors 123
6.2.3. Pathophysiology of Bullous Pemphigoid 124
6.2.4. Clinical Manifestations and Symptoms 124
6.2.5. Diagnostic Methods and Criteria 124
6.2.6. Treatment Options and Management Strategies 125
6.2.7. Prognosis and Potential Complications 126
6.3. Diagnosis and Differential Diagnosis 126
6.3.1. Importance of Accurate Diagnosis 126
6.3.2. Clinical Evaluation and Patient History 127
6.3.3. Laboratory Tests and Skin Biopsies 127
6.3.4. Immunofluorescence Studies 128
6.3.5. Differential Diagnosis of Vesiculobullous Diseases 128
6.3.6. Role of Dermatopathology 128
6.3.7. Challenges in Diagnosis 129
6.3.8. Emerging Diagnostic Techniques 130
6.4. Treatment and Management Strategies 130
6.4.1. Overview of Treatment Goals 131
6.4.2. Pharmacological Treatments (e.g., Corticosteroids and Immunosuppressants) 131
6.4.3. Non-pharmacological Management Strategies 132
6.4.4. Role of Patient Education and Support 132
6.4.5. Monitoring and Follow-up Care 132
6.4.6. Management of Complications 133
6.4.7. Impact of Lifestyle Changes on Disease Management 134
6.4.8. Multidisciplinary Approach to Treatment 134
Summary 135
References 137

CHAPTER 7

Connective Tissue Diseases 141

Introduction 141
7.1. Systemic Lupus Erythematosus (SLE) 142
7.1.1. Definition and Classification of Lupus 142
7.1.2. Etiology and Risk Factors 143
7.1.3. Common Symptoms and Manifestations 143

7.1.4. Diagnostic Criteria and Methods 144
7.1.5. Treatment Options and Management Strategies 144
7.1.6. Complications Associated with Lupus 145
7.1.7. Psychological Impact on Patients 145
7.1.8. Role of Lifestyle Modifications 146
7.2. Dermatomyositis 147
7.2.1. Definition and Classification of Dermatomyositis 147
7.2.2. Etiology and Potential Triggers 148
7.2.3. Characteristic Skin Rashes and Muscle Weakness 148
7.2.4. Diagnostic Approaches and Criteria 148
7.2.5. Treatment Modalities and Rehabilitation 149
7.2.6. Associated Conditions and Comorbidities 149
7.2.7. Long-term Prognosis and Outcomes 150
7.2.8. Importance of Patient Education 150
7.3. Scleroderma 151
7.3.1. Definition and Types of Scleroderma 151
7.3.2. Pathophysiology and Immune Response 152
7.3.3. Common Symptoms and Organ Involvement 152
7.3.4. Diagnostic Techniques and Challenges 153
7.3.5. Treatment Options and Management Approaches 153
7.3.6. Impact on Daily Living and Functionality 154
7.3.7. Psychological and Emotional Considerations 154
7.3.8. Support Systems and Resources for Patients 155
7.3.9. Emerging Research and Therapeutic Strategies 155
Summary 156
References 158

CHAPTER 8

Vasculitis and Purpura 161

Introduction 161
8.1. Types of Vasculitis 162
8.1.1. Large Vessel Vasculitis 162
8.1.2. Medium Vessel Vasculitis 162
8.1.3. Small Vessel Vasculitis 163
8.1.4. Primary vs. Secondary Vasculitis 163
8.1.5. Systemic vs. Localized Vasculitis 164
8.1.6. Common Types: Giant Cell Arteritis 164
8.1.7. Common Types: Takayasu arteritis 165
8.1.8. Common Types: ANCA-associated Vasculitis 165
8.1.9. Rare Forms of Vasculitis 165
8.2. Pathophysiology of Vasculitis 166
8.2.1. Immune System Involvement 166
8.2.2. Genetic Predispositions 167
8.2.3. Environmental Triggers 167
8.2.4. Inflammatory Processes 168
8.2.5. Vascular Damage Mechanisms 168
8.2.6. Role of Cytokines and Chemokines 168
8.2.7. Consequences of Vascular Inflammation 169
8.2.8. Interaction with Other Diseases 169
8.2.9. Diagnostic Challenges in Understanding Pathophysiology 170
8.3. Purpura: Causes and Types 170
8.3.1. Definition and Characteristics of Purpura 171
8.3.2. Thrombocytopenic purpura 171
8.3.3. Non-thrombocytopenic Purpura 172
8.3.4. Causes Related to Vasculitis 172
8.3.5. Causes Related to Infections 172
8.3.6. Causes Related to Medications 173
8.3.7. Causes Related to Systemic Diseases 173
8.3.8. Idiopathic Purpura 173
8.3.9. Diagnostic Criteria for Purpura 174
8.4. Diagnosis and Treatment 175
8.4.1. Clinical Evaluation and History Taking 175
8.4.2. Laboratory Tests for Vasculitis 176
8.4.3. Imaging Studies for Vascular Assessment 176
8.4.4. Biopsy Procedures and Their Significance 176
8.4.5. Treatment Options for Vasculitis 177
8.4.6. Treatment Options for Purpura 177
8.4.7. Role of Corticosteroids 177
8.4.8. Immunosuppressive Therapies 178
8.4.9. Monitoring and Follow-up Care 178
Summary 180
References 182

CHAPTER 9

Sarcoidosis and Granulomatous Skin Conditions 187

Introduction 187

9.1. Pathophysiology of Sarcoidosis 188

9.1.1. Immune Response in Sarcoidosis 188

9.1.2. Formation of Granulomas 189

9.1.3. Genetic Predisposition 189

9.1.4. Environmental Triggers 189

9.1.5. Role of Cytokines 190

9.1.6. Systemic Effects of Sarcoidosis 190

9.1.7. Differences between Localized and Systemic Sarcoidosis 191

9.1.8. Diagnostic Criteria for Sarcoidosis 191

9.1.9. Challenges in Understanding the Pathophysiology 192

9.2. Clinical Manifestations of Sarcoidosis 192

9.2.1. Common Symptoms of Sarcoidosis 193

9.2.2. Skin Manifestations of Sarcoidosis 193

9.2.3. Pulmonary Involvement 194

9.2.4. Ocular Complications 194

9.2.5. Cardiac Involvement 194

9.2.6. Neurological Symptoms 195

9.2.7. Musculoskeletal Symptoms 196

9.2.8. Variability in Presentation 196

9.2.9. Importance of Early Detection 196

9.3. Granulomatous Skin Conditions 198

9.3.1. Definition and Types of Granulomatous Skin Conditions 198

9.3.2. Common Granulomatous Diseases (e.g., Granuloma Annulare) 199

9.3.3. Pathophysiology of Granulomatous Skin Conditions 199

9.3.4. Clinical Features of Granulomatous Skin Conditions 200

9.3.5. Diagnostic Approaches for Granulomatous Skin Conditions 200

9.3.6. Treatment Options for Granulomatous Skin Conditions 201

9.3.7. Differential Diagnosis of Granulomatous Skin Conditions 201

9.3.8. Prognosis and Outcomes 202

9.4. Diagnosis and Management of Sarcoidosis 202

9.4.1. Diagnostic Imaging Techniques 203

9.4.2. Laboratory Tests for Sarcoidosis 203

9.4.3. Biopsy and Histopathological Examination 203

9.4.4. Treatment Options for Sarcoidosis 204

9.4.5. Role of Corticosteroids 204

9.4.6. Monitoring Disease Progression 205

9.4.7. Multidisciplinary Approach to Management 205

9.4.8. Patient Education and Support 205

Summary 207

References 209

CHAPTER 10

Genetic Skin Disorders 213

Introduction 213

10.1. Ichthyosis 214

10.1.1. Definition and Types of Ichthyosis 214

10.1.2. Genetic Mutations associated with Ichthyosis 214

10.1.3. Symptoms and Clinical Presentation 215

10.1.4. Diagnosis and Testing Methods 215

10.1.5. Treatment Options and Management Strategies 216

10.1.6. Psychological and Social Implications 217

10.2. Epidermolysis Bullosa 218

10.2.1. Definition and Classification of Epidermolysis Bullosa 218

10.2.2. Genetic Mutations Linked to Epidermolysis Bullosa 219

10.2.3. Symptoms and Clinical Manifestations 219

10.2.4. Diagnosis and Assessment Techniques 219

10.2.5. Treatment Options and Care Management 220

10.2.6. Impact on Daily Living and Mental Health 221

10.2.7. Future Perspectives in Epidermolysis Bullosa Treatment 221

10.3. Societal and Ethical Considerations 222

10.3.1. Stigmatization of Individuals with Skin Disorders 222

10.3.2. Access to Healthcare and Treatment Disparities 223

10.3.3. Ethical Implications of Genetic Testing 223

10.3.4. Role of Advocacy Groups and Support Networks 224
10.3.5. Public Awareness Campaigns and Education 224
10.3.6. Psychological Support for Affected Individuals 224
10.3.7. Employment and Social Integration Challenges 225
10.3.8. Insurance Coverage and Financial Burdens 225
10.3.9. Future Ethical Considerations in Genetic Research 226
Summary **227**
References **229**

CHAPTER 11

Pediatric Dermatology: Common Childhood Skin Conditions 233

Introduction **233**
11.1. Eczema (Atopic Dermatitis) **234**
11.1.1. Definition and Types of Eczema 234
11.1.2. Symptoms and Signs of Eczema 235
11.1.3. Common Triggers for Eczema Flare-ups 235
11.1.4. Diagnosis Methods for Eczema 235
11.1.5. Treatment Options for Eczema 236
11.1.6. Role of Moisturizers in Management 236
11.1.7. Long-term Management Strategies 237
11.1.8. Psychological Impact of Eczema on Children 237
11.1.9. Parental Education and Support Resources 238
11.2. Acne in Adolescents **238**
11.2.1. Definition and Types of Acne 239
11.2.2. Causes of Acne in Adolescents 239
11.2.3. Symptoms and Severity Classification 240
11.2.4. Diagnosis and Assessment of Acne 240
11.2.5. Treatment Options for Acne 241
11.2.6. Importance of Skincare Routines 241
11.2.7. Psychological Effects of Acne on Teenagers 241
11.2.8. Myths and Misconceptions About Acne 242
11.2.9. Role of Diet and Lifestyle in Acne Management 242
11.3. Psoriasis in Children **243**
11.3.1. Definition and Types of Psoriasis 243
11.3.2. Symptoms and Clinical Presentation 244
11.3.3. Causes and Risk Factors for Psoriasis 244
11.3.4. Diagnosis and Differential Diagnosis 245
11.3.5. Treatment Options for Pediatric Psoriasis 245
11.3.6. Importance of Early Intervention 246
11.3.7. Impact of Psoriasis on Children's Social Life 246
11.3.8. Long-term Management and Follow-up Care 247
11.3.9. Support Groups and Resources for Families 247
11.4. Infectious Skin Conditions **249**
11.4.1. Overview of Common Infectious Skin Conditions 249
11.4.2. Impetigo: Causes, Symptoms, and Treatment 250
11.4.3. Fungal Infections: Types and Management 250
11.4.4. Viral Infections: Warts and Molluscum Contagiosum 250
11.4.5. Scabies: Symptoms and Treatment Options 251
11.4.6. Importance of Hygiene in Prevention 251
11.4.7. Diagnosis Challenges in Pediatric Patients 252
11.4.8. Impact of Infections on School Attendance 252
11.4.9. Parental Guidance on Prevention and Care 252
Summary **254**
References **256**

CHAPTER 12

Neonatal Dermatology and Birthmarks 261

Introduction **261**
12.1. Types of Birthmarks **262**
12.1.1. Vascular Birthmarks: Definition and Examples 262
12.1.2. Pigmented Birthmarks: Definition and Examples 263
12.1.3. Differences between Congenital and Acquired Birthmarks 263

12.1.4. Common Types of Vascular Birthmarks (e.g., Hemangiomas) 264
12.1.5. Common Types of Pigmented Birthmarks (e.g., Café-au-lait Spots) 264
12.1.6. Rare Birthmarks and Their Implications 264
12.1.7. Genetic Factors Influencing Birthmark Development 265
12.1.8. Environmental Factors Affecting Birthmarks 265
12.1.9. Psychological Impact of Visible Birthmarks on Infants 266
12.2. Diagnosis and Assessment 267
12.2.1. Clinical Examination Techniques for Neonatal Skin 267
12.2.2. Importance of Patient History in Diagnosis 268
12.2.3. Use of Imaging Techniques in Assessment 268
12.2.4. Differentiating Between Benign and Concerning Birthmarks 269
12.2.5. Role of Pediatric Dermatologists in Diagnosis 269
12.2.6. Common Diagnostic Tools and Methods 270
12.2.7. Challenges in Diagnosing Skin Conditions in Neonates 270
12.2.8. Importance of Early Diagnosis for Treatment Outcomes 270
12.3. Treatment Options 271
12.3.1. Observation and Monitoring of Benign Birthmarks 271
12.3.2. Medical Treatments for Problematic Birthmarks 272
12.3.3. Surgical Interventions for Severe Cases 272
12.3.4. Laser Therapy for Vascular Birthmarks 273
12.3.5. Topical Treatments for Pigmented Birthmarks 273
12.3.6. Role of Pediatricians in Treatment Planning 274
12.3.7. Parental Education on Treatment Options 274
12.3.8. Ethical Considerations in Treating Birthmarks 275
12.3.9. Long-term Outcomes of Various Treatment Approaches 275
12.4. Prevention and Care 276
12.4.1. Importance of Skin Care in Newborns 276
12.4.2. Preventive Measures for Skin Conditions 277
12.4.3. Role of Nutrition in Skin Health 277
12.4.4. Educating Parents on Skin Monitoring 278
12.4.5. Recognizing Signs of Skin Infections 278
12.4.6. Importance of Regular Pediatric Check-ups 279
12.4.7. Cultural Perceptions of Birthmarks and Skin Care 279
12.4.8. Community Resources for Skin Health Education 279
Summary 281
References 283
Index 285

LIST OF FIGURES

Figure 1.1. The study of superficial mycoses, which encompass infections primarily affecting the skin, hair, and nails, provides critical insights into the prevalence and etiology of these fungal diseases

Figure 1.2. Superficial mycoses

Figure 1.3. Dermatophytes, such as *Trichophyton rubrum* and *Microsporum canis*, are commonly implicated in conditions like tinea pedis and tinea corporis, affecting keratinized tissues

Figure 1.4. Fungal infections present a variety of symptoms and clinical manifestations that can range from mild superficial conditions to severe deep mycoses

Figure 1.5. Azole antifungals

Figure 1.6. Cutaneous involvement in the deep mycoses

Figure 1.7. Eumycetoma

Figure 1.8. In immunocompromised individuals, such as those with HIV/AIDS, fungal infections can lead to atypical and more severe symptoms compared to immunocompetent individuals

Figure 1.9. Candida bloodstream infections in non-neutropenic patients without severe sepsis, whereas cases involving previous azole exposure necessitate alternatives such as amphotericin B deoxycholate or caspofungin

Figure 1.10. A map showing completed country estimates of fungal diseases by August 2017

Figure 1.11. Fungal infections exhibit a notable geographic distribution, influenced by environmental conditions, population behaviors, and the prevalence of specific fungal species

Figure 1.12. Elevated temperatures and altered precipitation patterns create favorable conditions for pathogens such as *Candida* and *Aspergillus*, which thrive in diverse environments as they adapt to a changing ecosystem

Figure 1.13. Effective surveillance and reporting systems are essential in combatting fungal infections, particularly invasive fungal diseases (IFD) that pose significant public health challenges

Figure 1.14. As *Candida* species, particularly those beyond *Candida* albicans, contribute significantly to the challenge of antifungal resistance, understanding the mechanisms behind biofilm formation has become increasingly critical

Figure 1.15. The role of immunotherapy in managing fungal infections is increasingly critical, given the rising incidence of both superficial and deep mycoses, which pose substantial threats to public health

Figure 1.16. Ecology of *Madurella mycetomatis*

Figure 1.17. Antifungal resistance presents a significant challenge in the management of fungal infections, including both superficial and deep mycoses

Figure 1.18. Role of technology in fungal infection management

Figure 2.1. Scabies

Figure 2.2. *Sarcoptes scabiei*

Figure 2.3. The clinical presentation of parasitic infestations is marked by a range of symptoms that vary depending on the specific parasite involved

Figure 2.4. Antiparasitic medications play a vital role, with drugs like ivermectin demonstrating a broad spectrum of activity against various parasites

Figure 2.5. The most concerning consequences are secondary bacterial infections, which can occur as a result of intense scratching, leading to conditions such as cellulitis and impetigo

Figure 2.6. World map of scabies age-standardised disability-adjusted life-years per 100 000 people

Figure 2.7. Head lice, scientifically known as *Pediculus humanus* capitis, are typically found on the scalp and are transmitted through direct head-to-head contact; they are particularly common among children in school settings

Figure 2.8. In human cases of leishmaniasis, cutaneous symptoms can include lesions, ulcers, and swelling, indicating the body's response to the parasite

Figure 2.9. Ivermectin

Figure 2.10. Effective prevention and control measures are vital in combating parasitic infestations such as scabies, lice, and leishmaniasis, all of which can significantly impact both individual and public health

Figure 2.11. Leishmaniasis

Figure 2.12. The transmission of parasitic infections through sandflies constitutes a significant public health concern, particularly in tropical and subtropical regions

Figure 2.13. Understanding the symptoms and clinical manifestations associated with parasitic infestations is paramount for accurate diagnosis and effective treatment

Figure 2.14. The impact of parasitic infestations, such as scabies, lice, and leishmaniasis, on affected populations is profound, particularly in regions with limited health resources

Figure 2.15. Scabies, caused by *Sarcoptes scabiei*, disproportionately affects populations in crowded living conditions, with higher prevalence rates reported in developing regions

Figure 3.1. Cutaneous tuberculosis

Figure 3.2. Mycobacterium tuberculosis, the causative agent of tuberculosis, can lead to the formation of localized granulomatous lesions on the skin when the immune system fails to contain the bacteria effectively

Figure 3.3. Cutaneous lesions manifest in several forms, including nodules, plaques, and ulcers, each with distinct characteristics that aid in differential diagnosis

Figure 3.4. *Tegumentary leishmaniasis*

Figure 3.5. Human leukocyte antigens (HLAs), which are pivotal to immune system function, play a crucial role in determining susceptibility

Figure 3.6. *Mycobacterium leprae* is a slow-growing bacterium that primarily targets peripheral nerves and skin, leading to the characteristic symptoms of the disease.

Figure 3.7. The immune response to cutaneous tuberculosis and leprosy is complex and varies significantly among individuals, influenced by factors such as genetic predisposition and the pathogenicity of the causative agents

Figure 3.8. Integrating clinical findings with robust laboratory techniques is crucial to distinguish leprosy from related pathologies effectively, ensuring timely and appropriate treatment

Figure 3.9. In the case of cutaneous tuberculosis, complications can manifest as chronic skin lesions that may lead to scarring and secondary infections, thereby affecting a person's quality of life

Figure 3.10. Molecular techniques, particularly polymerase chain reaction (PCR) and next-generation sequencing (NGS), have allowed researchers to detect Mycobacterium leprae at unprecedented precision, leading to more accurate diagnoses and insights into microbial genetic diversity

Figure 3.11. Standard treatment protocols for cutaneous tuberculosis (TB) primarily involve the use of antitubercular medications in accordance with guidelines established by the World Health Organization (WHO)

Figure 3.12. Antibiotics play a critical role in the treatment of cutaneous tuberculosis and leprosy

Figure 3.13. Erythema nodosum leprosum (ENL), a significant complication associated with leprosy, is characterized by painful nodules, fever, and systemic symptoms that may result in considerable morbidity

Figure 3.14. Public health initiatives play a crucial role in addressing the challenges posed by cutaneous tuberculosis and leprosy, particularly in resource-limited settings where these diseases flourish

Figure 3.15. Stigmatization can perpetuate cycles of poverty, as affected individuals often face discrimination in employment and social settings, leading to reduced capabilities and life choices

Figure 3.16. The impact of cutaneous tuberculosis and leprosy extends beyond physical manifestations, significantly affecting mental health and overall well-being

Figure 3.17. Advocacy and awareness campaigns play a pivotal role in addressing neglected tropical diseases (NTDs) like cutaneous tuberculosis and leprosy, which significantly affect public health, particularly in resource-limited settings

Figure 3.18. The integration of care into community health systems is pivotal for effectively addressing diseases such as cutaneous tuberculosis and leprosy, both of which disproportionately affect marginalized populations

Figure 4.1. Hyperpigmentation disorders

Figure 4.2. Melasma

Figure 4.3. Genetic factors influencing hyperpigmentation

Figure 4.4. Hormonal influences, particularly those occurring during pregnancy and due to contraceptive use, play a substantial role in the manifestation of hyperpigmentation disorders such as melasma and post-inflammatory hyperpigmentation (PIH)

Figure 4.5. Individuals frequently report a decline in self-esteem and body image, stemming from societal beauty standards that often stigmatize skin imperfections

Figure 4.6. Melasma is defined as a common skin condition characterized by the development of brown or gray-brown patches, primarily on sun-exposed areas such as the face

Figure 4.7. Dyschromias

Figure 4.8. Exposure to ultraviolet (UV) radiation is a primary trigger for hyperpigmentation, making it imperative for individuals at risk to adopt comprehensive sun protection measures, including the regular use of broad-spectrum sunscreens, protective clothing, and seeking shade during peak sunlight hours

Figure 4.9. Understanding the differences between melasma and other hyperpigmentation disorders, such as post-inflammatory hyperpigmentation (PIH), is crucial for effective diagnosis and treatment

Figure 4.10. Post-inflammatory hyperpigmentation (PIH)

Figure 4.11. Common conditions leading to post-inflammatory hyperpigmentation (PIH) include acne, eczema, psoriasis, and other inflammatory dermatoses, all of which can damage the skin barrier and result in increased melanocyte activity in response to injury

Figure 4.12. Accurate diagnosis is essential, as various factors like duration of the condition, associated symptoms, and patient history can influence clinical presentations

Figure 4.13. Effective skin care routines that focus on sun protection and the use of topical agents can significantly mitigate the risk of developing these conditions

Figure 4.14. Effective patient education is paramount in managing hyperpigmentation disorders such as melasma and post-inflammatory hyperpigmentation (PIH), as it equips individuals with the essential knowledge to understand their conditions and treatment options

Figure 4.15. Facial dyschromias

Figure 4.16. Nevus of Ota

Figure 4.17. Conditions like diabetes and endocrine disorders are known to impact melanin production, often exacerbating pigmentation issues in susceptible individuals

Figure 4.18. Effective management strategies, including education on the importance of sun protection, are essential, particularly since individuals with skin of color are often at a heightened risk due to disparities in photoprotection practices

Figure 5.1. Vitiligo is a complex acquired skin disorder characterized by the loss of functional melanocytes, leading to the development of depigmented patches on the skin

Figure 5.2. In vitiligo, patients typically exhibit patches of skin that lose pigment, leading to a contrast with surrounding areas, which can also result in emotional distress and social stigma

Figure 5.3. Individuals often experience stigma and discrimination due to the visible nature of their conditions, which can lead to anxiety, depression, and a diminished quality of life

Figure 5.4. Certain home remedies, such as the application of supportive topical agents, may help enhance skin appearance; however, their effectiveness varies widely among individuals

Figure 5.5. Albinism is a genetic condition characterized by a complete or partial absence of pigment in the skin, hair, and eyes due to the lack of functional melanocytes

Figure 5.6. In albinism, for instance, mutations in genes responsible for melanin synthesis lead to a significant reduction or complete absence of pigment in the skin, hair, and eyes, demonstrating a classic example of autosomal recessive inheritance

Figure 5.7. Albinism, characterized by a deficiency in melanin production, often results in ocular complications, including photophobia, nystagmus, and reduced visual acuity, primarily due to the lack of pigment in the retina that is essential for optimal light absorption and image clarity

Figure 5.8. The identification of key enzymes and genetic factors involved in pigmentation can aid in establishing a more accurate diagnosis

Figure 5.9. The advocacy and support for individuals with albinism are critical in combating the stigma and violence often associated with this condition

Figure 5.10. Individuals with hypopigmented conditions like vitiligo and albinism have historically been marginalized, viewed as other and often subjected to discrimination

Figure 5.11. Cultural beliefs and myths surrounding vitiligo and albinism significantly inform societal attitudes and treatment of individuals affected by these hypopigmentation disorders

Figure 5.12. Advocacy groups and organizations play a critical role in raising awareness and providing support for individuals affected by hypopigmentation and depigmentation disorders, such as vitiligo and albinism

Figure 5.13. Legal frameworks, such as the Americans with Disabilities Act (ADA) and the Rehabilitation Act, offer safeguards against employment discrimination and enable individuals to seek recourse in cases of unequal treatment in the workplace or public spaces

Figure 5.14. Increased awareness of the autoimmune nature of vitiligo, is fostering a more empathetic understanding of the condition and its psychological implications, as misconceptions and stigma often stem from a lack of knowledge

Figure 6.1. The pemphigus group of diseases represents a spectrum of autoimmune skin disorders characterized by the development of blisters in the epidermis due to the disruption of cell adhesion

Figure 6.2. Pemphigus is a group of autoimmune disorders characterized by the formation of vesicles and bullae, primarily affecting the skin and mucous membranes

Figure 6.3. The pathophysiology of pemphigus

Figure 6.4. Direct immunofluorescence (DIF)

Figure 6.5. Bullous pemphigoid is a significant autoimmune blistering disorder primarily characterized by the formation of large, tense blisters that typically occur on the skin and mucous membranes

Figure 6.6. Bullous pemphigoid involves the formation of autoantibodies against hemidesmosomes, notably BP230 and BP180

Figure 6.7. The erosive nature of these blisters poses significant morbidity, as they are prone to secondary infections and create discomfort that may hinder both dietary intake and overall quality of life

Figure 6.8. Dapsone has been shown to be effective in cases of linear IgA bullous dermatosis, achieving remission in a majority of patients

Figure 6.9. Clinical evaluation and patient history play critical roles in diagnosing vesiculobullous diseases, such as pemphigus and bullous pemphigoid

Figure 6.10. Immunofluorescence studies serve a crucial role in the diagnosis and differentiation of vesiculobullous diseases, particularly pemphigus and bullous pemphigoid

Figure 6.11. Dermatopathology plays a crucial role in the diagnosis and management of vesiculobullous diseases, such as pemphigus and bullous pemphigoid, by integrating clinical findings with histopathological and immunofluorescence studies

Figure 6.12. Corticosteroids for treatment and management strategies for vesiculobullous diseases

Figure 6.13. Mycophenolate mofetil

Figure 6.14. Effective patient education and support are crucial in managing vesiculobullous diseases such as pemphigus and bullous pemphigoid

Figure 6.15. The use of immunosuppressive agents to control disease activity while minimizing the potential for treatment-related complications

Figure 6.16. The treatment of vesiculobullous diseases, such as pemphigus and bullous pemphigoid, requires a multidisciplinary approach that integrates dermatological, immunological, and potentially rheumatological expertise

Figure 7.1. Systemic lupus erythematosus (SLE) represents one of the most complex and multifaceted autoimmune diseases within the category of connective tissue disorders

Figure 7.2. Dysregulation of the immune system contributes to the autoimmune nature of these conditions, whereby the body mistakenly attacks its own connective tissues

Figure 7.3. Nailfold capillaroscopy has emerged as an important tool, especially for its ability to reveal microvascular changes indicative of disease progression

Figure 7.4. Lupus, a prevalent form of autoimmune connective tissue disease, is associated with various complications that significantly impact patients' quality of life

Figure 7.5. Lifestyle modifications play a crucial role in the management of connective tissue diseases such as lupus, dermatomyositis, and scleroderma

Figure 7.6. Dermatomyositis is a rare autoimmune connective tissue disease characterized by muscle weakness and distinctive skin rashes, which distinguishes it from other inflammatory myopathies

Figure 7.7. Dermatomyositis, for instance, is often marked by skin changes such as periorbital erythema and Gottrons papules, which are significant diagnostic features alongside the profound muscle weakness that can ensue

Figure 7.8. Effective management of connective tissue diseases such as lupus, dermatomyositis, and scleroderma requires a comprehensive approach to treatment modalities and rehabilitation

Figure 7.9. The long-term prognosis and outcomes of patients with connective tissue diseases, such as lupus, dermatomyositis, and scleroderma, are influenced by various factors, including the presence of specific autoantibodies

Figure 7.10. Scleroderma, or systemic sclerosis, is a complex connective tissue disease characterized by the excessive accumulation of collagen, leading to skin thickening and organ fibrosis

Figure 7.11. Gastrointestinal complications are also prevalent, particularly dysphagia, which arises from the muscular dysfunction affecting the swallowing mechanism

Figure 7.12. Treatment strategies primarily involve immunosuppressive agents, with mycophenolate mofetil (MMF) emerging as a viable alternative to cyclophosphamide for patients with RD-related ILD, thanks to its lower side effect profile

Figure 7.13. The psychological and emotional ramifications of connective tissue diseases, such as lupus, dermatomyositis, and scleroderma, cannot be overstated, as these chronic conditions profoundly affect patients' quality of life

Figure 8.1. *Cryoglobulinaemic vasculitis*

Figure 8.2. Polyarteritis nodosa (PAN)

Figure 8.3. Granulomatosis with polyangiitis

Figure 8.4. Giant cell arteritis (GCA)

Figure 8.5. ANCA-associated vasculitis (AAV)

Figure 8.6. The immune system plays a pivotal role in the pathogenesis of vasculitis and purpura, characterized by inflammation of blood vessels and subsequent skin manifestations

Figure 8.7. Leukocytoclastic vasculitis (LCV)

Figure 8.8. Recent advances in neuroimaging techniques have improved our ability to distinguish inflammatory from non-inflammatory vascular lesions, enhancing diagnostic accuracy for conditions like primary central nervous system vasculitis (PCNSV)

Figure 8.9. Vascular inflammation, as seen in conditions such as vasculitis, leads to significant and multifaceted consequences that can severely impact an individual's health

Figure 8.10. Purpura, characterized by the appearance of purple spots on the skin due to bleeding underneath, can arise from various underlying conditions, primarily classified into non-thrombocytopenic and thrombocytopenic types

Figure 8.11. Thrombocytopenic purpura

Figure 8.12. Levamisole-adulterated cocaine

Figure 8.13. Medications can play a significant role in the onset of vasculitis and purpura, leading to notable inflammatory responses within the body

Figure 8.14. Idiopathic purpura

Figure 8.15. Effective clinical evaluation and thorough history taking are paramount in the diagnosis and management of conditions such as vasculitis and purpura

Figure 8.16. Techniques such as magnetic resonance angiography (MRA) and computed tomography angiography (CTA) are particularly useful in visualizing large vessel involvement, as seen in conditions like Takayasu arteritis

Figure 8.17. In cases of leukocytoclastic vasculitis, which presents with palpable purpura and may involve internal organs, treatment typically includes corticosteroids to reduce inflammation and suppress the immune response

Figure 8.18. Rapidly progressive glomerulonephritis (RPGN)

Figure 8.19. Regular follow-up visits not only enable clinicians to evaluate the progression of the disease but also allow for timely adjustments in treatment protocols

Figure 9.1. The pathophysiology of sarcoidosis

Figure 9.2. Granulomas are organized aggregates of immune cells, primarily macrophages, that arise in response to persistent antigens or irritants, a process often linked to chronic inflammation

Figure 9.3. Factors such as exposure to certain pathogens, organic dust, and industrial chemicals are thought to play pivotal roles in these conditions

Figure 9.4. The systemic effects of sarcoidosis extend well beyond its initial presentation, significantly impacting various organ systems and complicating the clinical landscape

Figure 9.5. Cutaneous sarcoidosis

Figure 9.6. Sarcoidosis is characterized by a diverse range of symptoms that can vary significantly among patients, complicating its diagnosis

Figure 9.7. Pulmonary involvement in sarcoidosis is one of the hallmark manifestations of this complex disease, often surpassing other organ systems in frequency and significance

Figure 9.8. Cardiac involvement in sarcoidosis represents a significant concern due to its potential for severe complications

Figure 9.9. Musculoskeletal symptoms are a frequently noted complication in patients with sarcoidosis, often presenting as arthralgia or arthritis that can significantly affect quality of life

Figure 9.10. The oral manifestations of Crohn's disease can serve as precursors to gastrointestinal involvement, highlighting how early symptoms can provide valuable insight into the patient's overall health status

Figure 9.11. Granulomatous skin conditions represent a diverse spectrum of dermatological disorders characterized by the formation of granulomas, which are organized clusters of macrophages that transform into epithelioid cells

Figure 9.12. The pathophysiology of granulomatous skin conditions

Figure 9.13. Initial assessments often include a thorough patient history and physical examination to identify characteristic skin lesions, which can appear as papules, plaques, or nodules

Figure 9.14. Tuberculosis, particularly in reactivated forms, can present with similar skin manifestations, making it crucial to rule out before confirming sarcoidosis

Figure 9.15. Management typically hinges on the severity of symptoms, with corticosteroids being the primary treatment for those with significant dermatological involvement or systemic symptoms

Figure 9.16. Elevated serum angiotensin-converting enzyme (ACE) levels are often associated with sarcoidosis and can serve as a supportive diagnostic marker; however, these levels may also be increased in other conditions, thereby limiting specificity

Figure 9.17. Corticosteroids play a pivotal role in managing sarcoidosis and associated granulomatous skin conditions, primarily due to their potent anti-inflammatory properties

Figure 9.18. Effective patient education and support are crucial components in managing sarcoidosis and granulomatous skin conditions, as they empower patients to actively participate in their treatment and care

Figure 10.1. Ichthyosis

Figure 10.2. Ichthyosis encompasses a diverse group of genetic conditions characterized by dry, scaly skin resulting from various mutations, most notably in keratin genes such as KRT1, KRT10, and KRT17

Figure 10.3. Genetic testing plays a crucial role in identifying specific mutations associated with these conditions, allowing for personalized diagnosis and treatment plans

Figure 10.4. Individuals affected by these conditions often face significant emotional distress, stemming from visible and sometimes painful symptoms that can lead to social isolation and stigmatization

Figure 10.5. Epidermolysis bullosa (EB) is a group of rare genetic skin disorders characterized by extreme fragility of the skin, leading to blistering and wounds resulting from minimal trauma

Figure 10.6. Common symptoms include intense itching and severe pain, affecting nearly half of the patients, which contributes to daily restrictions in activities and an overall diminished quality of life

Figure 10.7. The management of genetic skin disorders such as ichthyosis and epidermolysis bullosa (EB) requires a multifaceted approach that incorporates both treatment options and comprehensive care strategies

Figure 10.8. Advances in gene therapy, especially for severe subtypes such as Recessive Dystrophic Epidermolysis Bullosa (RDEB), present a forward-thinking approach by targeting the genetic mutations responsible for the disease

Figure 10.9. The stigmatization of individuals with genetic skin disorders, such as ichthyosis and epidermolysis bullosa, manifests profoundly in societal interactions and personal experiences, ultimately leading to significant psychological distress

Figure 10.10. With advancements in genomic technologies, such as next-generation sequencing, the ability to identify pathogenic variants has improved, providing opportunities for more accurate diagnoses and targeted therapies

Figure 10.11. Public awareness campaigns and education are vital in advancing the understanding and management of genetic skin disorders such as ichthyosis and epidermolysis bullosa (EB)

Figure 10.12. Individuals with genetic skin disorders, such as ichthyosis and epidermolysis bullosa, face significant employment and social integration challenges, largely stemming from the visible nature of their conditions

Figure 11.1. Eczema, or atopic dermatitis, is a prevalent chronic skin condition in children that significantly affects not only the skin but also the overall quality of life of patients and their families

Figure 11.2. In infants, eczema frequently appears on the face and scalp, while older children may develop lesions in the creases of the elbows and knees, a pattern that reflects the evolving nature of the condition

Figure 11.3. Given that eczema can present in varying forms, the dermatologist must assess specific symptoms such as pruritus, xerosis, and the characteristic distribution of lesions

Figure 11.4. Moisturizers play a critical role in the management of common childhood skin conditions, particularly in mitigating symptoms associated with atopic dermatitis and eczema

Figure 11.5. Children with severe atopic dermatitis often experience significant psychological distress, which can exacerbate their symptoms and lead to a vicious cycle of worsening skin issues and emotional turmoil

Figure 11.6. Acne in adolescents represents one of the most prevalent skin conditions encountered in pediatric dermatology, significantly impacting both physical appearance and psychological well-being

Figure 11.7. Adolescence is a critical period for the onset of acne, primarily due to the hormonal changes that occur during puberty

Figure 11.8. Clinicians typically begin with a thorough history and physical examination, assessing the type and severity of acne lesions, which range from comedones to inflammatory papules and cysts

Figure 11.9. Skincare routines play a pivotal role in managing various childhood skin conditions, emphasizing the necessity for proactive measures in pediatric dermatology

Figure 11.10. Many individuals associate the severity of acne with dietary choices, particularly the consumption of chocolate or greasy foods, although current research indicates that such dietary factors may have minimal influence on acne development

Figure 11.11. Psoriasis is an immune-mediated chronic inflammatory condition characterized by the rapid proliferation of skin cells, leading to the formation of thick, scaly plaques on the skin's surface

Figure 11.12. Genetic predisposition plays a significant role, with studies revealing that nearly 48.8% of affected children have a family history of psoriasis, indicating a strong hereditary component

Figure 11.13. Topical therapies, such as corticosteroids and vitamin D analogs, are often the first line of treatment, providing localized relief and reducing inflammation with minimal systemic effects

Figure 11.14. Children with psoriasis may experience feelings of embarrassment and social isolation due to the visible lesions associated with the condition

Figure 11.15. Support groups and resources play a pivotal role in alleviating this burden, providing essential emotional and practical assistance

Figure 11.16. In pediatric dermatology, various infectious skin conditions are prevalent, each presenting unique challenges and requiring tailored management strategies

Figure 11.17. Fungal infections represent a significant category of skin conditions in pediatric dermatology, with various types causing diverse clinical presentations

Figure 11.18. Scabies in pediatric populations

Figure 11.19. Atopic dermatitis (AD), a prevalent childhood condition, often intertwines with other atopic disorders, complicating its management and diagnostic clarity

Figure 11.20. Effective parental guidance plays a crucial role in the prevention and care of common childhood skin conditions, particularly atopic dermatitis

Figure 12.1. Birthmarks, which appear in various forms, can be classified into vascular and pigmented types, each bearing distinct characteristics and implications for neonatal health

Figure 12.2. Vascular birthmarks

Figure 12.3. Congenital birthmarks

Figure 12.4. Café-au-lait spots

Figure 12.5. Congenital pigmented nevi

Figure 12.6. Infants with noticeable birthmarks, such as hemangiomas or other vascular malformations, may face challenges in forming secure attachments and social relationships as they grow.

Figure 12.7. Pediatric practitioners should engage in meticulous observation, utilizing dermatoscopes for enhanced visualization of superficial skin structures, thereby facilitating better differentiation of benign from potentially malignant lesions.

Figure 12.8. Imaging techniques play a pivotal role in the assessment of neonatal dermatological conditions, particularly concerning the accurate diagnosis of congenital birthmarks and associated anomalies.

Figure 12.9. Diligent evaluation of skin lesions is vital, as many common manifestations like erythema toxicum and Mongolian spots are often benign.

Figure 12.10. Infantile hemangiomas, the most common vascular anomaly of infancy, can exhibit complex inheritance patterns and varying presentations that further obscure diagnosis.

Figure 12.11. Routine examinations allow for the assessment of changes in size, color, and texture, which can indicate the necessity for further evaluation or interventions.

Figure 12.12. Surgical procedures may be employed for a range of birthmarks and vascular anomalies, including hemangiomas and other malformations that could lead to complications, such as ulceration or functional impairment.

Figure 12.13. Topical treatments for pigmented birthmarks represent a significant advancement in the management of these common dermatological conditions in neonates.

Figure 12.14. Parents frequently experience anxiety upon learning about these benign tumors, necessitating clear and comprehensive communication from clinicians.

Figure 12.15. Infantile hemangiomas, prevalent among neonates, often undergo spontaneous regression, leading many clinicians to opt for a watchful waiting strategy.

Figure 12.16. Effective skin care in newborns is paramount for ensuring both their immediate comfort and long-term health, specifically within the context of neonatal dermatology.

Figure 12.17. Proper nutrition provides essential vitamins and minerals, which are critical for maintaining skin integrity and function.

Figure 12.18. Care providers and parents must understand that certain dermatological manifestations, such as café-au-lait spots or hypomelanosis of Ito.

Figure 12.19. Community resources for skin health education play a critical role in assisting parents and caregivers in understanding neonatal dermatology, particularly in relation to birthmarks and skin conditions.

PREFACE

Skin health is a paramount feature of overall well-being, not simply due to its protective function but also because of its value in the diagnosis of infectious and systemic disease. The skin is a preferred outward manifestation of internal pathology, immunity, and exterior contamination. Expertise in dermatologic lesions transcends issues of appearance; it is important in the identification of patterns of infection, patterns of imbalance of immunity, and genetic disease. Thus, the topic of dermatology is an essential component of medical professionals' studies, especially those in internal medicine, pediatrics, and primary care.

The diversity of skin conditions, ranging from infections and inflammatory disorders to birth defects and pigmentary changes, requires extensive and applied knowledge. A range of conditions can look the same, but the reasons are entirely different and require various approaches to diagnosis and management. The ability to appreciate fine differences in presentation, distribution, and evolution is a skill learned in formal education. Moreover, skin illnesses in neonates and children must receive special emphasis due to their typical characteristics, diagnostic challenges, and impact on development and growth.

The Textbook of Dermatology Volume 2 is designed to take forward the fundamental knowledge of the first volume by focusing on a wide range of individual dermatological conditions that demand clinical accuracy and practical utility. Volume 2 describes a range of diseases that not only occur commonly in everyday practice but are also of clinical significance due to their chronicity, complications, or public health significance. Each chapter introduces clinically relevant information in an organized, sequential format, set up to guide learners and practitioners to definitive diagnostic findings and effective treatment strategies.

Chapter 1 is about fungal infections, such as superficial and systemic mycoses, concerning diagnosis and treatment options in both resource-limited and hospital-based settings. Conditions like dermatophytosis, candidiasis, and deep fungal infections are explained with diagnostic hints and treatment suggestions.

Chapter 2 deals with parasitic infestations of the skin such as scabies, cutaneous larva migrans, and leishmaniasis. It emphasizes their identification in clinical practice, epidemiologic patterns of transmission, and modalities of treatment, particularly where these infections remain very much endemic.

Chapter 3 discusses cutaneous tuberculosis and leprosy, emphasizing their epidemiology, pathophysiology, clinical presentation, and evolving treatment regimens. The chapter attempts to elucidate the diagnostic criteria and long-term management of these traditionally significant but persistent infections.

Chapter 4 discusses hyperpigmentation disorders such as melasma, post-inflammatory hyperpigmentation, and drug-induced pigmentation. It aids in clarifying how to differentiate between benign and suspicious reasons for an excess of pigmentation and discusses information on pharmacologic and procedural management.

Chapter 5 discusses hypopigmentation and depigmentation diseases, including vitiligo, pityriasis alba, and albinism. In this chapter, diagnosis and treatment are discussed, including counseling of the patient, phototherapy, and emerging therapies.

Chapter 6 discusses vesiculobullous diseases, including autoimmune diseases such as pemphigus vulgaris, bullous pemphigoid, and epidermolysis bullosa. In this chapter, immunopathogenesis concepts, clinical diagnosis, and immunosuppressive therapy are discussed.

Chapter 7 covers connective tissue diseases presenting with cutaneous signs such as lupus erythematosus, dermatomyositis, and scleroderma. It covers systemic involvement, investigation, and current management, emphasizing multidisciplinary care.

Chapter 8 covers vasculitis and purpura, with classification into small, medium, and large vessel vasculitides. It covers diagnostic criteria, clues to systemic involvement in the clinic, and the role of biopsy, investigation, and imaging in making the diagnosis.

Chapter 9 presents sarcoidosis and granulomatous skin conditions. It stresses their systemic associations, clinical morphology, histopathology, and therapy, laying special emphasis on the exclusion of infectious diseases as etiological factors for granulomas.

Chapter 10 presents genetic skin conditions such as ichthyoses, genodermatoses, and epidermolysis bullosa. It provides an insight into modes of inheritance, clinical pointers, and recent advances in genetic research and management, including gene-based therapies.

Chapter 11 addresses pediatric dermatology with a focus on normal skin disease in children, such as atopic dermatitis, diaper dermatitis, viral exanthems, and acne in adolescents. The chapter attempts to provide useful clinical information relevant to early detection and management in primary and child care practice.

Chapter 12 concludes the book with neonatal dermatology and birthmarks, including normal skin changes in neonates and congenital lesions like hemangiomas, port-wine stains, and nevus sebaceous. The content enables differentiation of benign lesions from potentially serious ones among newborns, with referral and treatment recommendations.

The book is for undergraduate medical students, postgraduate dermatology students, and clinical practitioners who are handling dermatological issues in the context of general and specialist care. It is also a valuable source of reference for internists, pediatricians, infectious disease, and immunology health practitioners who will welcome a greater understanding of cutaneous presentation. The book deals in practical clinical observations backed by up-to-date guidelines and common sense considerations and is thus suitable for academic study as well as for daily clinical practice.

FUNGAL INFECTIONS

1

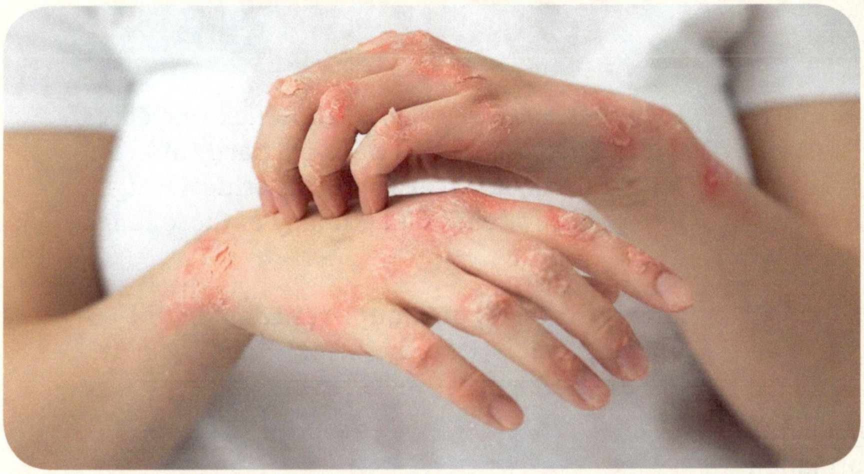

Introduction

Fungal infections, which can be classified as superficial and deep mycoses, are significant health issues all over the world with rising disease burden attributed to various factors, including the expansion of immunocompromised populations and environmental changes. The superficial mycoses, as typically seen in the skin and mucous membranes, predispose patients to present as localized infections, while deep mycoses infiltrate vital organs and systems to cause severe complications. Latest diagnostic techniques, such as reflectance confocal microscopy, have greatly improved recognition, enabling clinicians to differentiate between fungal infection and other cutaneous conditions effectively. This noninvasive imaging technique can see skin parasites, fungi, and other infecting agents with the same precision as histopathology (Pimenta et al., 2020). Also, diseases like eumycetoma, caused mainly by *Madurella mycetomatis* in the tropical regions, highlight the diverse ecological determinants and pathogenicity processes of such diseases, enhancing the need for proper knowledge and

LEARNING OBJECTIVES

After studying this chapter, you will be able to:

1. Understand Superficial Mycoses;
2. Explain Deep Mycoses;
3. Describe Epidemiology of Fungal Infections;
4. Focus on Advances in Research and Treatment.

prevention strategies (De Hoog et al., 2013). Recognition of these intricacies is essential to formulate proper therapeutic interventions and maximize patient outcomes.

1.1. Superficial Mycoses

Learning Outcome

1. Understand Definition and Characteristics;
2. Explain Common Types of Superficial Mycoses;
3. Focus on Causative Agents of Superficial Mycoses;
4. Describe Risk Factors for Superficial Infections;
5. Learn Symptoms and Clinical Manifestations;
6. Discuss Diagnosis of Superficial Mycoses;
7. Know Treatment Options for Superficial Infections;
7. Understand Prevention Strategies.

The progression of superficial mycoses, which are infections that predominantly happen in the skin, hair, and nails, provides valuable information regarding the transmission and etiology of the fungal infections. Superficial mycoses are caused most commonly by dermatophytes, yeasts, and non-dermatophytic molds, with tinea pedis and onychomycosis being notable examples. There is evidence that tinea pedis, the frequent foot infection, is regularly caused by *Trichophyton rubrum*, a dermatophyte, which thrives in wet conditions. The application of advanced diagnostic equipment like reflectance confocal microscopy (RCM) has improved the diagnosis and treatment of these infections significantly, offering a noninvasive approach through which the skin alterations caused by pathogens can be observed (Pimenta et al., 2020). Research also highlights the importance of studying epidemiological factors that influence these infections, and studies indicate that pet ownership, age, and environmental exposure affect susceptibility. Consequently, continued research into superficial mycoses continues to be necessary to provide proper public health interventions (Figure 1.1).

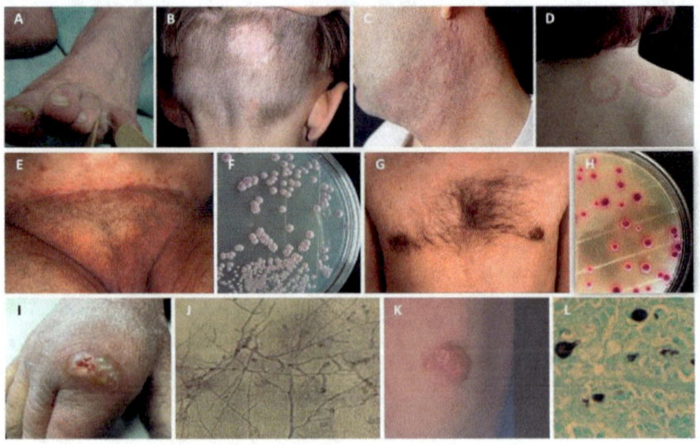

Figure 1.1. The study of superficial mycoses, which encompass infections primarily affecting the skin, hair, and nails, provides critical insights into the prevalence and etiology of these fungal diseases.

Source: https://pub.mdpi-res.com/jof/jof-09-00381/article_deploy/html/images/jof-09-00381-g002.png?1679394858.

1.1.1. Definition and Characteristics

Fungal infections, both superficial and deep mycoses, constitute a principal cause for concern with regard to health due to their varied presentations and pathogenic processes. Superficial mycoses tend to infect the outermost layers of skin, hair, and nails, characterizing diseases such as ringworm and athlete's foot, most often produced by dermatophytes. Deep mycoses infect deeper tissue structures and lead to systemic infections, most often among immunocompromised individuals. Among the most important characteristics of fungal infection is the adaptability of pathogenic fungi like the Candida species, which are renowned for their biofilm production, leading to enhanced resistance to antifungal therapy. Biofilms are not only protective against therapeutic drugs but also complicate the treatment of candidiasis, as other factors such as nutrient deprivation and cell density enhance antifungal resistance immensely (Silva et al., 2017). In addition, novel imaging techniques like reflectance confocal microscopy have been utilized as valuable diagnostic methods for these infections and allowed clinicians to observe fungal structures *in situ* (Pimenta et al., 2020) (Figure 1.2).

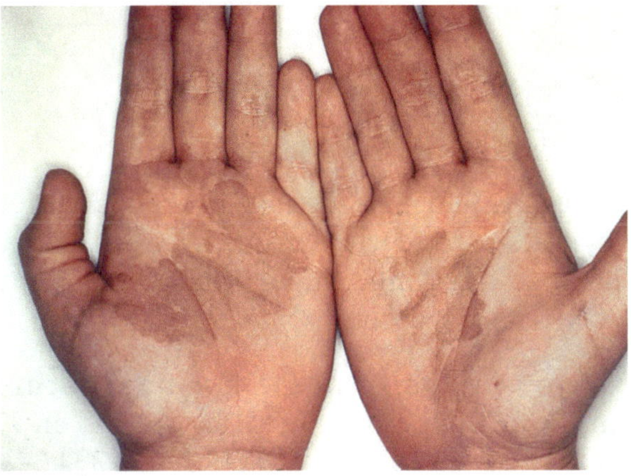

Figure 1.2. Superficial mycoses.

Source: https://www.adelaide.edu.au/mycology/sites/default/files/styles/ua_image_landscape/public/media/images/2021-09/mycoses-super.jpg?h=c4dd2c7b&itok=kb_Za_bj.

1.1.2. Common Types of Superficial Mycoses

Superficial mycoses are a significant category of fungal infections of important consequences to the skin and its appendages. These infections are usually caused by dermatophytes, with participation of such species as *Microsporum canis* and *Trichophyton mentagrophytes* quite frequently. *Microsporum canis*, indeed, is renowned for the causation of tinea capitis, particularly in children, where it prefers to manifest on the scalp, while *T. mentagrophytes* can infect both skin and nails in adults (Piorunek et al., 2024). Furthermore, superficial mycoses are of various types, including tinea corporis, tinea pedis, and tinea versicolor, all with their own clinical characteristics. Demographically, both age and gender have been found to be interestingly playing an important role in the prevalence of the infections; studies have shown that the female subjects are particularly susceptible to high rates of superficial mycoses compared to men (Mohammed et al., 2024). Knowledge of these more frequent superficial mycoses is required for successful diagnosis and treatment.

1.1.3. Causative Agents of Superficial Mycoses

The most frequent causative agents of superficial mycoses are a group of fungal species, the most relevant being dermatophytes and non-dermatophyte molds. Dermatophytes, such as *Trichophyton rubrum* and *Microsporum canis*, are the most frequent causative agents of diseases like tinea pedis and tinea corporis of keratinized tissues.

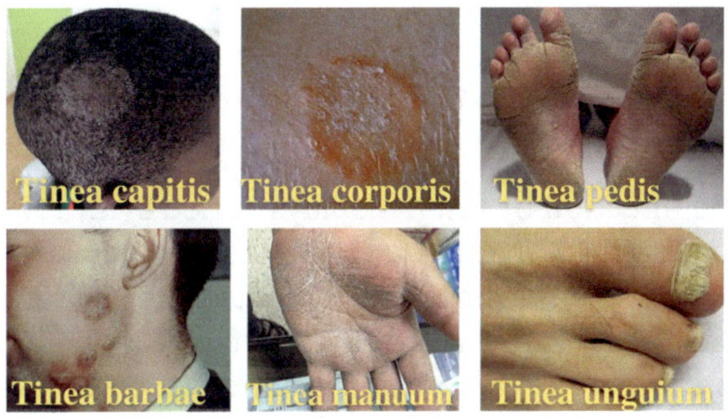

Figure 1.3. Dermatophytes, such as *Trichophyton rubrum* and *Microsporum canis*, are commonly implicated in conditions like tinea pedis and tinea corporis, affecting keratinized tissues.

Source: https://i0.wp.com/microbeonline.com/wp-content/uploads/2022/08/Tinea-.png?fit=1920%2C1080&ssl=1.

1.1.4. Risk Factors for Superficial Infections

Superficial fungal infections occur heavily based on various risk factors that predispose individuals to those pathogens. Individuals with compromised immunity, such as HIV/

AIDS patients, diabetes mellitus, and anticancer chemotherapy, are particularly vulnerable, with their immune levels reduced, allowing the growth of opportunistic fungi (Bhattacharyya et al., 2023). Environmental factors are also important; infections most commonly arise from contact with soil, plant, or water, which may serve as an access point for dermatophytes and new fungi (Bhattacharyya et al., 2023). Poor personal hygiene and the use of broad-spectrum antimicrobials can also alter the normal microbiota, creating a niche for fungal growth. The continuous exposure of healthcare facilities also contributes to these risks, such as long-term hospitalization that results in colonization by nosocomial pathogens like *Candida auris,* highlighting how the interaction among immunity, environment, and medical practice leads to superficial fungal infections (Bhattacharyya et al., 2023).

1.1.5. Symptoms and Clinical Manifestations

The infection by fungi displays varied symptoms and clinical manifestations that could range from mild superficial infections to deep mycoses with a severe nature. Superficial fungi such as dermatophytes primarily infect the stratum corneum, causing localized reactions of itching, redness, and scaling, and manifesting as tinea pedis or onychomycosis. Deep mycoses, on the other hand, can affect internal organs and the body at large, particularly in immunocompromised patients, leading to more severe manifestations of fever, malaise, and respiratory impairment. Dermatophytic granuloma, a severe expression of deep dermatophyte invasion, tends to be seen in patients with underlying conditions such as type 2 diabetes or those receiving immunosuppressive treatment, marking the multifaceted interaction between host factors and fungal pathogenicity (Bonifaz et al., 2021). It is therefore essential that such varied expressions be identified for effective diagnosis and management, a responsibility that ordinarily stems from the failure to place strong impetus on mycology in medical training (Figure 1.4).

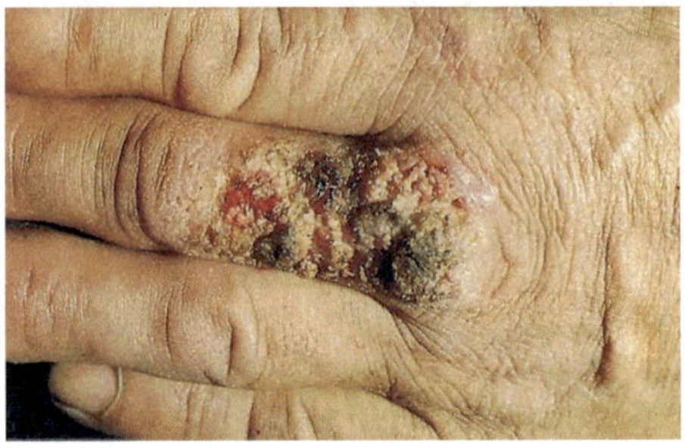

Figure 1.4. Fungal infections present a variety of symptoms and clinical manifestations that can range from mild superficial conditions to severe deep mycoses.

Source: https://media.springernature.com/lw685/springer-static/image/chp%3A10.1007%2F978-3-662-58713-3_16-1/MediaObjects/479707_0_En_16-1_Fig29_HTML.jpg.

1.1.6. Diagnosis of Superficial Mycoses

Diagnosis of superficial mycoses is usually characterized by the identification of typical fungal pathogens invading the skin, hair, and nails to produce a variety of dermatological presentations. Effective clinical diagnosis typically begins with adequate patient history and physical examination, followed by laboratory procedures such as direct microscopy, culture, and molecular diagnostics to detect the causative agents. Among common agents, dermatophytes, yeasts, including *Candida* spp., and mold including *Fusarium* spp., are not uncommon in cutaneous infection, particularly in immunocompromised individuals, as seen with the prevalence of infection in human immunodeficiency virus (HIV) patients presenting with a broad range of fungal infections with low CD4 levels (Muthanna & Jamil, 2022). Interestingly, appropriate treatment and control are based on accurate diagnosis with an organized approach involving microbiological studies and patient profile (Green et al., 1991). Therefore, proper diagnostic processes are important for intervention and patient success in superficial mycoses.

1.1.7. Treatment Options for Superficial Infections

Treatment options for superficial fungal infections, primarily those caused by dermatophytes, are evolving as traditional treatments face new challenges of growing drug resistance and decreasing efficacy. Current strategies are often centered around topical azoles, which are fungistatic from their inhibition of ergosterol synthesis in fungi, an important component of the fungal cell wall.

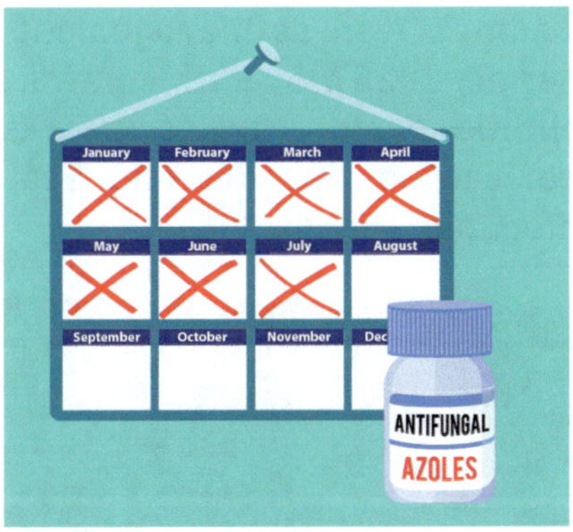

Figure 1.5. Azole antifungals.

Source: https://www.cdc.gov/aspergillosis/media/images/2024/04/347136-A_MDB_CleanSlate_AspergillusPatientCalendar.png.

However, the emergence of drug-resistant strains necessitates an exploration of novel therapeutic options, including the repurposing of bisphosphonates. Recent studies affirm that bisphosphonates have a synergistic effect with azole antifungals to enhance their antifungal activity as well as hinder resistance in many dermatophyte species (Kane et al., 2024). With the background of increasing incidence and severity of these infections, which can even arise in immunocompetent individuals due to prolonged hospitalization and indiscriminate use of antimicrobials (Bhattacharyya et al., 2023), new combinations that unite known therapies with newly identified agents are a hopeful remedy for improving patient treatment (Figure 1.5).

1.1.8. Prevention Strategies

Successful prevention of both deep and superficial fungal infections is crucial in avoiding the danger posed by pathogens such as *Candida* spp. One important method is to employ strict disinfection protocols, particularly within healthcare facilities where transmission risk is higher. For example, research has indicated that microbial loads on chiropractic treatment surfaces are reduced by a significant amount using standard hygiene procedures, underlining the imperative for regular monitoring and compliance with cleaning protocols (Kingham, 2019). Besides, an understanding of the adaptability processes of fungal pathogens, such as the excretion of proteolytic enzymes that enhance their infectivity, can inform prevention by underpinning directed interventions to preclude such strategies (Rapala-Kozik et al., 2010). Ultimately, an integrated strategy combining environmental hygiene, understanding fungal characteristics, and foresightful clinical policies can reduce the incidence of fungal infections significantly, effectively safeguarding public health.

Test Your Knowledge

1. Which skin layer is primarily affected in superficial fungal infections?
2. Which organism causes white piedra?

1.2. Deep Mycoses

Learning Outcome

1. Understand Definition and Characteristics;
2. Explain Common Types of Deep Mycoses;
3. Focus on Causative Agents of Deep Mycoses;
4. Describe Risk Factors for Deep Infections;
5. Learn Symptoms and Clinical Manifestations;
6. Discuss Diagnosis of Deep Mycoses;
7. Know Treatment Options for Deep Infections;
8. Understand Complications Associated with Deep Mycoses.

Deep mycoses represent an emergent subcategory of fungal infections that affect the majority of individuals who are immunocompromised, causing significant impairment of health and mortality. The infections, often caused by opportunistic pathogens such as Candida and Aspergillus species, are capable of disseminating systemically through the bloodstream to other organs, thus complicating clinical management. Evidence suggests that a significant proportion of deep mycoses patients harbor strains of Candida that are potentially resistant to first-line treatment like intravenous fluconazole, indicative of an alarming trend in antifungal resistance (Wissing et al., 2013). Besides, research identifies that while fluconazole may restrict the frequency of oropharyngeal candidiasis and febrile days, it neither significantly reduces the rate of deep mycoses nor improves patient outcomes, even with the existing challenges in effectively controlling these infections (Schaffner & Schaffner, 1995). Thus, controlling deep mycoses is an all-encompassing process that includes vigilant monitoring, targeted therapy, and research for new antifungal medications.

1.2.1. Definition and Characteristics

Fungal infections, whether they present in superficial or deep mycoses, are distinct in their presentation in various tissues, tending to result in distinctive clinical presentations. Superficial mycoses primarily affect the outer layers of skin, hair, and nails and tend to be distinguished by their superficial invasion and low potential to develop into systemic disease. On the other hand, deep mycoses extend to deeper tissue layers and can become systemic, making diagnosis and treatment protocols challenging because of their complex morphological characteristics. For example, chromoblastomycosis is typically diagnosed by verrucous plaques and can have various histopathological features, showing the complexity of deep fungal infections' diagnosis (Dhar et al., 2024). Additionally, emerging pathogens like *Chrysosporium* spp. represent the evolving situation of fungal pathogens, emphasizing their keratinophilic property and drug resistance, impacting both clinical presentation as well as management choices (Kukhar et al., 2025). Overall, an awareness of these definitions and characteristics is crucial for the correct identification and treatment of fungal infections (Figure 1.6).

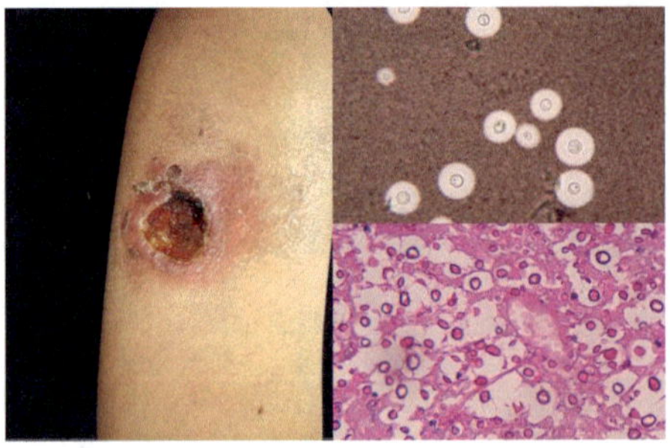

Figure 1.6. Cutaneous involvement in the deep mycoses.

Source: https://static.elsevier.es/multimedia/15782190/0000010700000010/v1_201611260103/S1578219016302414/v1_201611260103/en/main.assets/gr5.jpeg.

1.2.2. Common Types of Deep Mycoses

Deep mycoses, typically serious and sometimes even fatal, are primarily the result of pathogenic fungi infecting internal organs or deep tissues. Among the most common agents, Candida species, most notably *Candida albicans*, are frequently responsible for systemic infections, particularly in immunocompromised hosts, as evidenced by findings tending towards a high prevalence among patients seen in clinical settings (Devrari et al., 2018). Other significant pathogens include Aspergillus species, particularly *Aspergillus fumigatus,* that are responsible for aspergillosis of the lungs and more systemic forms in individuals with weakened immunity. *Cryptococcus neoformans*, responsible for fatal meningitis, most frequently infects the immunocompromised host, including HIV/AIDS patients. The rise in the occurrence of deep mycoses requires greater caution and diagnostic precision, particularly in clinical practice, where patients may present with predisposing factors, thus the need for ongoing research into cure strategies and prevention within public health facilities.

1.2.3. Causative Agents of Deep Mycoses

Understanding the etiologic agents of deep mycoses is central to the right diagnosis and care, particularly because of their association with high morbidity and mortality. Eumycetoma, caused primarily by *Madurella mycetomatis* and prevalent in hot deserts, is a case of the complex ecology surrounding the pathogens; its transmission might be contingent on environmental determinants such as contact with infected soil or animal dung, particularly cattle, in rural East Africa (De Hoog et al., 2013). In addition, emerging research points to the growing prevalence of deep fungal infections among immunocompromised patients, flagging comorbidities such as diabetes and post-transplantation as key determinants of susceptibility (Sivayogana, 2017). Among the many pathogens implicated in deep mycoses, *Madurella mycetomatis* is repeatedly the leading cause, underlining the value of targeted surveillance and intervention to lower the growing prevalence of such infection. Increased understanding of these agents is at the heart of advancing public health interventions against fungal infections (Figure 1.7).

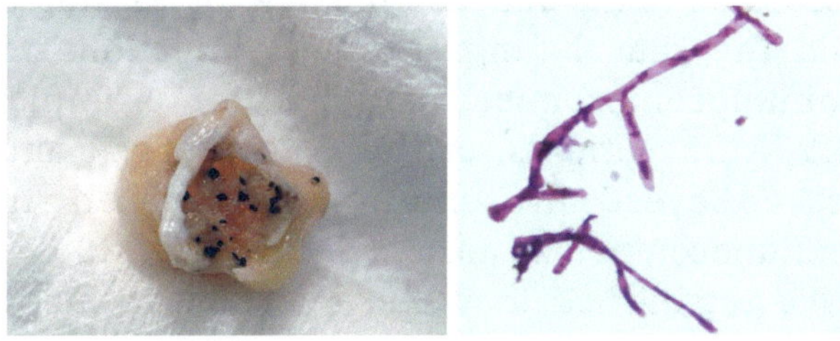

Figure 1.7. Eumycetoma.

Source: https://www.creative-biolabs.com/drug-discovery/therapeutics/images/Eumycetoma.jpg.

1.2.4. Risk Factors for Deep Infections

Deep infections, particularly those caused by fungal pathogens, are problematic in clinical practice due to many risk factors. Of these, immunosuppression is most important; those with impaired immune defenses, such as from baseline disease (e.g., HIV/AIDS) or immunosuppressive therapy for other illnesses, are at greater risk of opportunistic infections. In addition, prolonged hospitalization, particularly in intensive care units, increases exposure to potential pathogens, further heightening infection rates (Wissing et al., 2013). Secondly, invasive procedures such as surgery and catheter placement create further avenues for entry of infection. Literature regarding the use of intravenous (IV) fluconazole mentions the incidence of resistant Candida infection, which indicates even standard antifungal therapy can prove inadequate in certain populations (King et al., 2017). Knowledge about these risk factors is essential to effectively manage and prevent deep fungal infections among high-risk patients.

1.2.5. Symptoms and Clinical Manifestations

Fungal infections, whether superficial or deep, display a wide variety of symptoms and clinical presentation, which are very variable according to the patient's immunological status and the causal fungus. Fungal infections in immunocompromised patients, for example, HIV/AIDS patients, can lead to atypical and more severe presentations compared to immunocompetent hosts. For instance, studies have established that skin infection by fungi, particularly dermatophyte infection, is a relatively frequent occurrence in HIV patients (incidence reported as involving foot lesions in 33.3% of patients) (Gniadek et al., 2012). Conversely, deep mycoses, including invasive candidiasis, are life-threatening in intensive care environments where symptoms might be accompanied by fever and ongoing sepsis; these signs are frequently nonspecific and make it difficult to diagnose and treat in a timely fashion (Delaloye & Calandra, 2013). Familiarity with such presentations is important to maximize effective care and patient outcomes in fungal infection (Figure 1.8).

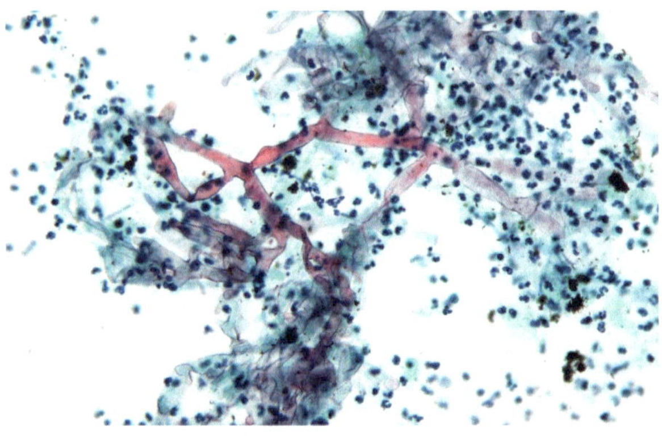

Figure 1.8. In immunocompromised individuals, such as those with HIV/AIDS, fungal infections can lead to atypical and more severe symptoms compared to immunocompetent individuals.

Source: https://upload.wikimedia.org/wikipedia/commons/3/3d/Zygomycosis.jpg.

1.2.6. Diagnosis of Deep Mycoses

Diagnosis of deep mycoses is a big challenge since clinical manifestations are nonspecific and conventional diagnostic tests are limited. Invasive fungal infections, particularly candidiasis, are being increasingly recognized as major causes of sepsis among hospital-admitted patients and contribute to 10%–15% of infections related to healthcare and exert significant impacts on patient outcomes. The diagnosis should occur early because treatment delay enhances mortality risk. Traditional culture methods are mostly unsuccessful, leading health professionals to adopt other diagnostics such as non-culture-based methods, for instance, mannan and β-d-glucan detection, and polymerase chain reaction assays (Pimenta et al., 2020). In addition, imaging techniques like reflectance confocal microscopy (RCM) are being evaluated for their potential to diagnose a range of fungal infections and provide real-time information on cutaneous presentations of deep mycoses, thus enabling better diagnosis and management of treatment (Pimenta et al., 2020).

1.2.7. Treatment Options for Deep Infections

Treatment of deep infections by fungal pathogens requires a personalized approach, particularly taking into account the unpredictable susceptibility of the various organisms. For instance, fluconazole is usually used as the initial therapy for proven *Candida bacteremia* in non-neutropenic patients with no severe sepsis, but those with a history of azole exposure necessitate alternatives like amphotericin B deoxycholate or caspofungin. In immunocompromised individuals, disease severity typically dictates treatment of choice; amphotericin B deoxycholate is used to treat neutropenic patients due to its broad activity and resistance against resistant strains (King et al., 2017). Moreover, the management of invasive aspergillosis depends on an assessment of clinical context, with voriconazole being the agent of choice for starting treatment, while combination regimens can be used in critically ill patients to maximize therapeutic outcomes (King et al., 2017). Thus, a general understanding of antifungal mechanisms and susceptibility patterns is required to maximize therapeutic strategies (King et al., 2017) (Figure 1.9).

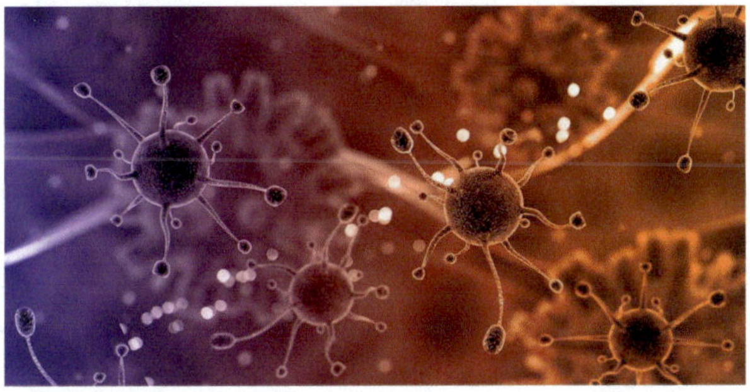

Figure 1.9. Candida bloodstream infections in non-neutropenic patients without severe sepsis, whereas cases involving previous azole exposure necessitate alternatives such as amphotericin B deoxycholate or caspofungin.

Source: https://hospitalpharmacyeurope.com/wp-content/uploads/2017/03/infectious-disease-965x500.jpg.

1.2.8. Complications Associated with Deep Mycoses

Deep mycoses have grave complications, particularly in immunocompromised individuals. These mycoses can cause serious systemic consequences as they are likely to affect essential organs such as the lungs and central nervous system. In AIDS patients, as a case in point, studies have found that mycoses can be remarkably prevalent, ranging in the estimates between 58% and 81% of infected individuals showing signs of fungal infection (Aluyi et al., 2010). These mycoses can manifest either as fatal meningitis or debilitating thrush, significantly decreasing the patient's quality of life. Curiously, the prevalence of dermatophytes also reflects the severity of skin infection among HIV-infected patients, where most of them develop strange and exacerbated symptoms compared to immunocompetent patients (Gniadek et al., 2012). In most cases, the intricacy of deep mycoses demands close monitoring and prompt intervention in a bid to prevent severe health outcomes.

Test Your Knowledge

1. Which fungal infection spreads via lymphatics from the site of inoculation?
2. What is the most common causative organism of eumycetoma?

1.3. Epidemiology of Fungal Infections

Learning Outcome

1. Understand Global Prevalence of Fungal Infections;
2. Explain Demographic Factors Influencing Infection Rates;
3. Focus on Geographic Distribution of Mycoses;
4. Describe Trends in Fungal Infection Outbreaks;
5. Learn Role of Climate Change in Fungal Infections;
6. Discuss Impact of Immunocompromised Populations;
7. Know Surveillance and Reporting Systems;
8. Understand Public Health Initiatives;
9. Explain Future Directions in Epidemiological Research.

The epidemiology of fungal disease, particularly superficial and deep mycoses, reveals impressive patterns and fluctuations governed by local and environmental conditions. Superficial infections, particularly the dermatophyte ones, worldwide account for 20%–30% of the population, with various prevalence rates in varying geographical areas; *T. rubrum*, for instance, is commonly isolated, although *T. tonsurans* is now a major pathogen in the focused populations, particularly among adults in upper-body infections (Galili et al., 2025).

Climate change has also played a big role in the alteration of the distribution of these pathogens, where regional research has come up with more cases of foot and hand mycoses in some Russian regions, where cases of trichophytia have grown immensely (Svirshchevskaya et al., 2024). This evolving epidemiology is testimony to the importance of continued surveillance and adaptive prevention mechanisms responsive to adjust to the evolving landscape of fungal disease.

1.3.1. Global Prevalence of Fungal Infections

Fungal infections are a significant global health issue, and their prevalence is diffuse across populations and age groups. Recent research evidence indicates that in children, dermatophytosis is exceedingly high; for instance, a survey of fungal growth among school children within the city of Kano revealed 91% of samples analyzed to be positive for growth, predominantly in males, with Trichophyton species and Microsporum species most commonly reported to be the leading dermatophytes (Ndako et al., 2012). In addition, the human toll of aggressive fungal infections extends far beyond superficial skin infections, with an estimated 1.8 million individuals in Turkey alone suffering from severe fungal infection annually, including invasive aspergillosis and allergic fungal rhinosinusitis (Hilmioğlu-Polat et al., 2018). These statistics underscore the urgent need for enhanced surveillance and public health interventions to curtail the global burden of fungal infections (Figure 1.10).

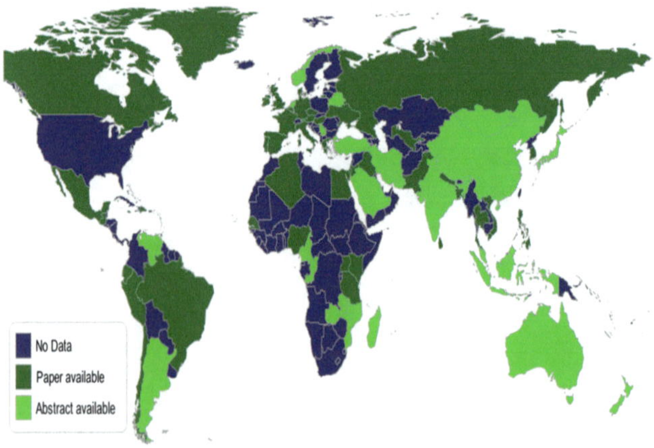

Figure 1.10. A map showing completed country estimates of fungal diseases by August 2017.

Source: https://pub.mdpi-res.com/jof/jof-03-00057/article_deploy/html/images/jof-03-00057-g001.png?1569609651.

1.3.2. Demographic Factors Influencing Infection Rates

Demographic factors influence the rates and patterns of fungal infections, particularly in various populations. Gender difference emerges since research indicates that males are disproportionately infected by fungal infections relative to females. This is accounted for by biological differences, such as variations in sex hormones and gene expression that are still poorly characterized (Rao et al., 2024). Some groups of the population, such as organ transplant recipients, are particularly vulnerable to invasive fungal infections. For instance, candidates for liver transplant are more susceptible to infections like candidiasis and aspergillosis, and certain prophylactic measures are needed to neutralize threats post-surgery (Senoner et al., 2023). The addition of age, economic status, and comorbidities makes the situation of fungal infections more complex, making it necessary to implement public health measures that are tailored to neutralize differences in demographics. By acknowledging this, medical professionals are able to develop more effective prevention and treatment methods for vulnerable populations.

1.3.3. Geographic Distribution of Mycoses

Fungal diseases have a high geographic distribution depending on environmental components, population behavior, and incidence levels of specific fungal organisms. For instance, dermatophytes, as they are often involved in superficial mycoses, have higher occurrences where there is high humidity and heat, and among populations with greater physical activity and close contact with animals.

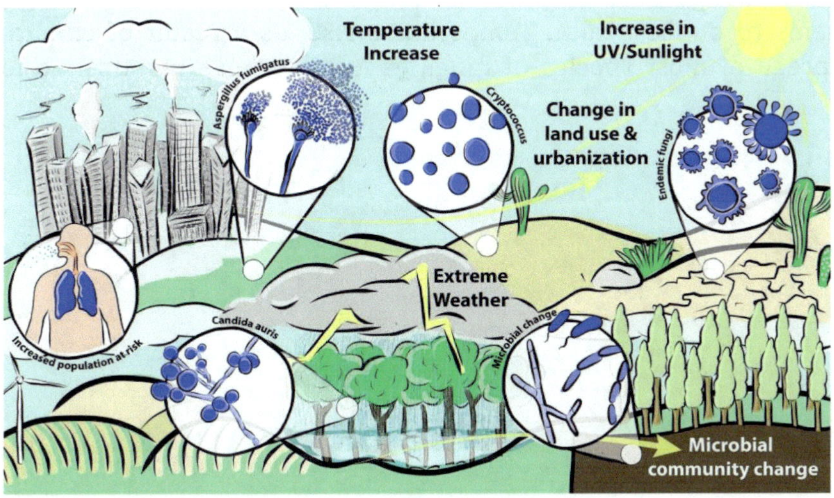

Figure 1.11. Fungal infections exhibit a notable geographic distribution, influenced by environmental conditions, population behaviors, and the prevalence of specific fungal species.

Source: https://www.mdpi.com/jof/jof-07-00367/article_deploy/html/images/jof-07-00367-g001.png.

In Nigeria's Kano city, a study indicated a school child prevalence of dermatophytosis, wherein 91 out of every 100 samples yielded positive fungal growth, predominantly reported in males who engage in outdoor play and come into contact with pets (Ndako et al., 2012). Moreover, modeling in Turkey puts the number of people with severe fungal infections annually at around 1.79 million, with significant superficial infection cases such as tinea pedis and onychomycosis (Hilmioğlu-Polat et al., 2018). The outcomes feature the complex interaction between geography and the epidemiology of mycoses (Figure 1.11).

1.3.4. Trends in Fungal Infection Outbreaks

Fungi infections are becoming more recognized as serious threats to health, exemplified by the dire trends of rising outbreaks for both deep and superficial mycoses. These serious infections, with high morbidity and mortality, most often originate from endogenous fungi such as Candida and Malassezia, and from external fungal origins. It is further exacerbated by the emergence of antifungal-resistant strains that need newer therapeutic interventions to combat the infections adequately (Ciociola et al., 2021). Lastly, zoonotic fungal infections, despite how much they are usually overlooked, also show a potential for transmission from pets to human beings in developing countries like Nigeria. The absence of appropriate attention given to such zoonoses is contrary to their capability to result in public health crises, mimicking the necessity for more information and prevention (Adebiyi & Oluwayelu, 2019). This convergence of factors indicates that the epidemiology of fungal infections is evolving, mirroring an imperative need for more research and intervention in public health.

1.3.5. Role of Climate Change in Fungal Infections

The effect of climate change on the spread of fungal infections is increasingly evident, posing widespread problems to public health. Temperature rise, as a result of climatic changes, favors the growth and spread of most species of fungi, especially those responsible for superficial and deep mycoses.

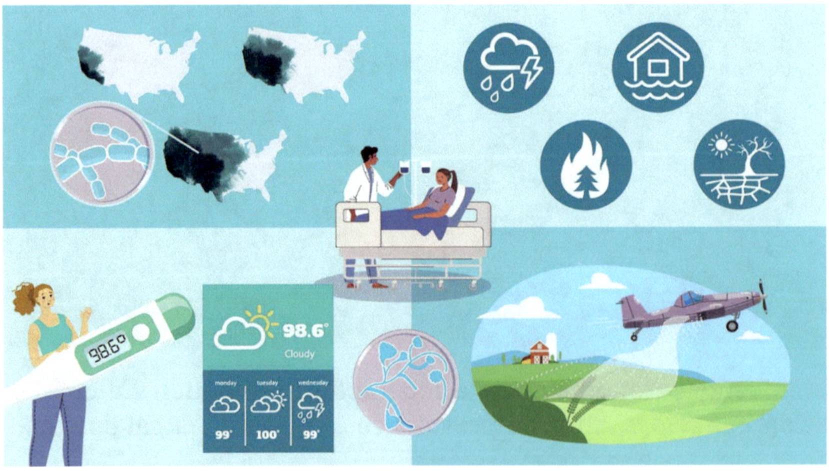

Figure 1.12. Elevated temperatures and altered precipitation patterns create favorable conditions for pathogens such as Candida and Aspergillus, which thrive in diverse environments as they adapt to a changing ecosystem.

Source: https://www.cdc.gov/fungal/media/images/2024/06/343286-A_MDB_INFO_ClimateChangeAndFungalDisease_NoText.jpg.

Hot environments and altered precipitation patterns favor the ecosystems for pathogens such as Aspergillus and Candida that exist in other habitats as they adapt to a changing ecosystem. Moreover, human activities and ecological degradation offer conditions that cause increased risk of exposure, particularly in vulnerable populations that live in areas that are deprived of hygiene and health services. This is an indication of the call for a multistakeholder global action to increase cases of fungal infections, as emphasized in an extensive review of the current situation at hand for fungal infections (Klimas et al., 2025). Also notable is awareness of how environmental factors synergize with the survival of fungi to facilitate effective preventive measures and hygienic practices in hospitals (Kingham, 2019) (Figure 1.12).

1.3.6. Impact of Immunocompromised Populations

The impact of immunocompromised populations on the prevalence and severity of fungal infections, particularly superficial and deep mycoses, is serious and multifaceted. Immunocompromised patients, such as those receiving cancer treatment or those who have received organ transplants, are particularly susceptible to invasive fungal diseases (IFD). Infections with species like *Candida albicans* and *Aspergillus fumigatus* tend to result in severe morbidity and mortality among affected patients. The implication of these conditions is further fueled by the growing population of immunocompromised patients globally, thus IFD is a priority for public health (Klimas et al., 20202025 Enhanced diagnostic methods have become imperative for the early detection and intervention to prevent complications since early treatment can radically improve outcomes (Fang et al., 2023). Moreover, the socioeconomic burden to healthcare systems is significant, which also lends support to the creation of more awareness and research on how to maximize management and prevention measures for this vulnerable group.

1.3.7. Surveillance and Reporting Systems

Effective surveillance and reporting systems are crucial in the battle against fungal infections, particularly invasive fungal diseases (IFD) that are of significant public health interest. The epidemiology of IFD necessitates the application of intensive data gathering methods in an effort to allow for accurate reporting of incidence and improved clinical outcomes. By studying intensive health data networks, as current research is presently illustrating, health care systems can identify trends and risk groups with an eye toward individualizing interventions.

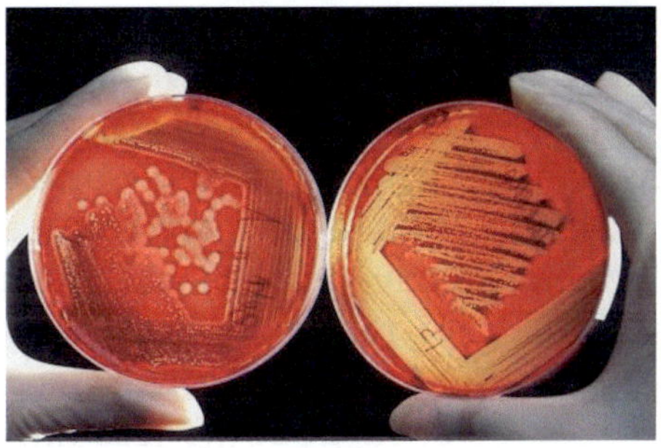

Figure 1.13. Effective surveillance and reporting systems are essential in combatting fungal infections, particularly invasive fungal diseases (IFD) that pose significant public health challenges.

Source: https://images.unsplash.com/photo-1631557677599-ee5fe0b3440b?crop=entropy&cs=tinysrgb&fit=max&fm=jpg&ixid=M3w3MDgyMDR8MHwxfHNlYXJjaHwxfHxmdW5nYWwlMjBkaXNlYXNlJTIwc3VydmVpbGxhbmNlJTJDJTIwc2tpbiUyMGZ1bmdhbCUyMGluZmVjdGlvbnMlMkMlMjBwdWJsaWMlMjBoZWFsdGh8ZW58MHwwfHx8MTc0OTkxNzU0OXww&ixlib=rb-4.1.0&q=80&w=500&?utm_source=numberanalytics&utm_medium=referral.

For instance, it has been shown through evidence that the most prevalent form of IFD is candidiasis, at 55% prevalence of all infections, and immunocompromised individuals are particularly vulnerable (Webb et al., 2018). Furthermore, as concerns broaden on morbidity and mortality due to such infections, improved surveillance assists in unveiling trends and potential outbreaks, lending further credence to allied public health interventions (Firacative, 2020). Finally, robust surveillance and reporting networks are essential in combating the increasing threat of fungal infection within hospital and community environments (Figure 1.13).

1.3.8. Public Health Initiatives

Public health action has a crucial role to play in bringing down the rising wave of fungal infections, particularly in terms of antimicrobial resistance. The release of the list of fungal priority pathogens (FPPL) by the World Health Organization in 2022 highlighted the necessity of developing effective public health responses to counter the drug-resistant fungal pathogens, having significant implications within clinical settings (Garvey et al., 2025). These initiatives will need to be directed at maximizing hygiene practice, especially in health care environments, for minimizing cross-transmission risk due to contaminated medical devices. Initiatives should also be focused on maximizing compliance with current cleaning and sterilization protocols, which are paramount in the prevention of infection due to these resilient pathogens. Also, additional studies and the use of new technologies, such as artificial intelligence in monitoring and diagnosis, can arm health systems with the necessary instruments to efficiently manage and prevent the transmission of fungi (Barnard & Carpenter, 2024). Public health action, coordinated through joint efforts, can significantly improve the fight against fungal infections.

1.3.9. Future Directions in Epidemiological Research

With the advancement of epidemiological studies, a key direction for future study is gaining knowledge about the environmental and social determinants of the incidence of fungal infection, particularly in vulnerable populations. Multidisciplinary approaches are particularly crucial in formulating a perspective on the emergence of new fungal pathogens, which was lately highlighted in studies emphasizing sophisticated interaction between host immunological function and pathogen virulence (Klimas et al., 2025). Moreover, solving the treatment of opportunistic mycoses, especially in immunocompromised patients, presents a solid research avenue since existing treatment measures fall short in effectively addressing such infections (Silva, 2013). Effective systems of surveillance, with a boost in genomics and data analysis technology, can provide a better platform for the study of epidemiological patterns and aid public health interventions. Finally, these focused research objectives attempt to refine prevention techniques and therapeutic strategies, aiming to realize better outcomes in the treatment of fungal diseases globally.

Test Your Knowledge

1. What is the most common fungal infection seen in HIV/AIDS patients?
2. Which public health practice is most effective in reducing superficial fungal infections?

1.4. Advances in Research and Treatment

Learning Outcome

1. Understand Recent Developments in Antifungal Therapies;
2. Explain Novel Drug Targets and Mechanisms;
3. Focus on the Role of Immunotherapy in Fungal Infections;
4. Describe Advances in Diagnostic Techniques;
5. Learn Research on Vaccine Development;
6. Discuss the Importance of Microbiome Studies;
7. Know Challenges in Antifungal Resistance;
8. Understand Role of Technology in Fungal Infection Management;
9. Explain Future Research Priorities.

The latest advances in research and treatment of candidiasis and other fungal infections have highlighted the intricacies of fighting such opportunistic pathogens. As Candida species, particularly those beyond *Candida albicans*, contribute significantly to the challenge of antifungal resistance, understanding the mechanisms behind biofilm formation has become increasingly critical.

Biofilms, by accumulating dense cell populations and exhibiting multifaceted resistance strategies, complicate treatment regimens for patients afflicted with candidiasis (Silva et al., 2017). At the same time, studies on the role of microbiomes in eye disease highlight the manner in which imbalances will lead to varied conditions, highlighting the necessity of learning more about microbial interactions within surface and deep mycoses (Su & Tighe, 2017). Furthermore, developments in antifungal therapy and inhibition of biofilms may become key to reducing efficacy losses and meeting resistance, portending improved patient care for these infections (Figure 1.14).

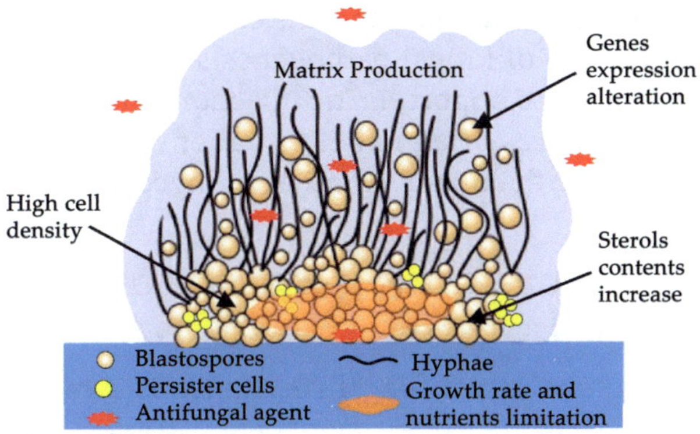

Figure 1.14. As Candida species, particularly those beyond *Candida albicans*, contribute significantly to the challenge of antifungal resistance, understanding the mechanisms behind biofilm formation has become increasingly critical.

Source: https://www.mdpi.com/jof/jof-03-00008/article_deploy/html/images/jof-03-00008-g001.png.

1.4.1. Recent Developments in Antifungal Therapies

The landscape of antifungal therapies is transforming dramatically, keeping up with the increasing incidence and severity of fungal infections. The recent developments encompass the introduction of novel delivery systems, with nanotechnology being at the forefront, enhancing the efficacy of antifungal medications. Liposomes and dendrimers are among the nanoarchitectures utilized as drug delivery systems (DDS), which offer improved bioavailability and targeted action against resistant fungal populations (Mishra et al., 2021). Further, ongoing research makes epidemiology and clinical presentation of various fungal pathogens a top priority to learn about, a justification that drives the development of novel treatments for infections specific (Klimas et al., 2025). These interdisciplinary approaches not only seek to treat already known pathogens but also for the future, forecasting threats ahead, which presents a pressing need for antifungal treatment innovation. With increased knowledge of fungal pathogenesis, our arsenal against these opportunistic infections increases, ultimately resulting in better patient outcomes with superficial as well as deep mycoses.

1.4.2. Novel Drug Targets and Mechanisms

The return of antifungal resistance is a major challenge to the management of fungal infections, and this indeed highlights the importance of new drug targets and mechanisms. Emerging research has unveiled the multifaceted adaptive responses of pathogenic fungi against antifungal agents, particularly their ability to modify cell structures and biochemical processes. For instance, studies on *Lomentospora prolificans* have demonstrated that the application of voriconazole causes basic changes in cell wall composition and structure with critical alterations in the level of glucan and mannan, which could represent useful targets for the creation of new therapeutic interventions (Pellon et al., 2017). Furthermore, biofilm development in Candida species makes treatment more difficult because such structures possess multifactorial resistance mechanisms, such as enhanced cell density and gene expression modification (Silva et al., 2017). Knowledge of these survival strategies forms the basis for designing targeted interventions that potentially could make currently available therapies more effective or lead to innovative drug development, ultimately resulting in better patient outcomes for superficial and deep mycoses.

1.4.3. Role of Immunotherapy in Fungal Infections

The application of immunotherapy in treating fungal diseases becomes all the more important with the growing prevalence of superficial and deep mycoses, which are serious threats to public health. Conventional antifungal therapy is often ineffective due to the development of drug-resistant microorganisms and the rising number of immunocompromised patients, raising the need for new therapeutic strategies. Immunotherapies provide a hopeful solution through the use of the body's immune response to fight fungal pathogens more efficiently. For instance, monoclonal antibodies and antifungal peptides were found to be promising in eliciting immune responses specifically against fungal antigens and lessening the severity of infections with greater precision. Such immunotherapeutic strategies not only aim to enhance the host's innate and adaptive immune response but also endeavor to minimize the toxicity of conventional antifungals, as highlighted by latest research (de Ullivarri et al., 2020; Qadri et al., 2023). Therefore, immunotherapy research is a very important frontier of fungal disease treatment with the potential to significantly change the treatment regimen (Figure 1.15).

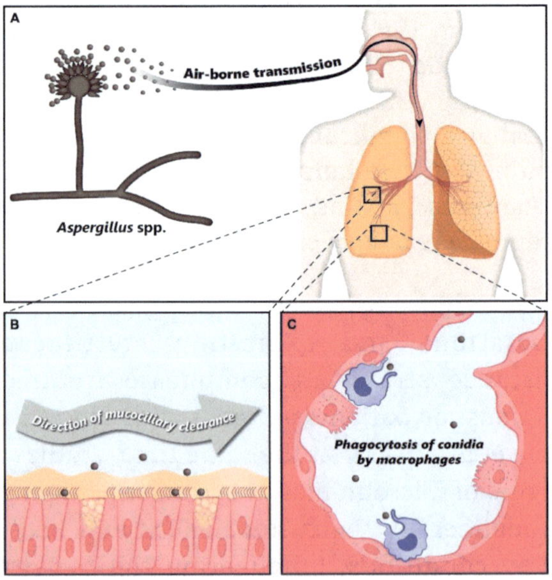

Figure 1.15. The role of immunotherapy in managing fungal infections is increasingly critical given the rising incidence of both superficial and deep mycoses, which pose substantial threats to public health.

Source: https://www.frontiersin.org/files/Articles/832510/fmed-09-832510-HTML/image_m/fmed-09-832510-g001.jpg.

1.4.4. Advances in Diagnostic Techniques

The evolving pattern of diagnostic instruments has shaped the management of fungal infections, both superficial and deep mycoses, significantly. The traditional methods, primarily microscopy and culture, have been supplemented more and more by newer methods that improve the accuracy and speed. Over all these years, advances such as polymerase chain reaction (PCR) assays and next-generation sequencing have revolutionized the identification of various fungal species, allowing earlier treatment and improved patient outcomes. Furthermore, the emergence of artificial intelligence, machine learning algorithms and biosensor technologies has facilitated the development of fast, highly sensitive, and specific tests for detecting fungal infections, addressing the drawbacks of conventional techniques. As evident from recent reviews, the intersection of these novel diagnostic methods can lead to enhanced clinical decision-making and individualized treatment protocols, significantly limiting morbidity due to invasive fungal infections (Fang et al., 2023). Such innovations are vital owing to the rising cases of diseases such as onychomycosis, which demonstrate a future possibility for enhanced resistance against traditional treatments (Bermudez et al., 2023).

1.4.5. Research on Vaccine Development

The development of effective vaccines to fight fungal infections remains a critical field of research against the background of the growing number of immunocompromised individuals vulnerable to severe mycoses. Current strategies are hampered by a poor understanding of host-fungal interactions and the complexities of immune responses triggered by vaccines. Significantly, the majority of studies indicate that advances in proteomics and glycomics have led to the identification of candidate antigens for subunit vaccines, along with better adjuvants to enhance immune responses against fungi (Carvalho et al., 2017). Despite this progress, no licensed vaccines are available, and this makes the case for innovative solutions. In addition, identification of environmental factors that may influence infection dynamics, such as the ecology of *Madurella mycetomatis*, illuminates potential strategies against preventing infection that are based on environmental control (in addition to vaccine development) (De Hoog et al., 2013). Thus, the intersection of basic science and applied science is key to the successful prevention of fungal infections (Figure 1.16).

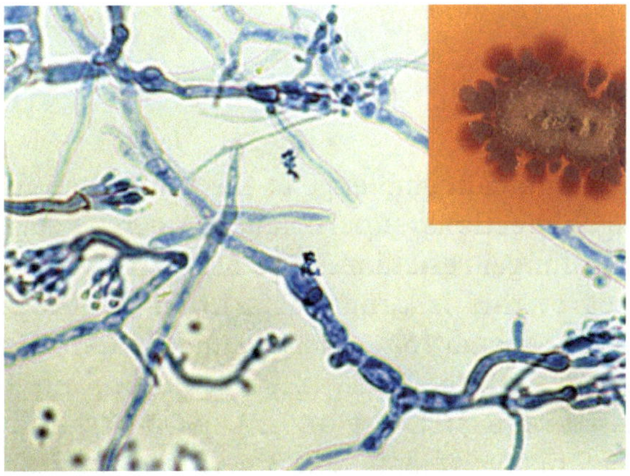

Figure 1.16. Ecology of *Madurella mycetomatis*.

Source: https://www.adelaide.edu.au/mycology/sites/default/files/styles/ua_image_landscape/public/media/images/2021-07/madurella.jpg?h=b7ccb692&itok=udZUHY9Y.

1.4.6. Importance of Microbiome Studies

The relevance of microbiome research has gained more interest, particularly on fungal infections, superficial mycoses, and deep mycoses. Explanation of the intricate relationship between the human microbiome and its fungal part is crucial in unraveling the dynamics of fungal pathogenesis. For instance, microbiome alterations, such as those caused by antibiotic treatment, can lead to opportunistic fungal infections, including candidiasis, particularly in immunocompromised individuals (Niño-Vega et al., 2024). Furthermore, it has been demonstrated that there are sex differences in fungal colonization and infection and that it is crucial to address a gender perspective for microbiome studies (Rao et al., 2024). By describing these complex interactions, researchers can enhance therapeutic interventions and public health interventions, essentially reducing the burden of fungal infection. Therefore, advancing microbiome research not only enhances our understanding of fungal infections, but it can also present potential paths to new therapies and prevention of these pathogens.

1.4.7. Challenges in Antifungal Resistance

One significant challenge to the management of fungal infections, superficial and deep mycoses, is antifungal resistance. One of the best-known cases of this is candidiasis, where pathogen biofilm formation, as by *Candida albicans*, makes it harder to treat. The complex biofilm structure assists in an intrinsic resistance mechanism against penetration by antifungal agents, ultimately leading to treatment failure (Silva et al., 2017). Besides, such species as *Trichosporon asahii*, which have been shown to be common pathogens in deep infections, exhibit heterogeneous resistance patterns, particularly to amphotericin B, and this is used to highlight the necessity for proper identification and susceptibility testing (Rodriguez-Tudela et al., 2005). The increasing incidence of resistant strains adds to the necessity for ongoing research into novel antifungal agents and therapy strategies that counter such obstacles. Without targeted treatment, the management of fungal infections will become progressively ineffective, and this will constitute a threat of serious proportions to public health (Figure 1.17).

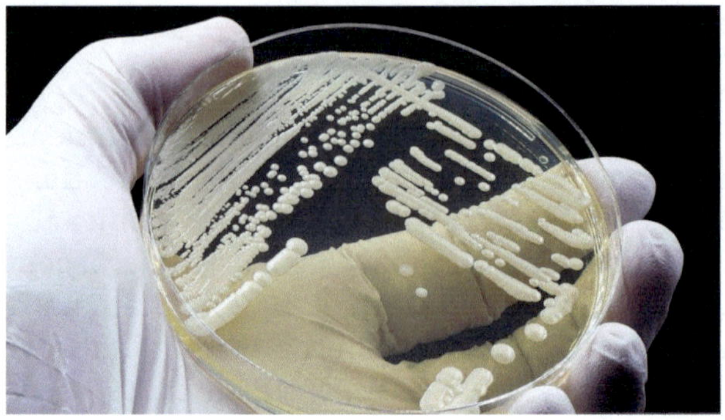

Figure 1.17. Antifungal resistance presents a significant challenge in the management of fungal infections, including both superficial and deep mycoses.

Source: https://images.theconversation.com/files/623917/original/file-20241007-18-a08o8p.jpg?ixlib=rb-4.1.0&rect=0%2C533%2C6560%2C3280&q=45&auto=format&w=1356&h=668&fit=crop.

1.4.8. Role of Technology in Fungal Infection Management

Technology is the key driver of enhanced diagnostics, efficacy of treatment, and understanding of fungal pathogens in clinical management today. Advanced molecular techniques, such as OMICS technologies, allow for the identification of fungal species and their resistance mechanisms, thereby informing clinical interventions on the management of infections like those of *Lomentospora prolificans,* a pathogen with considerable mortality in immunocompromised hosts (Konsoula et al., 2022). Further, the development of new diagnostic equipment enables rapid diagnosis of fungal infections and appropriate and timely antifungal therapies. These are significant advances in light of the complexity of the treatment of invasive mycoses, wherein resistance to existing antifungal agents poses significant challenges. With research continuing to unravel the sophisticated roles of fungi in human health, from the discovery of new drug candidates to potential use of fungi for biodegradation (Mapook et al., 2022), technological developments are ready to overhaul the status of fungal infection control significantly (Figure 1.18).

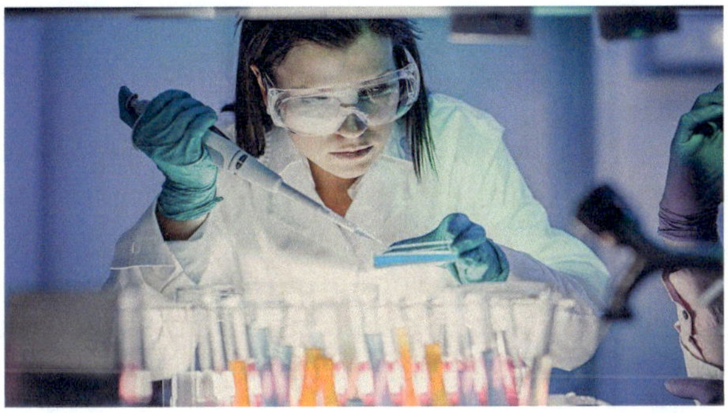

Figure 1.18. Role of technology in fungal infection management.

Source: https://assets.technologynetworks.com/production/dynamic/images/content/382793/global-deaths-from-fungal-disease-have-doubled-382793-960x540.jpg?cb=12645223.

1.4.9. Future Research Priorities

With the ongoing rise in fungal infections, it is crucial to determine future research priorities to learn more about and control these infections. Another significant area that needs further research is the development of improved diagnostic platforms using artificial intelligence and machine learning to enhance surveillance and monitor fungal pathogens more accurately. This new approach would be complemented by enhanced environmental surveillance to prevent medical device contamination—a key public health problem that has been recognized as particularly pertinent to drug-resistant pathogens (Garvey et al., 2025). Furthermore, it is essential to address the problems of biofilm development and persistence of drug-resistant fungi, which are significant clinical issues. Facilitating interdisciplinary interactions will develop a whole-system research culture that meets the requirements of contemporary public health and unites diverse perspectives in order to ultimately drive prevention, diagnosis, and treatment methods for fungal infections (Barnard & Carpenter, 2024).

Test Your Knowledge

1. Which antifungal has fungicidal action against dermatophytes?
2. Which antifungal is FDA-approved for onychomycosis treatment?

SUMMARY

Learning about fungal infections, with particular reference to superficial and deep mycoses, emphasizes the need for early diagnosis and effective therapeutic interventions. As depicted by various case studies, including those of severe aplastic anemia and associated complications, invasive fungal infections can complicate patient outcomes significantly, leaning towards serious morbidity and mortality (Krithinaki et al., 2025). The multifaceted pathological image of deep mycoses also underscores the significance of histopathological examination in arriving at accurate diagnoses, considering the varied morphological presentations that may complicate diagnosis (Dhar et al., 2024). This heterogeneity necessitates the application of a multidisciplinary model that integrates clinical experience with state-of-the-art diagnostic tests for the purpose of optimal management of both the hematology underlying disease and the fungal infections. In the end, future studies into the genetic and immunologic features of patients infected with such conditions will play an important role in formulating improved patient care and the design of targeted therapies for future therapy.

A comprehensive understanding of fungal infections entails a review of some key issues, including their epidemiology, clinical presentation, and treatment difficulties. As pointed out in existing literature, the growing epidemic of fungal infections poses significant public health risks, particularly among immunocompromised patients and those with predisposing underlying medical conditions (Klimas et al., 2025). Key pathogenic mechanisms, such as the ability of fungal pathogens to form biofilms and the various virulence factors that they have, underscore the complexity of their interaction with the host immune system, complicating treatment and management (Vila & Rozental, 2016). Furthermore, understanding the environmental and social determinants perpetuating these infections is crucial to ensuring successful public health interventions. Addressing such sophisticated issues requires a coordinated global effort focusing on developing diagnostic and treatment capabilities alongside an appreciation for the growing trends in antifungal resistance to counteract the rising threat of fungal infections worldwide.

KEY TERMS FROM THIS CHAPTER

- Adaptability
- Age
- Anticancer chemotherapy
- Antifungal activity
- Antimicrobials
- Appendages
- Athlete's foot
- Biofilm production
- Bisphosphonates
- Candida albicans
- Candida auris
- Candida species
- Cell density
- Clinicians
- Cryptococcus neoformans
- Culture
- Deep mycoses
- Dermatophytes

CRITICAL THINKING QUESTIONS

1. **Which of the following organisms is most commonly responsible for *Tinea corporis*?**
   a. *Candida albicans*
   b. *Trichophyton rubrum*
   c. *Malassezia furfur*
   d. *Epidermophyton floccosum*
2. **Which fungal infection presents with hypopigmented or hyperpigmented macules with fine scaling, commonly on the trunk?**
   a. *Tinea corporis*
   b. *Tinea versicolor*
   c. Candidiasis
   d. *Tinea capitis*
3. **Wood's lamp examination of *Tinea versicolor* shows fluorescence of which color?**
   a. Green
   b. Red
   c. Yellowish-green
   d. Coral red
4. **The term "satellite lesions" is most commonly associated with which condition?**
   a. Tinea capitis
   b. Cutaneous candidiasis
   c. Tinea cruris
   d. Onychomycosis
5. **Which of the following is the treatment of choice for onychomycosis?**
   a. Topical clotrimazole
   b. Oral terbinafine
   c. Oral fluconazole for 1 week
   d. Topical salicylic acid

Short Answer Questions

1. Which organism is the most common cause of *Tinea corporis*?
2. What is the classical microscopic appearance of *Malassezia furfur*?
3. Which deep fungal infection is known as "rose gardener's disease"?
4. Which organism causes chromoblastomycosis?
5. Which climatic condition promotes dermatophytosis?
6. Which age group is most affected by *Tinea capitis*?
7. Which antifungal class inhibits ergosterol synthesis?
8. What is the mechanism of action of terbinafine?

Answers to Critical Thinking Questions

1. (b); 2. (b); 3. (c); 4. (b); 5. (b)

REFERENCES

1. Adebiyi, A. I., & Oluwayelu, D. O. (2019). Zoonotic fungal diseases and animal ownership in Nigeria. https://core.ac.uk/download/478436841.pdf (accessed on 23rd July 2025).
2. de Hoog, G. S., Ahmed, S. A., Najafzadeh, M. J., Sutton, D. A., Keisari, M. S., Fahal, A. H., Eberhardt, U., Verkleij, G. J., Xin, L., Stielow, B., & van de Sande, W. W. (2013). Phylogenetic findings suggest possible new habitat and routes of infection of human eumyctoma. *PLoS neglected tropical diseases*, *7*(5), e2229. https://doi.org/10.1371/journal.pntd.0002229(accessed on 23rd July 2025).
3. Silva, S., Rodrigues, C. F., Araújo, D., Rodrigues, M. E., & Henriques, M. (2017). Candida Species Biofilms' Antifungal Resistance. *Journal of fungi (Basel, Switzerland)*, *3*(1), 8. https://doi.org/10.3390/jof3010008(accessed on 23rd July 2025).
4. Mishra, V., Singh, M., Mishra, Y., Charbe, N., Nayak, P., Sudhakar, K., Aljabali, A. A. A., Shahcheraghi, S. H., Bakshi, H., Serrano-Aroca, Á., & Tambuwala, M. M. (2021). Nanoarchitectures in Management of Fungal Diseases: An Overview. *Applied Sciences*, *11*(15), 7119. https://doi.org/10.3390/app11157119(accessed on 23rd July 2025).
5. Aluyi, HAS; Otajevwo, F D; Iweriebor, O. Incidence of pulmonary mycoses in patients with acquired immunedeficiency diseases. Nigerian Journal of Clinical Practice 13(1):p 78-83, Jan–Mar 2010. (accessed on 23rd July 2025).
6. Pellon, A., Ramirez-Garcia, A., Buldain, I., Antoran, A., Rementeria, A., & Hernando, F. L. (2017). Molecular and cellular responses of the pathogenic fungus Lomentospora prolificans to the antifungal drug voriconazole. *PloS one*, *12*(3), e0174885. https://doi.org/10.1371/journal.pone.0174885(accessed on 23rd July 2025).
7. Pimenta, R., Soares-de-Almeida, L., Arzberger, E., Ferreira, J., Leal-Filipe, P., Bastos, P. M., & Oliveira, A. L. (2020). Reflectance confocal microscopy for the diagnosis of skin infections and infestations. *Dermatology online journal*, *26*(3), 13030/qt9qz046f1.(accessed on 23rd July 2025).
8. Wissing, H., Ballus, J., Bingold, T. M., Nocea, G., Krobot, K. J., Kaskel, P., Kumar, R. N., & Mavros, P. (2013). Intensive care unit-related fluconazole use in Spain and Germany: patient characteristics and outcomes of a prospective multicenter longitudinal observational study. *Infection and drug resistance*, *6*, 15–25. https://doi.org/10.2147/IDR.S38945(accessed on 23rd July 2025).
9. Ndako, J.A., Osemwegie, O.O., Spencer, T.H., Olopade, B.K., Yunusa, G., & Banda, J.M. (2012). Prevalence of Dermatophytes and other associated Fungi among school children. https://core.ac.uk/download/32224884.pdf (accessed on 23rd July 2025).
10. Barnard, C. C., & Carpenter, E. (2024). *A Classification for Medical and Veterinary Libraries.* https://doi.org/10.56920/lshtmp-1 (accessed on 23rd July 2025).
11. Baumgardner, D. J. (2017). Freshwater fungal infections. https://digitalrepository.aurorahealthcare.org/cgi/viewcontent.cgi?article=1262&context=jpcrr (accessed on 23rd July 2025).
12. Rapala-Kozik, M., Karkowska-Kuleta, J., Ryzanowska, A., Golda, A., Barbasz, A., Faussner, A., & Kozik, A. (2010). Degradation of human kininogens with the release of kinin peptides by extracellular proteinases of Candida spp. *Biological chemistry*, *391*(7), 823–830. https://doi.org/10.1515/BC.2010.083(accessed on 23rd July 2025).

13. Bhattacharyya, S., A., K., Chakraborty, M., & Chatterjee, S. (2023). Emerging fungal infections of man. *MOJ Biology and Medicine*. https://www.semanticscholar.org/paper/a45b9004887a6bbbb29429028faa7be90f8d3267 (accessed on 23rd July 2025).

14. Bille, J., Calandra, T., Eggimann, P., et al. (2006). Treatment options of invasive fungal infections in adults. https://core.ac.uk/download/77158963.pdf (accessed on 23rd July 2025).

15. Bonifaz, A., Tirado-Sánchez, A., Mercadillo, P., Moreno-López, L. M., Fierro-Arias, L., Araiza, J., & González, G. (2021). Clinical and mycological study of 42 cases of dermatophyte granuloma (Majocchi granuloma). *JDDG: Journal der Deutschen Dermatologischen Gesellschaft, 19*. https://www.semanticscholar.org/paper/c5baa5b6479ae40baeccdc180a7cd7609c5445b9 (accessed on 23rd July 2025).

16. Delaloye, J., & Calandra, T. (2014). Invasive candidiasis as a cause of sepsis in the critically ill patient. *Virulence*, *5*(1), 161–169. https://doi.org/10.4161/viru.26187(accessed on 23rd July 2025).

17. Rodriguez-Tudela, J. L., Diaz-Guerra, T. M., Mellado, E., Cano, V., Tapia, C., Perkins, A., Gomez-Lopez, A., Rodero, L., & Cuenca-Estrella, M. (2005). Susceptibility patterns and molecular identification of Trichosporon species. *Antimicrobial agents and chemotherapy*, *49*(10), 4026–4034. https://doi.org/10.1128/AAC.49.10.4026-4034.2005(accessed on 23rd July 2025).

18. Carvalho, A., Duarte-Oliveira, C., Gonçalves, S.M. *et al.* Fungal Vaccines and Immunotherapeutics: Current Concepts and Future Challenges. *Curr Fungal Infect Rep* **11**, 16–24 (2017). https://doi.org/10.1007/s12281-017-0272-y (accessed on 23rd July 2025).

19. Ciociola, T., Giovati, L., Conti, S., & Magliani, W. (2021). Anti-Infective Antibody-Derived Peptides Active against Endogenous and Exogenous Fungi. *Microorganisms*, *9*(1), 143. https://doi.org/10.3390/microorganisms9010143(accessed on 23rd July 2025).

20. Hilmioğlu-Polat, S., Seyedmousavi, S., Ilkit, M., Hedayati, M. T., Inci, R., Tumbay, E., & Denning, D. W. (2019). Estimated burden of serious human fungal diseases in Turkey. *Mycoses*, *62*(1), 22–31. https://doi.org/10.1111/myc.12842 (accessed on 23rd July 2025).

21. Devrari, J. C., Pai, V., & Saxena, V. (2018). A mycological study of clinical samples from suspected mycoses in a tertiary care hospital. https://core.ac.uk/download/477854048.pdf (accessed on 23rd July 2025).

22. Dhar, S., Pradhan, S., Saha, A., Mazumder, G., Ghosh, S. K., Biswas, M., De, A., et al. (2024). Deep fungal infections of skin and role of histopathology in diagnosis. *Indian Journal of Dermatology, 69*, 442–452. https://www.semanticscholar.org/paper/0065daad03d1319017921e13507031ac8b9b259b (accessed on 23rd July 2025).

23. Fang, W., Wu, J., Cheng, M., Zhu, X., Du, M., Chang, C., Liao, W., et al. (2023). Diagnosis of invasive fungal infections: Challenges and recent developments. *Journal of Biomedical Science, 30*. https://doi.org/10.1186/s12929-023-00926-2 (accessed on 23rd July 2025).

24. Fernández de Ullivarri, M., Arbulu, S., García-Gutiérrez, E., & Cotter, P. D. (2020). Antifungal peptides as therapeutic agents. *Frontiers in Cellular and Infection Microbiology, 10*. https://doi.org/10.3389/fcimb.2020.00105 (accessed on 23rd July 2025).

25. Fernández Silva, F. V. (2013). Evaluation of virulence and new experimental therapeutic strategies for emerging and uncommon medically important fungal pathogens. https://core.ac.uk/download/19934802.pdf (accessed on 23rd July 2025).

26. Firacative, C. (2020). Invasive fungal disease in humans: Are we aware of the real impact? *Memórias do Instituto Oswaldo Cruz, 115*. https://doi.org/10.1590/0074-02760200430 (accessed on 23rd July 2025).

27. Galili, E., Taieb, A., Shemer, A., Leor, G., Lyakhovitsky, A., Barzilai, A., & Baum, S. (2025). Epidemiology and trends of cutaneous fungal infections (2019–2022) in Israel: A single tertiary-center study. *Journal of Fungi, 11*. https://www.semanticscholar.org/paper/bae3778124ae0163881b4c4f2e4d61dad3332df1 (accessed on 23rd July 2025).

28. Gniadek, A., Garlicki, A., Gądek, A., et al. (2012). Prevalence of dermatophytes in interdigital spaces in HIV patients. https://core.ac.uk/download/344346889.pdf (accessed on 23rd July 2025).

29. Garvey, M., Kremer, T. A., & Rowan, N. J. (2025). Efficacy of cleaning, disinfection and sterilization modalities for addressing infectious drug-resistant fungi: A review. *Journal of Applied Microbiology*. https://doi.org/10.1093/jambio/lxaf005 (accessed on 23rd July 2025).

30. Green, M., Wald, E. R., Tzakis, A., Todo, S., & Starzl, T. E. (1991). Aspergillosis of the CNS in a pediatric liver transplant recipient: case report and review. *Reviews of infectious diseases, 13*(4), 653–657. https://doi.org/10.1093/clinids/13.4.653(accessed on 23rd July 2025).

31. Muthanna, A., & Jamil, A. (2022). Cutaneous infections among Human Immunodeficiency Virus (HIV) - infected patients in a single center in Kuala Lumpur, Malaysia. *Microbes and Infectious Diseases, 3*(1), 55–61. Retrieved from https://www.ajol.info/index.php/mid/article/view/219975(accessed on 23rd July 2025).

32. Kane, A., Rothwell, J., Guttentag, A., Hainsworth, S., & Carter, D. A. (2024). Bisphosphonates synergistically enhance the antifungal activity of azoles in dermatophytes and other pathogenic molds. *mSphere, 9*. https://www.semanticscholar.org/paper/dc195e668b4e9d4cbb37633729d338ef412766c8 (accessed on 23rd July 2025).

33. King, J., Pana, Z. D., Lehrnbecher, T., Steinbach, W. J., & Warris, A. (2017). Recognition and Clinical Presentation of Invasive Fungal Disease in Neonates and Children. *Journal of the Pediatric Infectious Diseases Society, 6*(suppl_1), S12–S21. https://doi.org/10.1093/jpids/pix053 (accessed on 23rd July 2025).

34. Kingham, M. C. (2019). Monitoring treatment table hygiene in a chiropractic training clinic. https://core.ac.uk/download/323341146.pdf (accessed on 23rd July 2025).

35. Klimas, F., Zatłoka-Mazur, D., Rusiński, K., Zając, P., Pawłowski, B., Sienkiewicz, M., ... Pudełko, I. (2025). Fungal Infections: Epidemiology, Clinical Challenges, and Advances in Diagnosis and Treatment - a review. *Quality in Sport, 38*, 57928. https://doi.org/10.12775/QS.2025.38.57928(accessed on 23rd July 2025).

36. Konsoula, A., Tsioutis, C., Markaki, I., Papadakis, M., Agouridis, A. P., & Spernovasilis, N. (2022). *Lomentospora prolificans*: An emerging opportunistic fungal pathogen. *Microorganisms, 10*, 1317–1317. https://doi.org/10.3390/microorganisms10071317 (accessed on 23rd July 2025).

37. Krithinaki, M. I., Kokkinakis, I., Markatzinou, S., Masaoutis, C., Solomou, E., Papakitsou, I., Xirouchaki, N., et al. (2025). Severe aplastic anemia complicated with fatal invasive fungal infections in a young patient harboring perforin gene polymorphism. *Hematology Reports, 17*. https://www.semanticscholar.org/paper/1d8acbbd665cca331c8750719f4b91ee95f3017c (accessed on 23rd July 2025).

38. Kukhar, Y., Bailina, G., Smagulova, A., Uakhit, R., & Kiyan, V. (2025). Characteristics of *Chrysosporium* spp. pathogens causing skin mycoses in horses. *Journal of Fungi, 11*. https://www.semanticscholar.org/paper/78a433b90eb945a3189815087dbdc78e64e85b1a (accessed on 23rd July 2025).

39. Vila, T. V. M., & Rozental, S. (2016). Biofilm Formation as a Pathogenicity Factor of Medically Important Fungi. InTech. doi: 10.5772/62768(accessed on 23rd July 2025).

40. Mapook, A., Hyde, K. D., Hassan, K., Matio Kemkuignou, B., Čmoková, A., Surup, F., Kuhnert, E., et al. (2022). Ten decadal advances in fungal biology leading towards human well-being. *Fungal Diversity, 116*, 547–614. https://doi.org/10.1007/s13225-022-00510-3 (accessed on 23rd July 2025).

41. Maskan Bermudez, N., Rodriguez-Tamez, G., Perez, S. M., & Tosti, A. (2023). Onychomycosis: Old and new. *Journal of Fungi, 9*, 559–559. https://doi.org/10.3390/jof9050559 (accessed on 23rd July 2025).

42. Mitchell, T. G. (2016). Fungal pathogens of humans. https://www.semanticscholar.org/paper/91c3e75691f77c6d45235fbabd74dbd8c85ac342 (accessed on 23rd July 2025).

43. Mohammed, N. A., Fadhil, N. M., & Ahmed, A. D. (2024). Prevalence of fungal infections that isolated from different sites in Diyala Province/Iraq. *Al-Kufa University Journal for Biology*. https://www.semanticscholar.org/paper/aae1ff182abab4850f28529f9e688995b668f873 (accessed on 23rd July 2025).

44. Niño-Vega, G. A., Padró-Villegas, L., & López-Romero, E. (2024). New ground in antifungal discovery and therapy for invasive fungal infections: Innovations, challenges, and future directions. *Journal of Fungi, 10*, 871–871. https://doi.org/10.3390/jof10120871 (accessed on 23rd July 2025).

45. Piorunek, M., Kubisiak-Rzepczyk, H., Dańczak-Pazdrowska, A., Trafas, T., & Walkowiak, J. (2024). Superficial zoonotic mycoses in humans associated with cats. *Journal of Fungi, 10*. https://www.semanticscholar.org/paper/46e7ed95c93f014019483867b4134d9cc9b76440 (accessed on 23rd July 2025).

46. Qadri, H., Shah, A. H., Alkhanani, M., Almilaibary, A., & Mir, M. A. (2023). Immunotherapies against human bacterial and fungal infectious diseases: A review. *Frontiers in Medicine, 10*. https://doi.org/10.3389/fmed.2023.1135541 (accessed on 23rd July 2025).

47. Rao, H. H., & McClelland, E. E. (2024). A new overview of sex bias in fungal infections. *Journal of Fungi, 10*, 607–607. https://doi.org/10.3390/jof10090607 (accessed on 23rd July 2025).

48. Schaffner, A., & Schaffner, M. (1995). Effect of prophylactic fluconazole on the frequency of fungal infections, amphotericin B use, and health care costs in patients undergoing intensive chemotherapy for hematologic neoplasias. *The Journal of infectious diseases, 172*(4), 1035–1041. https://doi.org/10.1093/infdis/172.4.1035(accessed on 23rd July 2025).

49. Senoner, T., Breitkopf, R., Treml, B., & Rajšić, S. (2023). Invasive fungal infections after liver transplantation. *Journal of Clinical Medicine, 12*, 3238–3238. https://doi.org/10.3390/jcm12093238 (accessed on 23rd July 2025).

50. Sivayogana, R. (2017). Clinic-epidemiological, mycological and mycopathological study of deep mycoses. https://core.ac.uk/download/327695974.pdf (accessed on 23rd July 2025).

51. Su, C. W., & Tighe, S. (2017). Microorganisms and common ophthalmic diseases. Int J Ophthalmol Eye Res. 5(1), 272-276. https://core.ac.uk/download/144775814.pdf (accessed on 23rd July 2025).

52. Svirshchevskaya, E., Matushevskaya, E., Ivanova, M., Vladimirova, E. V., & Matushevskaya, Y. I. (2024). Epidemiology, therapy and prevention of superficial skin mycoses. *Meditsinskiy sovet = Medical Council*. https://www.semanticscholar.org/paper/50ab7f9cae5b4e28f7b30dcb3487eaa2a6bb9338 (accessed on 23rd July 2025).

53. Webb, B., Ferraro, J. P., Rea, S., Kaufusi, S., Goodman, B., & Spalding, J. (2018). Epidemiology and clinical features of invasive fungal infection in a US health care network. *Open Forum Infectious Diseases, 5*. https://doi.org/10.1093/ofid/ofy187 (accessed on 23rd July 2025).

PARASITIC INFESTATIONS

2

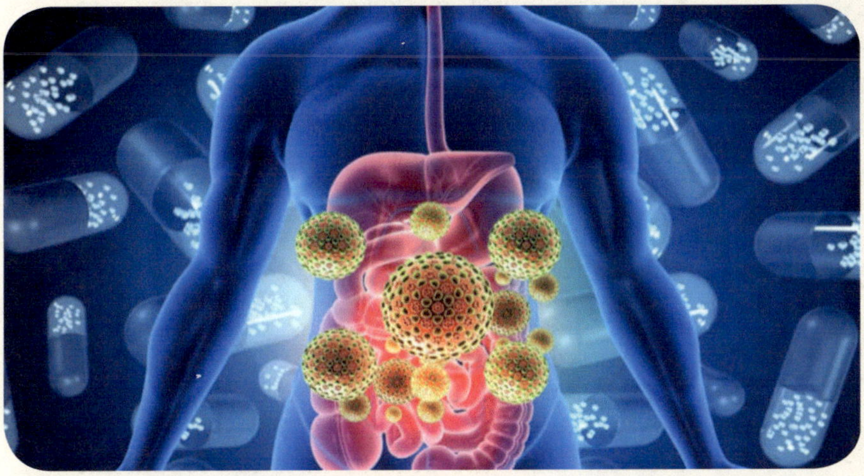

LEARNING OBJECTIVES

After studying this chapter, you will be able to:

1. Understand Scabies;
3. Explain Lice;
4. Describe Leishmaniasis.

Introduction

Parasitic infestations are a significant global public health issue, affecting millions and most critically vulnerable populations in low-income economies. The most prevalent are scabies, lice, and leishmaniasis, each with its particular issue and impact on human health. The seriousness of these ailments emphasizes the imperative necessity of effective treatment modalities, as evidenced by the research into antiparasitic medication such as ivermectin, which has proven a broad spectrum of activity against a variety of parasites (Sulik et al., 2023). Notably, the prevalence of parasitic skin infections also occurs in animals, where studies have indicated that parasitic diseases like sarcoptic mange and leishmaniasis have an endemic prevalence among dogs, which illustrates the interconnectedness of zoonotic disease and its projected influence on veterinary medicine (Zahri et al., 2024). An awareness of such parasitic infestations is crucial to planning specific interventions and promoting health outcomes for both animal and human populations.

2.1. Scabies

Learning Outcome

1. Understand Causative Agent: Sarcoptes scabiei;
2. Explain Transmission and Risk Factors;
3. Focus on Symptoms and Clinical Presentation;
4. Describe Diagnosis Methods;
5. Learn Treatment Options;
6. Discuss Prevention Strategies;
7. Know Complications Associated with Scabies;
8. Understand Scabies in Different Populations;
9. Explain Global Prevalence and Epidemiology.

Scabies caused by the *Sarcoptes scabiei* mite is still a significant public health concern, considering the high degree of contagion and prevalence among various populations. This cutaneous infestation by scabies parasites is transmitted by direct skin contact, quickly reaching epidemic proportions within populations, particularly with close living conditions or in vulnerable groups such as refugees and asylum seekers.

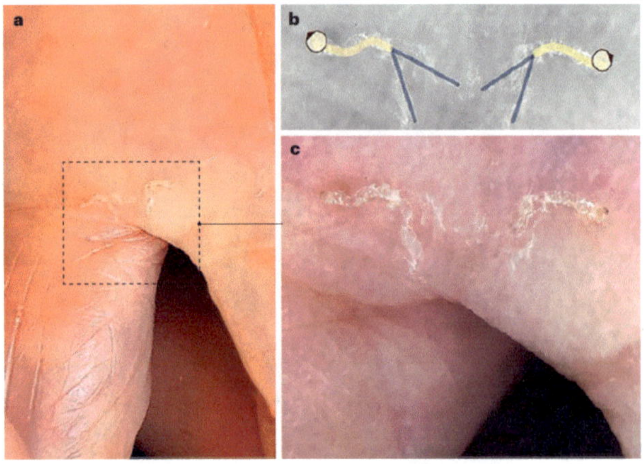

Figure 2.1. Scabies.

Source: https://media.springernature.com/lw685/springer-static/image/art%3A10.1038%2Fs41572-024-00552-8/MediaObjects/41572_2024_552_Fig6_HTML.png.

Presentation is typically that of intense itching and a characteristic rash, which may progress to secondary infections without treatment. Successful control of scabies, however, involves not only the application of topical or systemic scabicides but also active public health action. Innovations such as the Identify-Isolate-Inform (3I) Tool enable healthcare workers to quickly recognize symptoms, isolate the impacted and include local health authorities, hence enabling an organized response to outbreaks and diminishing the impact on the general population (Cheng et al., 2020). Therefore, the management of scabies requires a two-pronged strategy with a focus on prevention and treatment (Figure 2.1).

2.1.1. Causative Agent: Sarcoptes scabiei

A principal parasitic cause of widespread discomfort and disease is *Sarcoptes scabiei*, the scabies mite. An ectoparasite that tunnels into the skin, the scabies mite is responsible for intense pruritus and scratching-induced secondary infections. *S. scabiei* transmission is primarily spread by widespread skin-to-skin contact and thus occurs commonly among groups in close living quarters, e.g., residents of care homes or crowded families.

Additionally, its effects reach beyond man; these mites infest animals, making diagnosis and treatment of infected species challenging, as exemplified by a study on canines showing that Sarcoptic mange is a prevalent etiology of dermatitis (*Sarcoptes* spp.). Scabies management includes antiparasitic drugs, among which ivermectin is particularly effective owing to its broad-spectrum efficacy against diverse parasitic infections (Sulik et al., 2023). This emphasizes the importance of active public health interventions to curtail its spread (Figure 2.2).

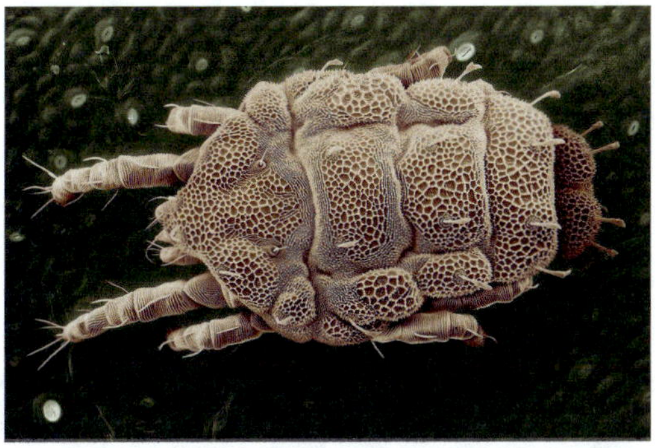

Figure 2.2. *Sarcoptes scabiei.*

Source: https://microbiotics.com.ng/wp-content/uploads/2024/01/scabies.jpg.

2.1.2. Transmission and Risk Factors

Understanding the transmission and risk factors of parasitic infestations is important for effective prevention and control strategies. Human causative conditions like scabies and lice primarily spread by direct contact, usually in crowded or unsanitary conditions, emphasizing the role of social determinants in their spread. Similarly, leishmaniasis is transmitted by sandfly bites and environmental determinants such as urbanization and land cover change have a significant impact on the parasite and its vector distribution. Host factors like age and immunity also contribute to susceptibility; for instance, children, undernourished children, or immunocompromised patients are more susceptible. Recent studies point to the necessity of treating these conditions in low-income nations, whose prevalence is compounded by the unavailability of healthcare, and indicate the need for targeted interventions (Sulik et al., 2023; Zahri et al., 2024). Their identification is important for the development of proper public health interventions and educational programs.

2.1.3. Symptoms and Clinical Presentation

The course of parasitic infestations is one of many varied symptoms depending on the specific parasite involved. For instance, scabies, which is caused by the *Sarcoptes scabiei* mite, would classically manifest with intense itch and rash on areas of skin folds that, if left untreated, would become secondarily infected. Infestations like those by leeches produce pruritus and observable nits or lice on the body and scalp, and thus state that proper treatment is indicated. Leishmaniasis, however, can be cutaneous and present in varying forms of lesions, but frequently ulcerated. By identifying these signs, each parasite will need specific treatments. While typical conventional anti-parasitic treatment generally tends to go towards eliminating the parasite as such, antibiotic treatment may also be necessary in cases where secondary infections develop, as observed with the intricacies of treating such infestations (Man et al., 2022; Sulik et al., 2023) (Figure 2.13).

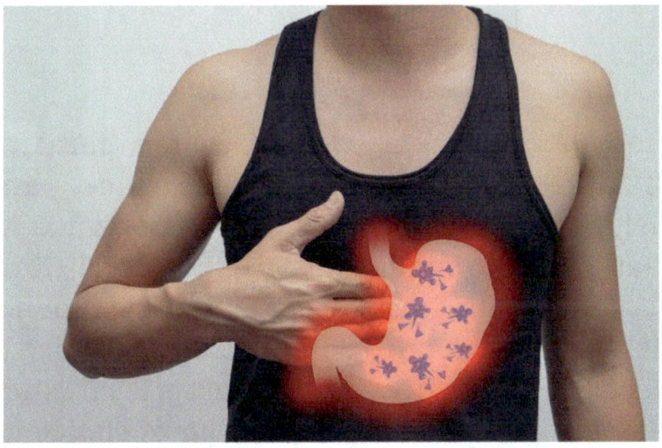

Figure 2.3. The clinical presentation of parasitic infestations is marked by a range of symptoms that vary depending on the specific parasite involved.

Source: https://sydneygutclinic.com/wp-content/uploads/2020/02/shutterstock_462525766.jpg.

2.1.4. Diagnosis Methods

Effective diagnosis of parasitic infestations such as scabies, lice, and leishmaniasis involves an integrated process of clinical evaluation, laboratory tests, and taking history. Initial assessment may only give symptomatic evidence, such as pruritus, which can be a pointer to multiple parasitic infections. Scabies and infestation by lice, for instance, are frequent presentations with severe itching and palpable skin lesions, compelling healthcare providers to examine the skin of the patient in minute detail. Laboratory diagnosis may involve microscopic examination of skin scrapings or hair samples for the presence of parasites, as has been mentioned in Zahri et al. (2024). Moreover, serological investigations can also be involved in the diagnosis of leishmaniasis, wherein antibody detection provides evidence of infection and determines the appropriate treatment strategy. The correlation between laboratory and clinical findings is important in the rendering of accurate diagnoses, and ultimately, the success of therapy protocols for these parasitic infestations.

2.1.5. Treatment Options

Effective treatment modalities for parasitic infestations such as scabies, lice, and leishmaniasis are of utmost importance to treat these common but niggling conditions. Antiparasitic drugs are essential, with compounds such as ivermectin demonstrating a broad spectrum of activity against multiple parasites. Its non-toxicity has made it the go-to choice for treating infestations in animals and humans alike, curing ailments such as river blindness and strongyloidiasis (Sulik et al., 2023). Treatment protocols may also involve the administration of antibiotics where secondary infections occur due to parasitic infection, making the use of an integrated approach the way forward (Man et al., 2022). Whereas mounting resistance to existing therapy is increasingly becoming the rule, continued research into both pharmacological and non-pharmacological therapy is still crucial. Through tailoring interventions to align with the individual parasite's life cycles and symptoms, the effectiveness of treatment as well as patient outcomes can be maximized in response to the evolving epidemiology of parasitic diseases (Figure 2.4).

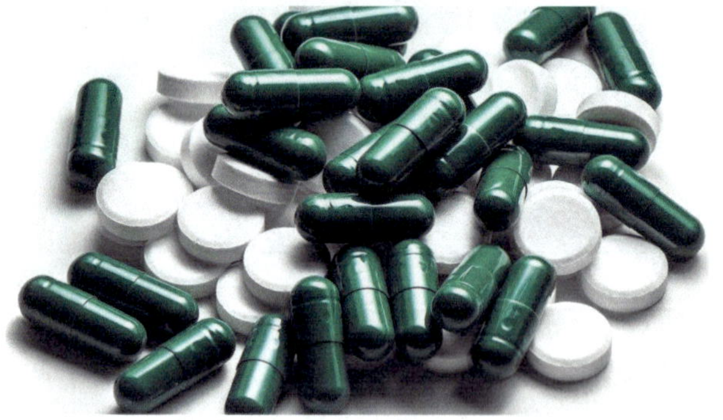

Figure 2.4. Antiparasitic medications play a vital role, with drugs like ivermectin demonstrating a broad spectrum of activity against various parasites.

Source: https://my.klarity.health/wp-content/uploads/2024/03/What-are-antiparasitic-drugs-featured-image.jpg.

2.1.6. Prevention Strategies

Successful prevention measures play a vital role in reducing the impact of parasitic infestations such as scabies, lice, and leishmaniasis. Public health measures should include education and awareness programs to inform communities on the mode of transmission and symptoms of these parasitic infestations. For instance, promoting regular hygiene practices, such as, regular bathing and home cleaning, can significantly reduce the incidence of scabies and lice infestation. Furthermore, the deployment of targeted treatment measures, for instance, the use of ivermectin, which has been proven to be effective in curing various parasitic infections, plays a significant role in controlling outbreaks among affected communities (Sulik et al., 2023). Secondly, lifestyle requirements and environmental concerns have to be met, as in the case of canine leishmaniasis, the link between pets and the environment plays a key role in multiplicative transmission risks (Zahri et al., 2024). With a more extensive strategy of education, treatment, and environmental management, such parasitic outbreaks may be significantly minimized.

2.1.7. Complications Associated with Scabies

Scabies, a very contagious skin infestation by the *Sarcoptes scabiei* mite, is often complicated by numerous complications apart from sheer discomfort and pruritus. Most distressing among them is secondary bacterial infection, which can arise through vigorous scratching and lead to cellulitis and impetigo. Secondly, in densely populated environments, especially among vulnerable groups such as refugees, scabies can facilitate the spread of other infectious diseases, thereby exacerbating public health crises, such as the epidemics in Lebanon due to the Syrian refugee influx (Kawa et al., 2019).

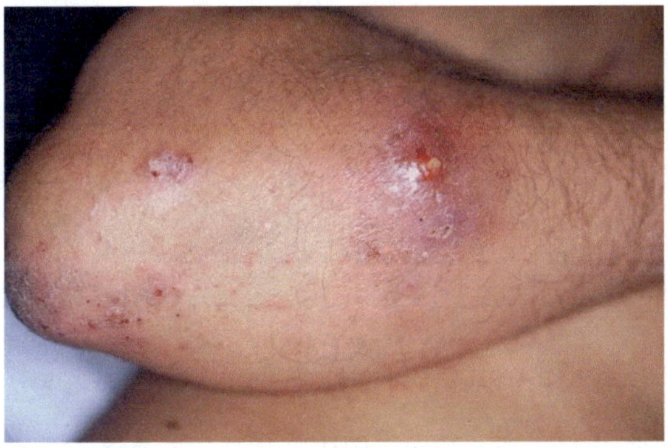

Figure 2.5. The most concerning consequences are secondary bacterial infections, which can occur as a result of intense scratching, leading to conditions such as cellulitis and impetigo.

Source: https://media.springernature.com/lw685/springer-static/image/art%3A10.1007%2Fs40257-024-00856-1/MediaObjects/40257_2024_856_Fig4_HTML.jpg.

Furthermore, the psychosocial impact of suffering from scabies, by way of stigma and, in some cases, extreme psychological distress, can significantly affect an individual's quality of life. The convergence of these complications necessitates a comprehensive treatment strategy and public health measures to mitigate the wider impacts of scabies infestations (Figure 2.15).

2.1.8. Scabies in Different Populations

Scabies is a severe public health concern that, in most instances, impacts vulnerable populations in various populations and geographical regions. In Aboriginal Australians residing in Central Australia, for instance, cultural contact between people and their dogs may influence the prevalence of scabies because zoonotic transmission may exist in conjunction with traditional human-to-human transmission among the human population (Gaskin et al., 2007). Furthermore, socioeconomic status generally exacerbates scabies spread in densely populated residential zones with resultant augmented infection among vulnerable communities. The association of scabies with other conditions, such as dermatitis and otitis in canines, highlights the interlinked nature of human as well as animal health. This intricate association calls for specialized education and intervention strategies aimed at targeted community requirements in a bid to reverse the outcome of scabies as well as overall public health outcomes in multicultural populations with parasitic infestation.

2.1.9. Global Prevalence and Epidemiology

Global prevalence of parasitic infestations such as scabies, lice, and leishmaniasis has emerged as a global public health concern, primarily among low- and middle-income countries. These infestations are likely caused by factors such as overcrowding and housing conditions, especially among the displaced population. For instance, the Syrian refugee crisis in Lebanon experienced an increase in leishmaniasis, scabies, and infestation of lice during outbreaks, increasing the burden on the public health system of the nation based on recent skin condition assessments among Syrian refugees (Kawa et al., 2019). While treatment successes like ivermectin have been effective to counter various parasitic diseases, including those in the human and animal populations, ongoing surveillance and novel interventions are required to contain these outbreaks and their influence on community health (Sulik et al., 2023). Eradicating the epidemiology of infestations requires coordinated action by health authorities and non-governmental actors to improve standards of living and healthcare access (Figure 2.6).

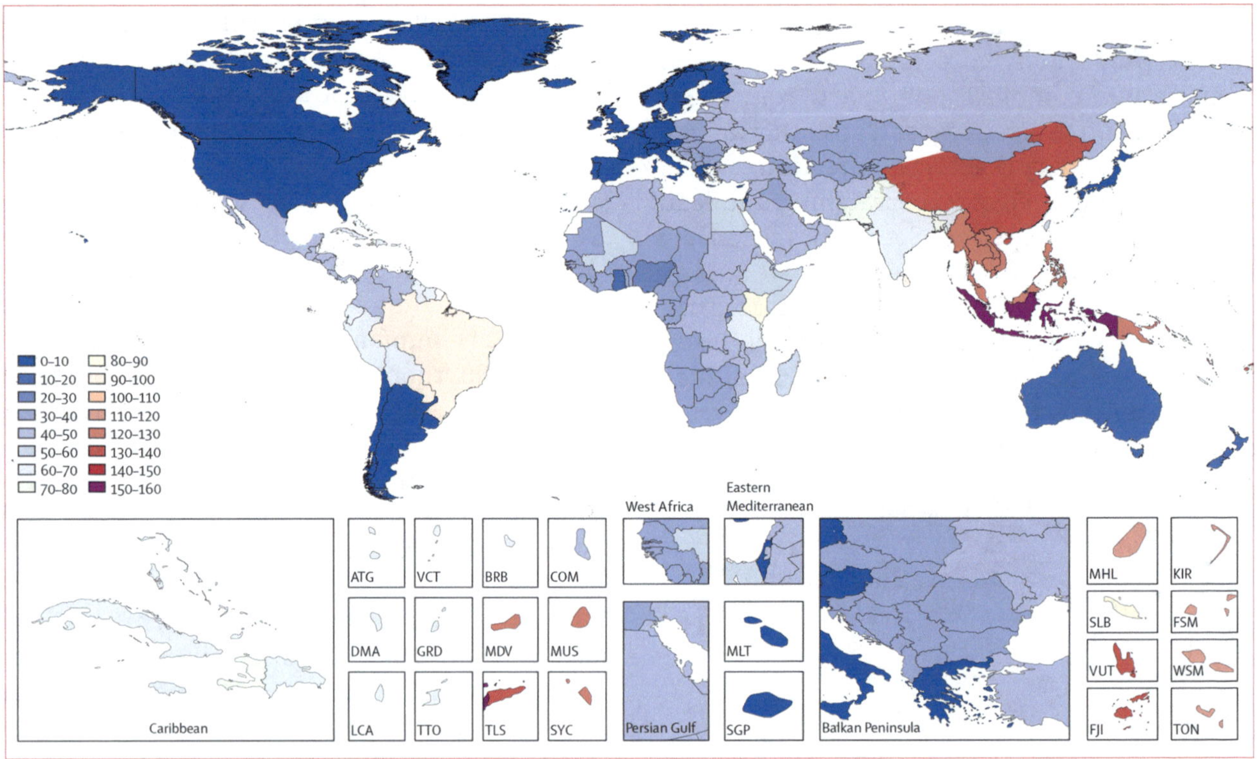

Figure 2.6. World map of scabies age-standardised disability-adjusted life-years per 100 000 people.

Source: https://www.thelancet.com/journals/laninf/article/PIIS1473-3099%2817%2930483-8/fulltext.

Test Your Knowledge

1. In infants, which area is most likely to be affected by scabies?
2. What is the first-line treatment for classic scabies?

2.2. Lice

Learning Outcome

1. Understand Types of Lice;
2. Explain the Life Cycle of Lice;
3. Focus on Symptoms and Signs of Infestation;
4. Describe Diagnosis and Identification;
5. Learn Treatment and Management Strategies;
6. Discuss Social Stigma and Psychological Impact;
7. Know Prevention and Control Measures;
8. Understand Lice in Various Demographics.

Of the various ectoparasitic invertebrates, lice (order Phthiraptera) are a significant public health issue due to their omnipresence and discomfort that they cause. Small, wingless insects, lice are obligatory parasites that live off human hosts by deriving sustenance from blood. Lice infections, also known as pediculosis, comprise three primary types: head, body, and pubic lice, each of which occurs in a particular region of habitat on the human host. Transmission of lice is most likely to occur in close-contact environments, such as schools and shared residential spaces, and thus increases the likelihood of outbreaks. Infestation is not only physically painful; secondary bacterial infection is possible through scratching, which is discussed in contemporary dermatological studies addressing the issue, such as pieces situating infestations within broader public health frameworks (Adaskevich, 2016; Barros-Battesti et al., 2024). Thus, the treatment of infestation with lice is crucial at both the individual and community levels.

2.2.1. Types of Lice: Head Lice, Body Lice, and Pubic Lice

Lice, parasitic insects infesting human beings, are generally categorized into three primary categories: head lice, body lice, and pubic lice, with distinct features and modes of transmission. Head lice, or *Pediculus humanus* capitis, are typically found on the scalp and transmitted through direct head-to-head contact; they are particularly common in children in school-going groups. Body lice, or *Pediculus humanus* corporis, reside in clothing and bedding and emerge to feed on the host's blood and are generally associated with insanitary lifestyles and close living conditions. Lastly, pubic lice or crab lice occur most often in coarse body hair, such as the pubic area, and spread through sexual contact. Recent studies have also suggested potential associations between head louse infestations and bacterial pathogens, including *Acinetobacter baumannii*, with public health significance (Larkin, 2022; Sulik et al., 2023). It is crucial to get to know these three types of lice so that infestations can be controlled and prevented effectively (Figure 2.7).

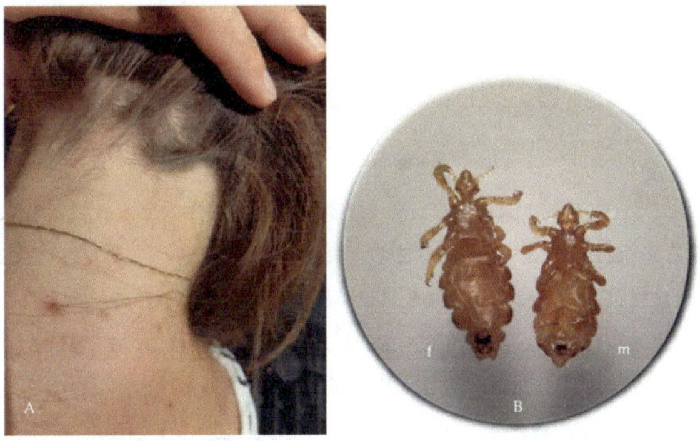

Figure 2.7. Head lice, scientifically known as *Pediculus humanus* capitis, are typically found on the scalp and are transmitted through direct head-to-head contact; they are particularly common among children in school settings.

Source: https://www.mdpi.com/jcm/jcm-11-00783/article_deploy/html/images/jcm-11-00783-g001.png.

2.2.2. Life Cycle of Lice

The lice lifecycle is a multistage process and underscores the resilience of these parasitic infestations, as commonly known in public health. The lifecycle of lice is a three-stage one, including egg (nits), nymph, and adult. Eggs are typically laid near the hair follicle and mature after a week and become nymphs, which mature into adults within approximately 7–10 days under ideal situations.

Adult lice live up to 30 days on the human host, during which they breed prolifically and lead to heavier infestations if left untreated. High reproduction and transmission rates account for their resilience in human populations, particularly in crowded environments such as schools and childcare centers, where there is close contact to facilitate transmission (Savona-Ventura, 2002). Effective management of lice infestations is crucial since they can lead to secondary bacterial infections and thus the need for ongoing research into effective treatments such as ivermectin, which has promise against other parasitic infections (Sulik et al., 2023).

2.2.3. Symptoms and Signs of Infestation

Parasite infestations manifest in an array of signs and symptoms necessary for timely identification and intervention. For instance, infestations such as scabies and lice result in intense itching where the parasites nest or burrow. Itching typically results in secondary infections from scratching. In a study of parasitic dermatitis in dogs, pruritus and erythema were identified as frequent symptoms and a high percentage of the infested animals presented with these signs of infestation. Similarly, skin manifestations in human leishmaniasis can also include swelling, ulcers, and lesions, which are indicators of the body's immune system reacting to the parasite (Sulik et al., 2023). Early identification of these symptoms is important since they can be determinants of the extent of infestation and inform treatment to avoid further complications (Figure 2.8).

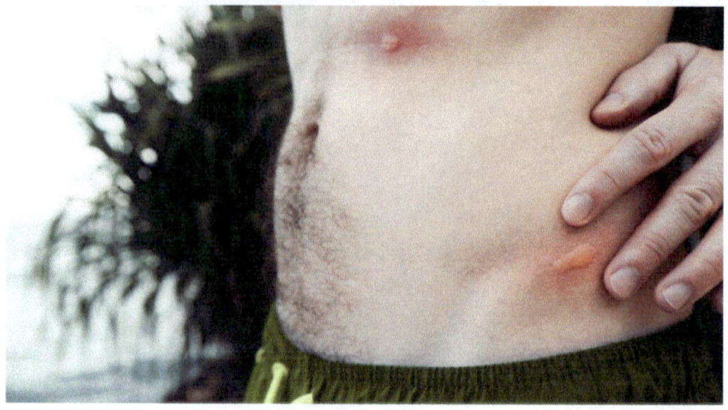

Figure 2.8. In human cases of leishmaniasis, cutaneous symptoms can include lesions, ulcers, and swelling, indicating the body's response to the parasite.

Source: https://media.post.rvohealth.io/wp-content/uploads/sites/3/2024/02/Skin-reaction-to-mosquito-bites-header-1024x575.jpg.

2.2.4. Diagnosis and Identification

Successful identification and diagnosis of parasitic infestations are crucial in limiting their impact on public health. Diagnostic procedures are usually a combination of clinical evaluation and laboratory testing for confirmation of parasites. For instance, scotch tests and skin scrapings are typically employed to identify routine ectoparasites such as lice and scabies mites, as demonstrated in a study among dogs, whereby methods such as microscopy and skin scraping revealed a high incidence of otitis externa as well as parasitic dermatitis. Besides, drugs like ivermectin have not only proven effective against a broad spectrum of parasites but also simplified the diagnosis of the resistant ones (Sulik et al., 2023). As the dynamics of parasitic infections change, the efficacy of diagnostic procedures must be maintained to promote timely diagnosis and effective treatment, thereby protecting vulnerable communities from the mass risk of such infections.

2.2.5. Treatment and Management Strategies

Effective treatment and management choices of parasitic infestations such as scabies, lice, and leishmaniasis are required to avoid their impact on public health. Ivermectin has been among the pivotal therapeutic drugs due to its wide-spectrum antiparasitic effect and low toxicity level, for which it is prescribed for various infestations in humans and animals (Sulik et al., 2023). In addition to pharmacological treatment, critical management strategies consist of educating involved communities about hygiene as well as the timely identification of infestation.

For instance, awareness of risk factors associated with some conditions may enhance prevention; parasitic conditions like leishmaniasis tend to have associations with aspects such as lifestyle and age (Zahri et al., 2024). These interrelated strategies underpin the need for effective medicine as well as good public health practice to halt the spread of parasitic infestations. Hence, treating both biologic and environmental aspects is vital for successful cure and control of such infestations (Figure 2.9).

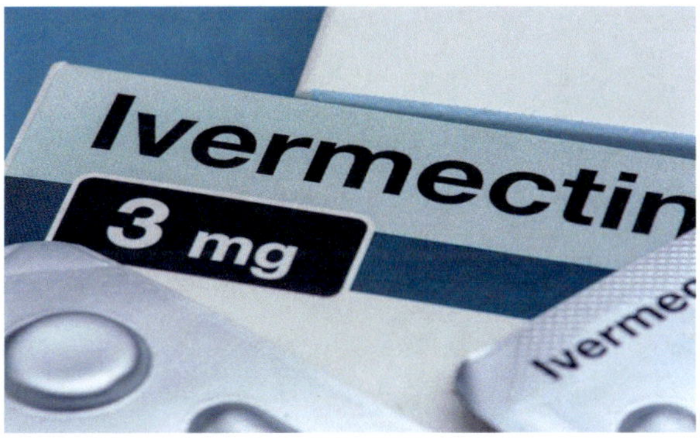

Figure 2.9. Ivermectin.

Source: https://www.leehealth.org/getattachment/434e9884-775b-4021-b16b-efbf25d602de/Ivermectin-NEW-1.jpg?lang=en-US&width=800&height=500.

2.2.6. Social Stigma and Psychological Impact

Social stigma related to parasitic infestations such as scabies and infestation by lice is the main source of psychological impact endured by the sufferers. Widespread social perception that links the disorders with poor hygiene or poverty gives rise to feelings of shame and isolation from society. Stigma tends to aggravate mental health, inducing anxiety and depression in the sufferers. According to research, whereas millions suffer from vector-borne and neglected tropical diseases, their accompanying shame and stigma can deter individuals from seeking adequate treatment (Bauer, 2023). Furthermore, ignorance and illiteracy regarding such infestations have a propensity for fueling ill stereotypes and maintaining stigma (Adaskevich, 2016). Addressing such social factors is critical not only to promote public health initiatives but also to minimize the psychological burden of those afflicted by such diseases. Ultimately, creating a more empathetic public discourse on parasitic infestations is necessary in minimizing their broader psychological impact.

2.2.7. Prevention and Control Measures

Effective prevention and control are important in the combat against parasitic infections such as scabies, lice, and leishmaniasis, all of which have important individual and public health consequences. Amongst such measures, promoting improved living standards is crucial, particularly in densely populated areas where outbreaks are common, like the impact of the Syrian refugee crisis in Lebanon, which has seen an upsurge in skin conditions due to congestion and poor sanitation (Kawa et al., 2019). Additionally, early treatment and diagnosis play a vital role in controlling such infestations; ivermectin, for instance, has been found effective against most parasites and is increasingly applied not only to humans but also in veterinary medicine to avoid infestations (Sulik et al., 2023). Coordination among non-governmental organizations and health organizations can similarly enhance the efficacy of such approaches, enabling timely action that minimizes the risks associated with parasitic diseases (Figure 2.10).

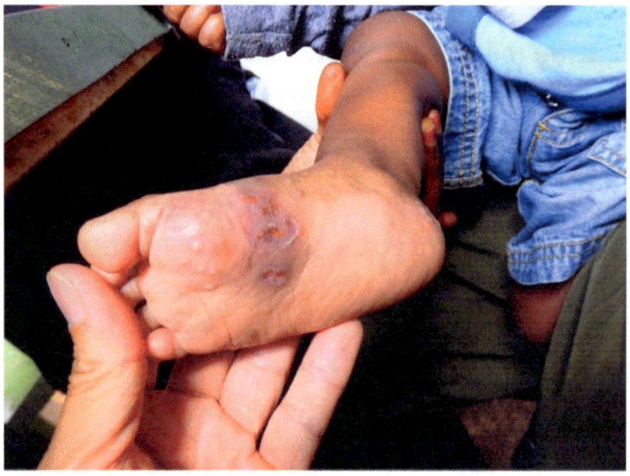

Figure 2.10. Effective prevention and control measures are vital in combating parasitic infestations such as scabies, lice, and leishmaniasis, all of which can significantly impact both individual and public health.

Source: https://www.who.int/images/default-source/departments/ntd-library/scabies-and-other-ectoparasites/scabies-rie2-(tanzania).tmb-1200v.jpg?Culture=en&sfvrsn=6bb1d4d2_18.

2.2.8. Lice in Various Demographics

Prevalence of lice infestation differs significantly among populations based on socio-economic status and access to healthcare. In poverty-stricken regions, particularly in the developing world, lice infestations are more prevalent due to situations such as overcrowding of living spaces and limited resources for hygiene. The effect of these parasitic infections is greatly increased in poor communities with co-endemic neglected illnesses. These populations are not only socially disadvantaged but also economically disadvantaged, which increases the risk of the health implications associated with lice infestation. Research has indicated that successful interventions addressing individual demographic requirements can have a considerable impact in decreasing the number of lice cases by encouraging improved hygiene habits and comprehensive health education programs (Ehrenberg & Ault, 2005). Without these targeted strategies that include socio-economic factors, the issue of treating lice infestations continues to be insufficiently tackled (Daniel & Justin-Temu, 2011). These strategies need to be employed to establish healthier populations and mitigate the effects of neglected diseases.

Test Your Knowledge

1. What is the typical mode of transmission of pubic lice?
2. Which lice infestation is most commonly associated with poor hygiene and overcrowding?

2.3. Leishmaniasis

Learning Outcome

1. Understand Causative Agents such as Leishmania species;
2. Explain Transmission Through Sandflies;
3. Focus on Types of Leishmaniasis;
4. Describe Symptoms and Clinical Manifestations;
5. Learn Diagnosis Techniques;
6. Discuss Treatment Options and Challenges;
7. Know Impact on Affected Populations;
8. Understand Prevention and Control Strategies;
9. Explain Global Distribution and Epidemiological Trends.

Leishmaniasis, a protozoan parasite of the Leishmania genus-induced neglected tropical disease with significant public health issues in most regions of the globe, particularly in tropical and subtropical regions. The disease manifests in cutaneous, muco-cutaneous, and visceral types of leishmaniasis, the latter being most dangerous and potentially fatal when not treated.

This disease is primarily transmitted by bites from infected sandflies, which thrive under unhygienic conditions and low standards of housing. The growing human-animal bond, particularly with household animals like dogs, has been linked to leishmaniasis transmission patterns, since such household pets can serve as reservoirs of parasites (Chomel, 2014). Besides, laboratory precautions are emphasized by the requirement for handling *Leishmania* spp. with precaution in research settings to prevent laboratory-associated infections (Sini et al., 2023). Public health interventions aimed at vector control and improved socio-economic status are important to regulate the spread of this parasitic disease (Figure 2.11).

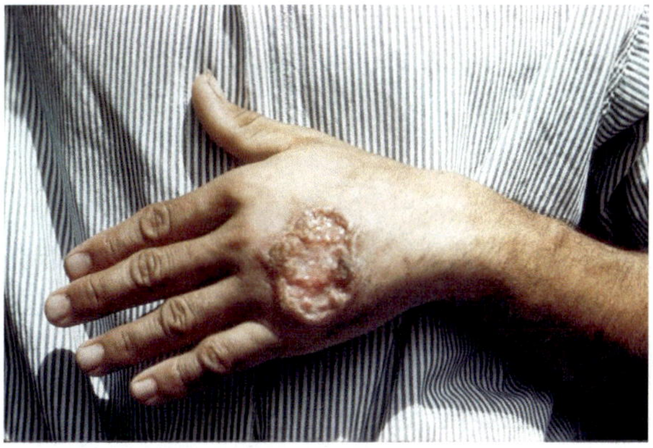

Figure 2.11. Leishmaniasis.

Source: https://upload.wikimedia.org/wikipedia/commons/thumb/6/67/Skin_ulcer_due_to_leishmaniasis%2C_hand_of_Central_American_adult_3MG0037_lores.jpg/1200px-Skin_ulcer_due_to_leishmaniasis%2C_hand_of_Central_American_adult_3MG0037_lores.jpg.

2.3.1. Causative Agents: Leishmania Species

Leishmaniasis, a protozoan parasite infection caused by Leishmania species, is a health burden to many regions of the world, with more severity observed in the tropical and subtropical areas. The parasites spread to humans through the bite of the infected females of phlebotomine sandflies, and they bring about a variety of clinical presentations, such as cutaneous, mucocutaneous, and visceral leishmaniasis. The pathobiology of Leishmania species is highly correlated with the immune response they provoke in the host, leading to severe tissue destruction in the visceral forms of the disease. An understanding of Leishmania transmission dynamics and environmental risk factors is crucial, according to research indicating that housing can predispose animals, including canines, to leishmaniasis, affecting their health as well as that of the humans that come into contact with them (Zahri et al., 2024). Better monitoring and treatment practices, including the use of antiparasitic medication, remain a valuable recourse in combating this parasitic infestation (Sulik et al., 2023).

2.3.2. Transmission Through Sandflies

Parasitic disease transmission by sandflies is a significant public health consideration in the tropics and subtropics. These small, blood-feeding flies are vectors for a number of pathogens, including the Leishmania species that cause leishmaniasis, a long-term disease characterized by skin ulcers and systemic signs. Sandflies, particularly species in the Phlebotomus and Lutzomyia genera, serve as intermediates, transferring parasites between host species while feeding in cycles. The dynamics of such transmission are complemented by extrinsic influences such as habitat alteration and climatic conditions, which influence sandfly populations and their interaction with animals and humans.

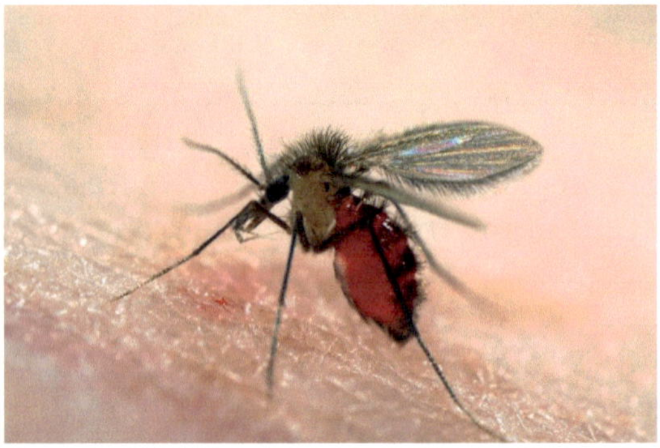

Figure 2.12. The transmission of parasitic infections through sandflies constitutes a significant public health concern, particularly in tropical and subtropical regions.

Source: https://media.npr.org/assets/img/2023/10/31/sciencesourceimages_2226824_custom-ee0f26078f8bc8379462d5b9164fe5a743c8c116.jpg.

The ongoing research on antiparasitic medications, including the application of ivermectin, offers potential choices for such prevention of infestation (Sulik et al., 2023). Therefore, one should be aware of the role of sandflies as a vector for such parasitic transmission so that effective public health interventions may be planned (Travis & Labadan, 1967) (Figure 2.12).

2.3.3. Types of Leishmaniasis: Cutaneous, Visceral, and Mucocutaneous

The Leishmania genus harbors a sequence of species responsible for the various leishmaniasis types, which are primarily classified as cutaneous, visceral, and mucocutaneous leishmaniasis, each presenting specific health challenges. Cutaneous leishmaniasis is usually marked by skin lesions, which, even though painful and deforming, are not necessarily fatal. On the other hand, visceral leishmaniasis, or kala-azar, attacks internal organs and, if left untreated, is fatal; it disproportionately finds support in regions with less developed health infrastructure. Mucocutaneous leishmaniasis, though rarer, encompasses severe tissue damage to mucous membranes and severely deteriorates the quality of life. An understanding of these distinctions is crucial for best practices in diagnosis and treatment protocols, and priority continues in combating parasitic diseases globally. Recent literature highlights the urgent need for the development of antiparasitic drugs to treat the heterogeneous forms of leishmaniasis (Adaskevich, 2016; Sulik et al., 2023).

2.3.4. Symptoms and Clinical Manifestations

Symptoms and clinical manifestations in relation to parasitic infestations have to be well known to make a correct diagnosis and an effective intervention. For instance, scabies, caused by infestation with *Sarcoptes scabiei*, is characterized by intense pruritus and erythema, often accompanied by secondary bacterial infections due to scratching. Infestation with lice, on the other hand, might result in scalp irritations and sleep disturbances attested in children. Infection manifests in the presence of visible nits and crawling lice, which are evidence of active infestation. Also, leishmaniasis presents as cutaneous, mucocutaneous, or visceral types, with vastly different symptoms; cutaneous leishmaniasis can result in painful ulcers and swelling in a localized area. Lastly, as already stated, definitive clinical signs will lead medical professionals to diagnose each infestation, ultimately making it easier for treatments to be rendered. Apart from this, it must be borne in mind that factors such as potential secondary infections need to be taken into consideration, emphasizing the necessity of specific treatment of individual parasites to improve the patient's prognosis (Man et al., 2022) (Figure 2.13).

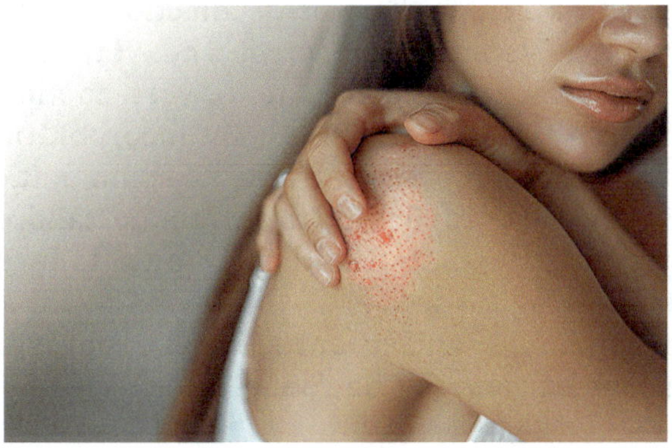

Figure 2.13. Understanding the symptoms and clinical manifestations associated with parasitic infestations is paramount for accurate diagnosis and effective treatment.

Source: https://assets.truemeds.in/tm-cms-prod/parasitic_infection_disease_banner_61d94f786d.png?width=640.

2.3.5. Diagnosis Techniques

Correct identification of parasitic infestations such as scabies, lice, and leishmaniasis aids in the provision of proper treatment and management. Various techniques are employed for detecting such parasites, and these include skin scrapings, scotch tape tests, trichograms, and ear swabs. For instance, skin scrapings are commonly employed in order to detect *Sarcoptes scabiei*, the causative agent of scabies, by observing specimens under a microscope for the presence of mites. Likewise, the scotch tape method helps diagnose lice by encasing adult insects and eggs to look at them visually. Studies prove the value of employing a combination of these diagnostic techniques in order to increase accuracy, especially since multiple parasitic ailments have overlapping symptoms. Besides, drugs such as ivermectin have been found to be effective against a wide range of parasites and enhance the clinical management of infestations with a focus on the importance of precise diagnosis methods in public health (Sulik et al., 2023).

2.3.6. Treatment Options and Challenges

Parasitic infestations such as scabies, lice, and leishmaniasis have treatment options alongside many challenges in treatment. While classical antiparasitic medicines like ivermectin have wide-spectrum activity against a large variety of parasites, their application is made difficult by the onset of drug resistance among populations. For instance, ivermectin has been widely used in the treatment of river blindness and strongyloidiasis, but ongoing research serves to highlight the importance of alternative therapeutic strategies as resistance patterns evolve (Sulik et al., 2023). Additionally, the treatment typically involves the use of antibiotics to manage secondary infections from cutaneous parasites, as with leishmaniasis infections. Cutaneous variations and the distinctive life cycles of these parasites pose distinct challenges, which require individualized therapeutic approaches involving drug and non-drug interventions (Man et al., 2022). This multifaceted nature of parasite treatment underscores the need for ongoing research and ingenuity in solutions to help fight such endemic infestations.

2.3.7. Impact on Affected Populations

The impact of parasitic infestations, for instance, scabies, lice, and leishmaniasis, on infected populations is considerable, particularly in regions with weak health infrastructure. In Lebanon, for instance, the influx of Syrian refugees into the nation has also grown such infestations exponentially, placing a tremendous burden on the domestic health system. With the displaced individuals being brought into crowded and poorly equipped facilities, they become highly susceptible to infectious diseases, including scabies and leishmaniasis, further exacerbating public health challenges (Kawa et al., 2019). Furthermore, such infestations are capable of leading to social stigmatization and emotional distress, with affected individuals facing not only the bodily expressions but also the social frame of mind that accompanies these infestations. Eliminating these issues through improved living standards, early diagnosis, and effective preventive measures is crucial in an effort to minimize the adverse effects on such marginalized populations and guarantee their health and well-being (Sulik et al., 2023) (Figure 2.14).

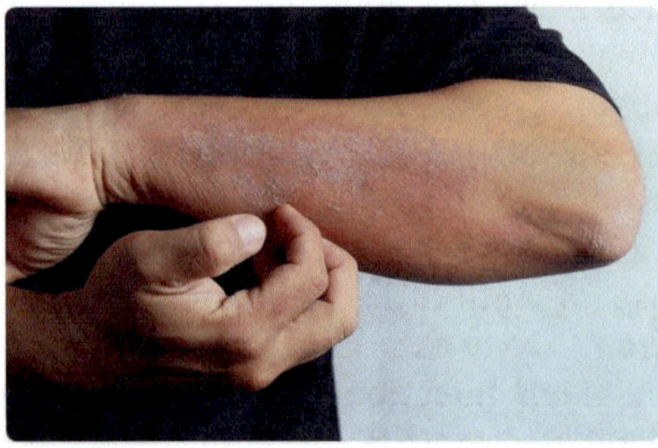

Figure 2.14. The impact of parasitic infestations, such as scabies, lice, and leishmaniasis, on affected populations is profound, particularly in regions with limited health resources.

Source: https://www.news-medical.net/image-handler/picture/2021/5/shutterstock_1066262183.jpg.

2.3.8. Prevention and Control Strategies

Effectively preventing and controlling parasitic infestations such as scabies, lice, and leishmaniasis is critical to their minimization of impact on public health. Important interventions include promoting personal hygiene, environmental sanitation, and early infection diagnosis. Education also plays an important role since the education of the populace regarding transmission modes can significantly lower the rate of infection. Antiparasitic medications, most notably ivermectin, have come into the limelight due to their broad-spectrum activity against most parasites, reasserting their place in veterinary and human medicine (Sulik et al., 2023). In addition, dermatological conditions, which are typically linked with parasitic infection, require intensive veterinary control and veterinary public health initiatives to thwart zoonotic threats (Zahri et al., 2024). By incorporating these multi-component strategies, communities will have the capability to formulate tailored interventions that tackle their own tailored epidemiological scenarios, fostering a healthier environment, and eventually, the parasitic disease burden will be reduced.

2.3.9. Global Distribution and Epidemiological Trends

The worldwide dissemination of parasitic infestations such as scabies, lice, and leishmaniasis mirrors striking epidemiological trends influenced by environmental, socioeconomic, and demographic determinants. Scabies caused by *Sarcoptes scabiei* shows high burdens in populations with high living density, with high prevalence rates in the Third World. Infestation by lice is also frequent in school children, particularly in regions with limited access to healthcare and sanitary facilities. Leishmaniasis, being transmitted by sandflies, is geographically very heterogeneous, and endemic areas are largely located in subtropical and tropical environments (Barros-Battesti et al., 2024). Understanding these trends is crucial for the deployment of effective public health measures and resource prioritization. Lastly, the onset of drug resistance and changing climate patterns exacerbate the transmission of such infestations, which is challenging for global health programs combating eradication and control. Therefore, it is necessary to address these wide-ranging health dangers on a holistic basis (Figure 2.15).

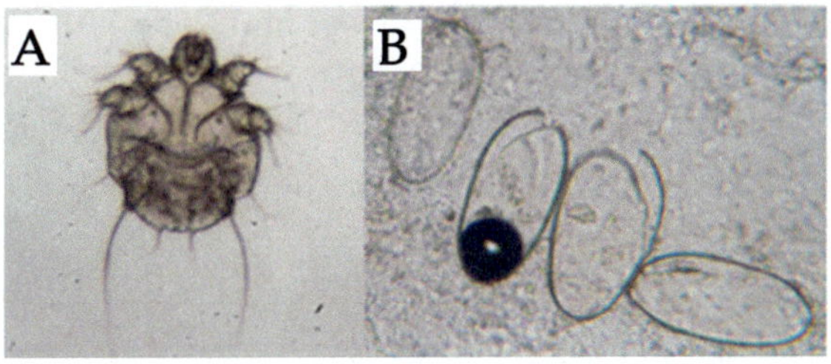

Figure 2.15. Scabies, caused by *Sarcoptes scabiei*, disproportionately affects populations in crowded living conditions, with higher prevalence rates reported in developing regions.

Source: https://www.mdpi.com/pathogens/pathogens-10-00868/article_deploy/html/images/pathogens-10-00868-g001.png.

Test Your Knowledge

1. What is the drug of choice for treating visceral leishmaniasis?
2. Which Leishmania species causes mucocutaneous leishmaniasis?

SUMMARY

The pervasiveness of parasitic infestations—such as scabies, lice, and leishmaniasis—underscores the imperative for an integrated approach in treatment and prevention strategies. The prevalence of dermatological parasitic disease among dogs has some dominant trends and correlates that are crucial to the effective assault of these diseases. For instance, one study highlighted how parasitic dermatoses accounted for 44.10% of dermatological cases seen in a veterinary clinic and how aspects such as age, lifestyle, and environmental factors were significant factors in their prevalence (Zahri et al., 2024). Moreover, the prevalence of conditions such as dermatitis and otitis externa in dogs also indicates the importance of awareness regarding predisposing factors such as living conditions and breed. Therefore, a comprehensive understanding of these parasitic infestations not only improves treatment but also guides research and public health interventions in the future.

The study of parasitic infestations, including scabies, lice, and leishmaniasis, provides relevant information that establishes the complex relationship between socio-economic determinants and public health. Above all, the poor populations are disproportionately affected by such underprivileged diseases, putting excessive social and economic loads on families and individuals (Ehrenberg & Ault, 2005). The ecological and biological features of ectoparasites such as mites and lice also contribute to the transmission dynamics and public health concerns (Barros-Battesti et al., 2024). Integrated, multi-disease intervention plans become indispensable to effective control, which necessitates certain methods targeting the specific risk factors prevalent in diverse community settings. Strategies involving multidisciplinary action could enhance public health success and encourage sustainable development within marginalized populations, ultimately benefiting broader programs directed towards controlling these prevalent diseases. The findings suggest an immediate appeal for novel combat models against parasitic infestations' resilience in vulnerable populations.

KEY TERMS FROM THIS CHAPTER

- Scabies
- Human health
- Medication
- Parasites
- Sarcoptic mange
- Veterinary medicine
- Sarcoptes scabiei
- Identify-Isolate-Inform (3I) Tool
- Health authorities
- Leishmaniasis
- Treatment modalities
- Ivermectin
- Parasitic skin infections
- Zoonotic disease
- Parasitic infestations
- Scabicides
- Symptoms
- Prevention

CRITICAL THINKING QUESTIONS

1. **What is the causative organism of scabies?**
   a. *Sarcoptes scabiei* var. hominis
   b. *Demodex folliculorum*
   c. *Pediculus humanus*
   d. *Leishmania donovani*
2. **The pathognomonic lesion of scabies is:**
   a. Papule
   b. Nodule
   c. Burrow
   d. Vesicle
3. **Norwegian scabies is commonly seen in which group of patients?**
   a. Immunocompetent children
   b. Diabetic patients
   c. Immunocompromised or debilitated individuals
   d. Athletes
4. **Which of the following is NOT a typical site for scabies lesions?**
   a. Interdigital spaces
   b. Waistline
   c. Scalp in adults
   d. Axillae
5. **Which of the following parasites causes Cutaneous Larva Migrans?**
   a. *Ancylostoma braziliense*
   b. *Strongyloides stercoralis*
   c. *Taenia solium*
   d. *Wuchereria bancrofti*

Short Answer Questions

1. What is the causative organism of scabies?
2. What is the typical incubation period of scabies after first exposure?
3. What is the causative organism of head lice?
4. Nits are most commonly found attached to which part of the hair?
5. What is the causative agent of cutaneous leishmaniasis?
6. Which insect transmits Leishmania species?

Answers to Critical Thinking Questions

1. (a); 2. (c); 3. (c); 4. (c); 5. (a)

REFERENCES

1. Zahri A, Bouslikhane M, El Mazini S, Lemrani M, El Berbri I, Abouelkaram MA, Balenghien T, and Bourquia M (2024). Survey on Dermatological Disorders of Dogs during 2020-2022 in Rabat, Morocco. World Vet. J., 14(3): 449-460. DOI: https://dx.doi.org/10.54203/scil.2024.wvj52(accessed on 23rd July 2025).
2. Adaskevich, V. P. (2016). *Skin Diseases and Sexually Transmitted Infections*. https://core.ac.uk/download/80150454.pdf (accessed on 23rd July 2025).
3. Cheng, T. A., Mzahim, B., Koenig, K. L., Alsugair, A., Al-Wabel, A., Almutairi, B. S., Maysa, E., & Kahn, C. A. (2020). Scabies: Application of the Novel Identify-Isolate-Inform Tool for Detection and Management. *The western journal of emergency medicine, 21*(2), 191–198. https://doi.org/10.5811/westjem.2020.1.46120(accessed on 23rd July 2025).
4. Sulik, M., Antoszczak, M., Huczyński, A., & Steverding, D. (2023). Antiparasitic activity of ivermectin: Four decades of research into a "wonder drug". *European journal of medicinal chemistry, 261*, 115838. https://doi.org/10.1016/j.ejmech.2023.115838(accessed on 23rd July 2025).
5. Sini, M. F., Tamponi, C., Mehmood, N., Dessì, G., Ariu, F., Carta, C., Coghetto, A., Pentcheva, P., Gabrielli, S., Scala, A., & Varcasia, A. (2023). Laboratory associated zoonotic parasitic infections: a review of main agents and biosecurity measures. *Journal of infection in developing countries, 17*(6), 762–781. https://doi.org/10.3855/jidc.9428(accessed on 23rd July 2025).
6. Darci Moraes Barros-Battesti, Valeria Castilho Onofrio, and Filipe Dantas-Torres Part V: Ectoparasites, chapters 60–67, pages 732–841, in Concepts in Animal Parasitology. 2024. Scott L. Gardner and Sue Ann Gardner, editors. Zea Books, Lincoln, Nebraska, United States; part V doi: 10.32873/unl.dc.ciap075(accessed on 23rd July 2025).
7. Bauer, I. L. (2023). The oral repellent–Science fiction or common sense? Insects, vector-borne diseases, failing strategies, and a bold proposition. https://core.ac.uk/download/577868641.pdf (accessed on 23rd July 2025).
8. Gaskin, S., Bentham, R., Cromar, N., & Fallowfield, H. (2007). The Zoonotic Potential of Dogs in Aboriginal Communities in Central Australia. Environmental Health, 7(4), 36–45. https://search.informit.org/doi/10.3316/informit.997869549509147(accessed on 23rd July 2025).
9. Ehrenberg, J. P., & Ault, S. K. (2005). Neglected diseases of neglected populations: thinking to reshape the determinants of health in Latin America and the Caribbean. *BMC public health, 5*, 119. https://doi.org/10.1186/1471-2458-5-119(accessed on 23rd July 2025).
10. Kawa, Nisrine; Hanna, Edith; and Bizri, Abdul Rahman (2019) "Transmissible Dermatological Diseases Affecting Syrian Refugees in Lebanon," *Journal of Refugee & Global Health*: Vol. 2 : Iss. 2 , Article 4. https://core.ac.uk/download/223224052.pdf (accessed on 23rd July 2025).
11. George DR, Finn RD, Graham KM, et al. Should the poultry red mite Dermanyssus gallinae be of wider concern for veterinary and medical science?. *Parasit Vectors*. 2015;8:178. Published 2015 Mar 25. doi:10.1186/s13071-015-0768-7(accessed on 23rd July 2025).
12. Chomel, B. B. (2014). Emerging and re-emerging zoonoses of dogs and cats. https://core.ac.uk/download/323070120.pdf (accessed on 23rd July 2025).
13. Gardner, S. A. (2023). *Concepts in Animal Parasitology: Master Bibliography*. https://core.ac.uk/download/590237251.pdf (accessed on 23rd July 2025).

14. Man, E., Price, H. P., & Hoskins, C. (2022). Current and future strategies against cutaneous parasites. *Pharmaceutical research*, *39*(4), 631–651. https://doi.org/10.1007/s11095-022-03232-y (accessed on 23rd July 2025).
15. Travis, B. V., & Labadan, R. M. (1967). Arthropods of medical importance in Asia (and the European USSR), Part II: Data on arthropods other than mosquitoes. Technical report 67-65-ES. Project reference 1V025001A120, Series ES-32
16. United States Army Materiel Command, Natick Laboratories, Natick, Massachusetts
17. https://core.ac.uk/download/620961592.pdf (accessed on 23rd July 2025).
18. Larkin, K. (2022). *Pediculus humanus capitis* as a potential vector for *Acinetobacter baumannii*. https://core.ac.uk/download/532572445.pdf (accessed on 23rd July 2025).
19. Daniel, K., & Justin-Temu, M. (2011). Poverty, Parasitosis and HIV/AIDS - Major Health Concerns in Tanzania. InTech. doi: 10.5772/23159 (accessed on 23rd July 2025).
20. Savona-Ventura, C. (2002). Parasites and pests of medical significance in the Maltese environment: A historical review of culprit species. https://core.ac.uk/download/83020397.pdf (accessed on 23rd July 2025).

CUTANEOUS TUBERCULOSIS AND LEPROSY

3

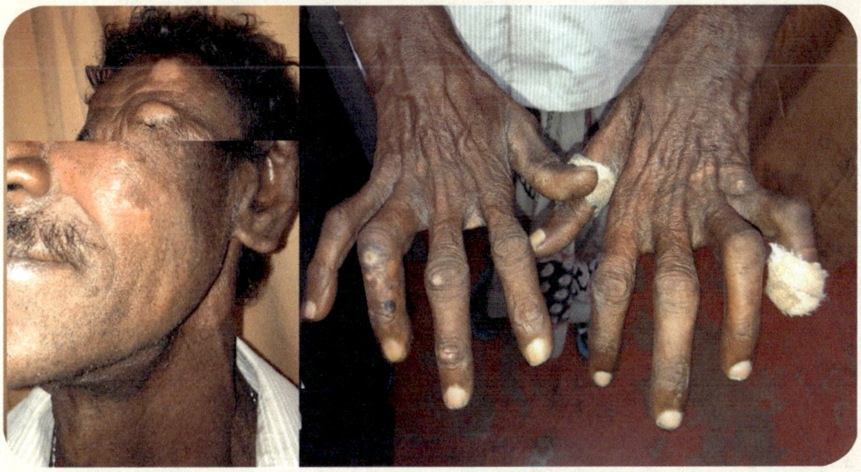

LEARNING OBJECTIVES

After studying this chapter, you will be able to:

1. Understand Pathophysiology of Cutaneous Tuberculosis;
2. Explain Pathophysiology of Leprosy;
3. Describe Treatment and Management;
4. Focus on Societal and Cultural Implications.

Introduction

Cutaneous tuberculosis and leprosy are significant public health concerns, primarily in regions where socio-economic standards are the cause of the epidemiology of these diseases. These two diseases are caused by mycobacterial species, with cutaneous tuberculosis caused by *Mycobacterium tuberculosis* and leprosy caused by *Mycobacterium leprae.* Human beings get exposed to mycobacterial species because they are found in different environmental niches, leading to infections that might exceed the innate immune system. In the majority of individuals, pathogenic mycobacterial species can invade our first-line barrier defenses and control phagocyte activation, leading to disease in the respiratory tract or skin and soft tissues, and, in some cases, resulting in disseminated infection (Franco-Paredes et al., 2018). Understanding the pathogenesis of these diseases is crucial, especially in view of the current burden of antimicrobial resistance, which complicates the control of these diseases (Murray et al., 2022). The implication of cutaneous tuberculosis and leprosy calls for practices focusing on early diagnosis and adequate treatment.

3.1. Pathophysiology of Cutaneous Tuberculosis

Learning Outcome

1. Understand the Causative Agent;
2. Explain Mechanisms of Skin Involvement;
3. Focus on Immune Response to Infection;
4. Describe Types of Cutaneous Lesions;
5. Learn Diagnostic Methods for Cutaneous Tuberculosis;
6. Discuss Differential Diagnosis with Other Skin Conditions;
7. Know Complications Associated with Untreated Cases;
8. Understand the Role of Genetics in Susceptibility.

Cutaneous tuberculosis, a manifestation of *Mycobacterium tuberculosis* infection, develops when the bacteria infect the skin, the most frequent ones being ulcerative or nodular, which can seriously impair the integrity of the skin. Pathophysiology is a complex immune reaction wherein macrophages and T-lymphocytes are involved in granuloma formation, attempting to encapsulate the infection. This local immune response can lead to caseation necrosis, which forms the characteristic lesions of the disease. Notably, the disease is aggravated by etiologies such as malnutrition, immunosuppression, and coinfection with other organisms, including those responsible for leprosy, so it becomes more difficult to treat and for recovery (Perez et al., 2024). Moreover, the use of BCG vaccination, while highly preventive in character, can cause undesirable inflammatory responses at injection sites, thereby revealing the intricate interaction between therapeutic interventions and cutaneous tuberculosis pathophysiological effects (Bernini et al., 2015). Demystifying this intricate interaction is important to the manufacture of effective management plans for those who have been affected by it (Figure 3.1).

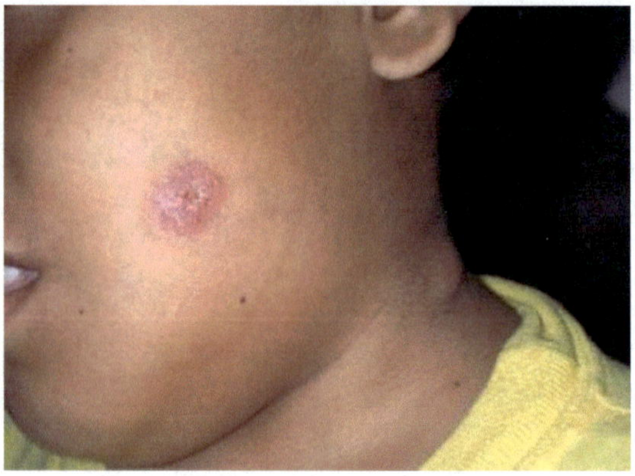

Figure 3.1. Cutaneous tuberculosis.

Source: https://ars.els-cdn.com/content/image/1-s2.0-S0738081X06000678-gr1.jpg.

3.1.1. Causative Agent: Mycobacterium tuberculosis

Mycobacterium tuberculosis, the etiologic agent of cutaneous tuberculosis, is an extremely versatile pathogen more commonly seen in its pulmonary manifestations. Although classically tuberculosis is seen to present through the lungs, cutaneous tuberculosis has also gained attention for its polymorphism of presentation, thereby highlighting the bacterium's power to infect the skin. Recent evidence regarding microbial virulence highlights the complex interactions between *Mycobacterium tuberculosis* and the host immune system. Clarification of such interactions sheds light on the pathogenesis of cutaneous lesions in immunocompromised individuals or disease-exposed persons. Advances in microbiology also continue to refine our knowledge of *Mycobacterium tuberculosis* as a simple pathogen, hypothesizing that elements of its interaction with human hosts may encompass elements of mutualism under certain circumstances, as in the case of other cutaneous microbes (Moore et al., 2003). Hence, the understanding of the intricate function of this bacterium is most important for the proper planning of treatment protocols.

3.1.2. Mechanism of Skin Involvement

Cutaneous tuberculosis and leprosy skin involvement mechanisms rely mainly on the immune response generated by the pathogens inducing these diseases. Mycobacterium tuberculosis, the causative organism of tuberculosis, can induce the formation of localized granulomatous skin lesions if the immunity is not able to control the bacteria effectively. Immune evasion in such cases is usually a result of the coordination of numerous host factors, i.e., pre-existing immunosuppression or concurrent infection, e.g., those occurring in leprosy patients. In fact, cutaneous leishmaniasis has been reported to coinfect other diseases, influencing clinical manifestations and complicating diagnosis and treatment protocols, as seen in TL coinfections studies (Martínez et al., 2018). Furthermore, the bacillus Calmette-Guérin (BCG) vaccine, though a protective measure against tuberculosis, can inadvertently precipitate inflammatory skin symptoms and autoimmune responses (Bernini et al., 2015). Understanding these complex mechanisms is important for optimizing therapeutic interventions in the cutaneous presentation of such diseases (Figure 3.2).

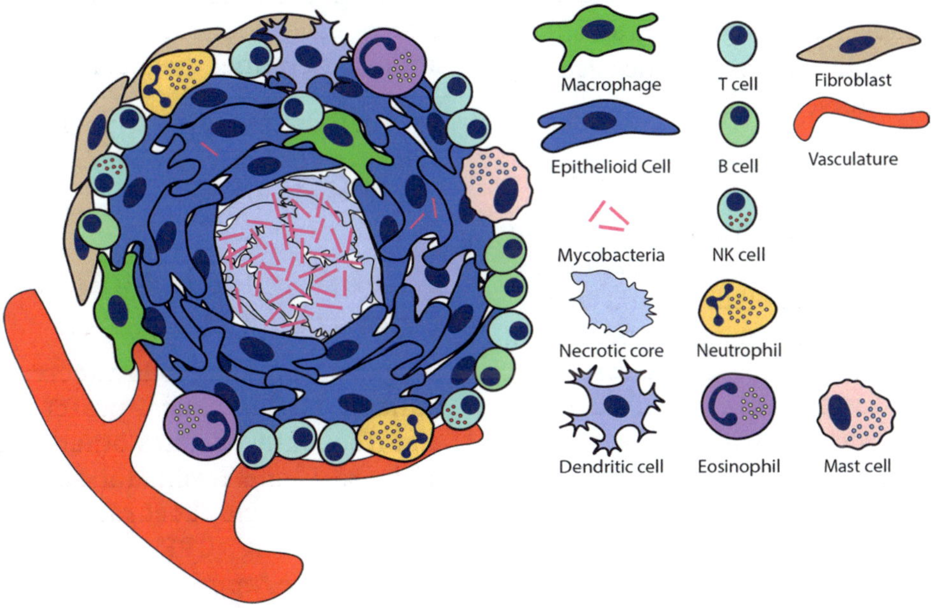

Figure 3.2. *Mycobacterium tuberculosis*, the causative agent of tuberculosis, can lead to the formation of localized granulomatous lesions on the skin when the immune system fails to contain the bacteria effectively.

Source: https://images-provider.frontiersin.org/api/ipx/w=1200&f=png/https://www.frontiersin.org/files/Articles/820134/fimmu-13-820134-HTML/image_m/fimmu-13-820134-g001.jpg.

3.1.3. Immune Response to Infection

Immunity against infection by cutaneous leprosy and tuberculosis is a multifaceted interaction between adaptive and innate mechanisms that are designed to eliminate the pathogen. In cutaneous tuberculosis, the macrophages play a crucial role in recognizing the antigens of *Mycobacterium tuberculosis*, thereby triggering a chain reaction of immunity involving the activation of T cells and the formation of granulomas to contain the infection. Interestingly, immuno-histochemical studies found that 68% of the cases showed detectable mycobacterial antigens, pointing to immune system activation against the infection (Padmavathy & Rao, 2005).

Leprosy, on the other hand, is difficult because it is able to evade immune detection and, therefore, tends to cause multi-organ co-infections complicating clinical presentation. Research has shown that co-infections can modulate the immune response, possibly lowering the success rate of treatments (Martínez et al., 2018). Hence, knowledge of these effects is important for improving diagnostic accuracy and therapeutic interventions.

3.1.4. Types of Cutaneous Lesions

Knowledge of the various types of cutaneous lesions is vital in the diagnosis and treatment of diseases like cutaneous tuberculosis and leprosy. Cutaneous lesions are recognized to present in the form of nodules, plaques, and ulcers, with features that vary to allow differential diagnosis. Leprosy can be associated with granulomatous lesions, where studies have established that leprosy accounts for a significant proportion of granulomatous cutaneous lesions in certain regions, illustrated by statistics indicating that 82.46% of cases of the study were due to leprosy (Kevadiya & Shah, 2024). Cutaneous tuberculosis, on the other hand, can manifest in erythematous nodular or ulcerative forms and mimic leprosy in presentation and chronicity. This overlap in diagnosis requires a heightened index of suspicion of both conditions in the setting of atypical cutaneous lesions by clinicians, thereby facilitating prompt and effective therapeutic interventions (Figure 3.3).

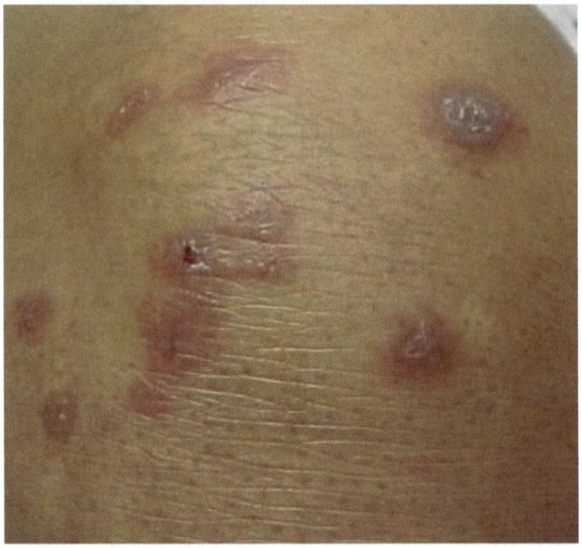

Figure 3.3. Cutaneous lesions manifest in several forms, including nodules, plaques, and ulcers, each with distinct characteristics that aid in differential diagnosis.

Source: https://www.dermatologyadvisor.com/wp-content/uploads/sites/20/2019/03/ch1407.fig1_.jpg.

3.1.5. Diagnostic Methods for Cutaneous Tuberculosis

Diagnosis of cutaneous tuberculosis (CTB) is difficult as the clinical presentation is varied and frequently imitates other dermatoses such as leprosy and leishmaniasis. It is important that diagnostic accuracy be achieved in differentiating CTB from such imitators to facilitate appropriate management. The traditional method is the tuberculin skin test and the detection of *Mycobacterium tuberculosis* by culture or PCR. Though skin biopsy can be a valuable tool for histopathological examination and can present caseating granulomas that diagnose TB, coinfections complicate the diagnosis. For instance, coinfection with leishmania pathogens can lead to overlapping signs that can impede correct diagnosis, as shown by Martínez et al. (2018). In addition, O'Brien et al. (2008) highlight the importance of knowing the epidemiological history, given that patients' travel history has a direct influence on the likelihood of CTB diagnosis and, therefore, merits thorough clinical evaluation.

3.1.6. Differential Diagnosis with Other Skin Conditions

Differential diagnosis for cutaneous tuberculosis and leprosy is difficult to a greater degree, because other skin conditions tend to share similar clinical manifestations. Diseases such as leishmaniasis and sporotrichosis present with identical cutaneous lesions, which complicate acquiring a proper diagnosis with subsequent treatment.

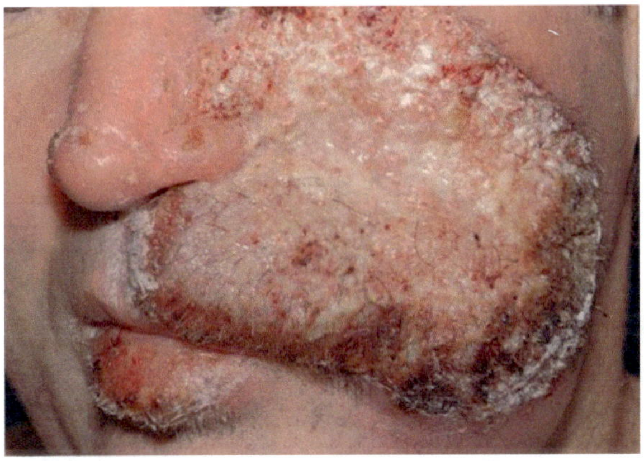

Figure 3.4. *Tegumentary leishmaniasis.*

Source: https://static.elsevier.es/multimedia/03650596/0000009400000003/v1_202012010801/S036505962030619X/v1_202012010801/en/main.assets/gr1.jpeg.

An example is *Tegumentary leishmaniasis*, which may present in the form of diagnostic overlap, since both leishmaniasis and leprosy have granulomatous skin lesions that cannot be differentiated clinically without further evaluation (Martínez et al., 2018). Moreover, in tuberculosis, especially in tuberculous lymphadenitis, identification of *Mycobacterium tuberculosis* in tissue is significant since it can make the diagnosis and signify the complex interaction of the humoral immunity factors that will mimic other dermatoses (Ramanathan, 1998). Thus, a careful clinical evaluation supplemented with selected diagnostic testing will be needed to differentiate these conditions best (Figure 3.4).

3.1.7. Complications Associated with Untreated Cases

Untreated cases of cutaneous tuberculosis and leprosy may lead to serious complications that significantly disrupt the patient's health and quality of life. In cutaneous tuberculosis patients, chronic inflammation may progress to extreme skin necrosis and deformity, significantly disrupting self-esteem and social relationships. The progressive condition of untreated leprosy might result in nerve damage and loss of sensation, muscle weakness, and subsequent physical disabilities. To this effect, secondary infections are a common risk in such untreated states, worsening the condition and making treatment more complex. Notably, the rising prevalence of neglected tropical diseases such as tuberculosis and leprosy poses a significant threat to health systems, especially in developing nations where access to effective interventions remains low (Boffa et al., 2004). Thus, early intervention and diagnosis are central to preventing the causative debilitating impacts of such diseases and promoting better health outcomes among sufferers.

3.1.8. Role of Genetics in Susceptibility

The genetics of susceptibility to cutaneous tuberculosis and leprosy is a significant area of study, as particular genetic factors can significantly influence how people respond to such diseases. Human leukocyte antigens (HLAs), which form the focal point of immune function, play a significant role in determining susceptibility. The genes that encode these HLAs, on the major histocompatibility complex

(MHC) region of chromosome 6, are also involved in presenting antigens to T lymphocytes, thereby orchestrating the response to infection. Variation in HLA genes has the potential to cause differential susceptibility or resistance to mycobacterial infections because the variation may affect T-cell activation and response efficacy (Singh et al., 1997). In addition, understanding the genetic basis of diseases, particularly in the case of such neglected tropical diseases, uncovers prospects for targeted therapeutic intervention and vaccine development as underscored by recent genomics studies (Croft, 2016) (Figure 3.5).

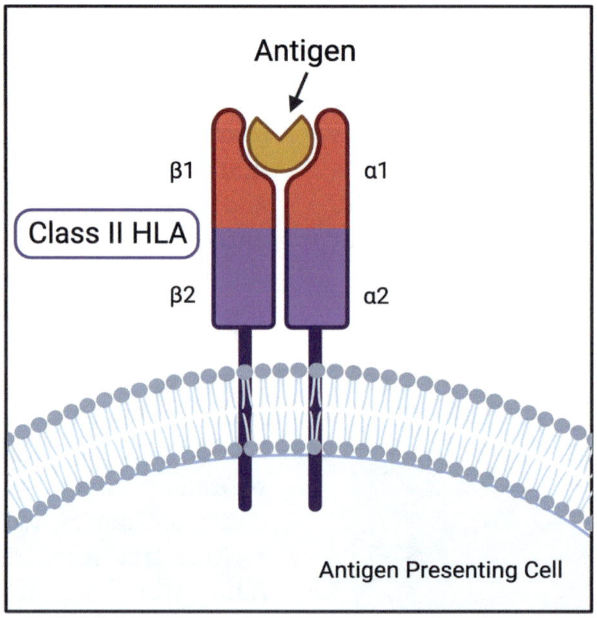

Figure 3.5. Human leukocyte antigens (HLAs), which are pivotal to immune system function, play a crucial role in determining susceptibility.

Source: https://images-provider.frontiersin.org/api/ipx/w=1200&f=png/https://www.frontiersin.org/files/Articles/1270488/fimmu-14-1270488-HTML-r1/image_m/fimmu-14-1270488-g001.jpg.

Test Your Knowledge

1. What distinguishes tuberculosis verrucosa cutis from other forms?
2. Which type of cutaneous TB reflects high immunity and low bacterial load?

3.2. Pathophysiology of Leprosy

Learning Outcome

1. Understand the Causative Agent;
2. Explain Mechanism of Skin and Nerve Involvement;
3. Focus on Immune Response and its Variations;
4. Describe Types of Leprosy and Their Clinical Features;
5. Learn Diagnostic Methods for Leprosy;
6. Discuss Differential Diagnosis with Other Dermatological Diseases;
7. Know Complications and Long-term Effects;
8. Understand Genetic Factors Influencing Disease Progression;
9. Explain Recent Advancements in Understanding Leprosy.

The pathophysiology of leprosy, caused by the intracellular bacterium *Mycobacterium leprae*, is a reflection of the intricate interaction between microbial virulence and host immune response. After transmission, the bacillus infects peripheral nerves and skin and causes diverse clinical presentations ranging from superficial cutaneous lesions to extensive nerve damage. This pathogenesis is also underscored by the bacterium's capacity to evade the immune system, forming a spectrum of disease that encompasses tuberculoid leprosy with good immunity through to lepromatous leprosy with suppressed immunity and uncontrolled bacterial proliferation.

Furthermore, the socioeconomic factors of leprosy's prevalence, particularly in low- and middle-income countries, contribute to its public health relevance in that compromised access to treatment worsens disease outcome. Understanding such dynamics is pertinent, especially when confronting other intracellular pathogens of the same type, like those applied in examples concerning tuberculosis, as both harbor cross-cutting social and biological factors in controlling disease (Bernini et al., 2015; Perez et al., 2024).

3.2.1. Causative Agent: Mycobacterium leprae

The bacterium responsible for causing leprosy, *Mycobacterium leprae*, is a slow-growing bacillus that mainly infects peripheral nerves and skin, thus imparting the disease its characteristic features. As compared to more prevalent pathogens, its specific adaptations provide it protection within the host's immune space, making it an interesting study topic.

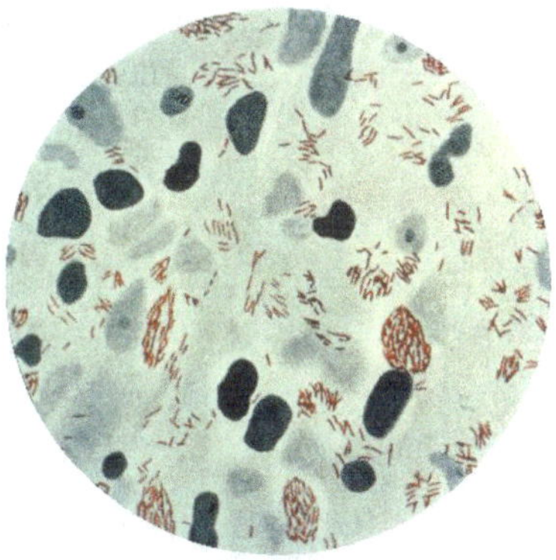

Figure 3.6. *Mycobacterium leprae* is a slow-growing bacterium that primarily targets peripheral nerves and skin, leading to the characteristic symptoms of the disease.

Source: https://upload.wikimedia.org/wikipedia/commons/d/da/Mycobacterium_leprae.jpeg.

The interaction of *M. leprae* with its human host is a classic example of a dynamic interplay of pathogenicity and host defense, as advances in immunology clarify how this bacterium escapes detection and treatment. Recent findings suggest that the body's response to infection with *M. leprae* is regulated by the presence of some immune mediators, such as TNF-alpha, showing similar responses in other bacterial infections, highlighting the importance of understanding immune dynamics for effective leprosy control (Moore et al., 2003). In addition, recent studies of human cutaneous microbiota suggest the potential for beneficial interactions impacting the disease process, suggesting a dynamic interplay between the presence of microbes and host well-being (Figure 3.6).

3.2.2. Mechanism of Skin and Nerve Involvement

Skin and nerve involvement in cutaneous tuberculosis and leprosy is a multidimensional process due to the host immune reaction against the pathogens *Mycobacterium tuberculosis* and *Mycobacterium leprae.* With leprosy, and particularly the lepromatous form, skin and nerve damage is due to inflammation with foamy macrophages and dense inflammatory cell infiltrate, leading to necrotizing vasculitis and epidermal thinning histopathologically observed (Fiqnasyani et al., 2023). The inflammation disrupts the nerves' normal functioning, predisposing to loss of sensation and deformities due to the delay in treatment and diagnosis. For instance, patients suffering from pure neuritic Hansen's disease experience some major challenges of diagnosis because the skin is free of lesions, which in turn postpones intervening and causes permanent damage to nerves (Jayaraman, 2012). Therefore, it is important to understand the pathogenesis of these diseases to come up with efficient diagnosis and treatment measures that can help contain their effects on individuals.

3.2.3. Immune Response and Its Variations

The immune response to cutaneous tuberculosis and leprosy is complex and extremely variable between individuals, based on variables such as genetic susceptibility and pathogenicity of the etiologic organisms.

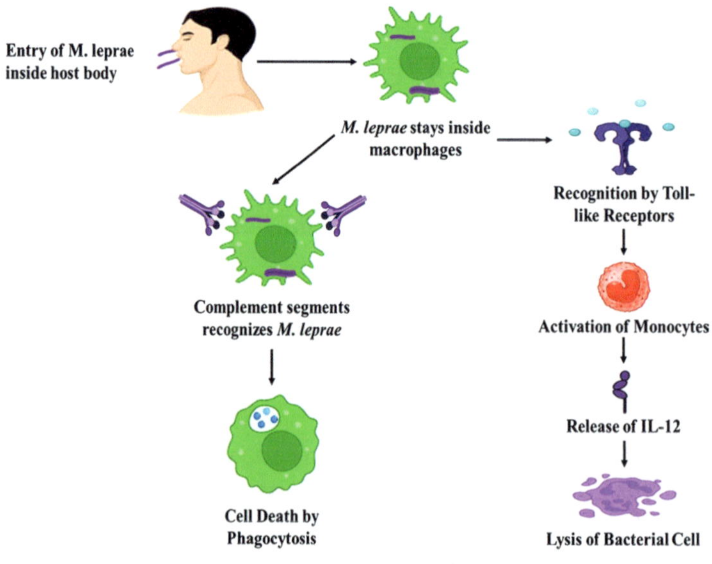

Figure 3.7. The immune response to cutaneous tuberculosis and leprosy is complex and varies significantly among individuals, influenced by factors such as genetic predisposition and the pathogenicity of the causative agents.

Source: https://www.frontiersin.org/files/Articles/1361641/fphar-15-1361641-HTML-r1/image_m/fphar-15-1361641-g004.jpg.

Both conditions feature the formation of granulomas, which are indicative of the body's effort to sequester and wall off the causative infectious agents. In some, however, the immune system may fail to clear the agent effectively, leading to residual lesions and gradations of tissue damage, such as in the formation of infectious granulomatous reactions with mycobacterial infections like leprosy and tuberculosis (Rota & Emeksiz, 2020). Also, studies on *Mycobacterium ulcerans*, the causative agent of Buruli ulcer, show that the pathogen may be able to down-regulate essential inflammatory mediators, hinting at a broader immunological modulation that has effects possibly on healing and immunity (Phillips et al., 2014). Such an understanding of these immune response variations is critical in developing effective treatments for such crippling diseases (Figure 3.7).

3.2.4. Types of Leprosy and Their Clinical Features

Leprosy, a chronic infectious disease produced by the *Mycobacterium leprae* bacterium, manifests in various forms with varying clinical manifestations. Two major forms of leprosy include tuberculoid and lepromatous leprosy. Tuberculoid leprosy is characterized by limited lesions that may be anesthetic to a small degree and the immune reaction sufficient to localize the disease and lead to final healing of the cutaneous lesions.

Lepromatous leprosy consists of numerous skin lesions that are often smooth, multiple, and more anesthetic and show an abnormal immune reaction. Of particular interest is the differentiation between these categories because lepromatous leprosy can lead to widespread morbidity from nerve destruction and secondary infections, complicating clinical treatment (Kodnani & Shah, 2016). The spectrum of leprosy clinical presentation underscores the necessity for correct diagnosis and effective management strategies, as mimicking signs with diseases like cutaneous tuberculosis can lead to diagnostic challenges (Martínez et al., 2018).

3.2.5. Diagnostic Methods for Leprosy

The diagnostic methods of leprosy present unique challenges, mostly due to the inability to culture the causative pathogen, *Mycobacterium leprae*, from clinical specimens. Classical methods, such as histopathology, cannot prove acid-fast bacilli and therefore present a challenge in making a definitive diagnosis. As an additional methodology, immunohistochemical staining has been promising, particularly in revealing mycobacterial antigens in tissue specimens, as reported by studies illustrating positivity in a good proportion of cases of cutaneous tuberculosis, where cross-reactivity can also be observed in cases of leprosy (Padmavathy & Rao, 2005).

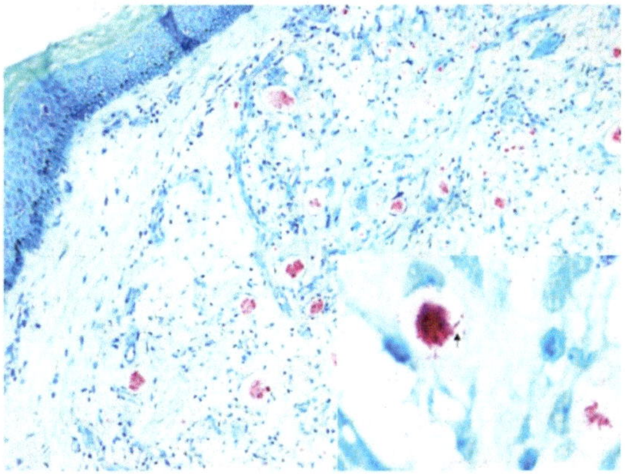

Figure 3.8. Integrating clinical findings with robust laboratory techniques is crucial to distinguishing leprosy from related pathologies effectively, ensuring timely and appropriate treatment.

Source: https://media.springernature.com/lw685/springer-static/image/art%3A10.1186%2Fs12879-024-09937-2/MediaObjects/12879_2024_9937_Fig4_HTML.jpg.

Such an observation suggests a multifaceted interaction among the diagnostic methods in such mycobacterial infections. Besides, leprosy in the tropics can manifest in many other conditions, and therefore diagnostic confusion arises (Richens, 2004). Thus, combining clinical observations with good laboratory practices is crucial to differentiating leprosy from related pathologies efficiently so that proper treatment can be administered on time (Figure 3.8).

3.2.6. Differential Diagnosis with Other Dermatological Diseases

Differential diagnosis between cutaneous tuberculosis and leprosy is challenging because of the shared clinical manifestations of both infections with other dermatoses. Differential diagnosis usually requires a combination of clinical examination and histopathological examination. For example, skin lesions that occur with leprosy can be similar to lesions present in other dermatoses, so it is necessary to be careful to differentiate them from each other. A paper noted that biopsies of leprosy patients had significant histopathological findings which were not always in concordance with clinical diagnoses, underscoring the influence of histopathology in confirming or excluding diagnoses (Bisht et al., 2020). Besides, the application of advanced diagnostic techniques such as quantitative polymerase chain reaction (qPCR) assays has been shown to improve specificity for leprosy, but one should consider cross-reactivity with other cutaneous diseases (Martinez et al., 2011). This demands utilizing a multidisciplinary strategy to arrive at a definitive diagnosis in such challenging cases.

3.2.7. Complications and Long-term Effects

The long-term sequelae and complications of leprosy and cutaneous tuberculosis are significant challenges for patients. For cutaneous tuberculosis, the complications can be in the form of chronic skin lesions with potential for scarring and secondary infection, hence affecting an individual's quality of life. In addition, the BCG vaccine, as a model of effective prevention of tuberculosis, can induce deleterious autoimmune reactions, such as acute inflammatory polyarthritis and granulomatous pneumonia, demonstrating the complexity of treatment (Bernini et al., 2015). Similarly, leprosy is complicated by erythema nodosum leprosum (ENL), a severe disease that can induce recurrent painful nodules along with systemic manifestations, necessitating long-term corticosteroid treatment. This prolonged usage is typically preceded by severe morbidity and has been associated with increased mortality rates, especially in vulnerable populations (Walker et al., 2014). The two diseases thus mirror the multifaceted implications of their long-term expression (Figure 3.9).

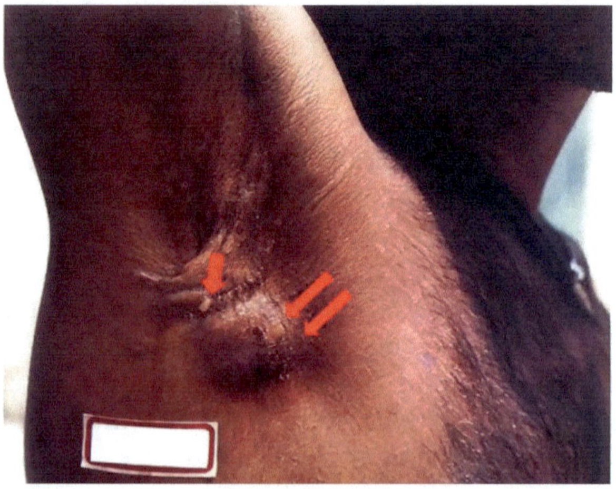

Figure 3.9. In the case of cutaneous tuberculosis, complications can manifest as chronic skin lesions that may lead to scarring and secondary infections, thereby affecting a person's quality of life.

Source: https://www.mdpi.com/pathogens/pathogens-12-00920/article_deploy/html/images/pathogens-12-00920-g004.png.

3.2.8. Genetic Factors Influencing Disease Progression

The interaction between genetic determinants and disease progression is a very important area of research in making sense of cutaneous tuberculosis as well as leprosy. Human leukocyte antigens (HLAs), central elements of the immune system, have a great impact on people's susceptibility to these diseases. HLAs, which are controlled by MHC genes, are essential in the activation of T lymphocytes and consequently the mediation of immune responses to *Mycobacterium tuberculosis* and *Mycobacterium leprae*. These antigenic variations can affect the effectiveness of pathogen recognition and immune activation, pointing out how genetic predispositions affect disease susceptibility (Singh et al., 1997). Apart from these, shared biological and sociodemographic determinants in low-resource settings emphasize the contributions of genetic determinants to disease outcomes. Implications of these genetic determinants extend beyond patient susceptibility, prompting an interdisciplinary workforce to intervene and offer a greater insight into the diagnosis and treatment of cutaneous tuberculosis and leprosy (Perez et al., 2024).

3.2.9. Recent Advancements in Understanding Leprosy

The new insights into the understanding of leprosy have significantly helped elucidate the multifaceted nature of disease pathogenesis and host-parasite interactions. Molecular tools, particularly polymerase chain reaction (PCR) and next-generation sequencing (NGS), have provided scientists with the ability to identify *Mycobacterium leprae* with unparalleled specificity, leading to better diagnoses and insight into microbial gene diversity.

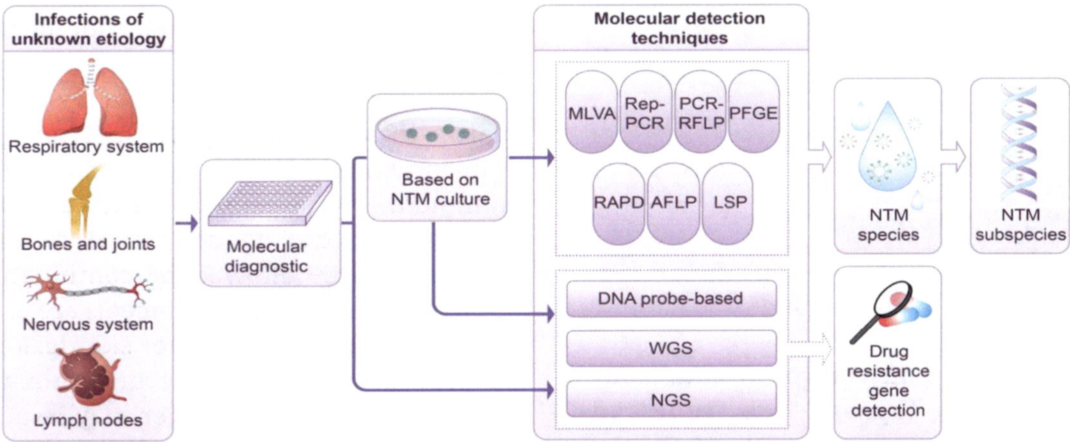

Figure 3.10. Molecular techniques, particularly polymerase chain reaction (PCR) and next-generation sequencing (NGS), have allowed researchers to detect *Mycobacterium leprae* at unprecedented precision, leading to more accurate diagnoses and insights into microbial genetic diversity.

Source: https://www.frontiersin.org/files/Articles/1410672/fpubh-12-1410672-HTML/image_m/fpubh-12-1410672-g001.jpg.

These developments shed light on the natural history of the disease and the long-term influence of the disease on human health, especially in cutaneous manifestations. In addition, studies on the role of immunological processes, such as dysregulated levels of Immunoglobulin E, have demonstrated how immune processes can alter susceptibility and severity of leprosy, as is observed in other dermatoses (Pate et al., 2010; Gabriel et al., 2024). Taken together, these developments not only enhance the accuracy of diagnosis but also give rise to targeted therapeutic options that promise to revolutionize the treatment of leprosy and its complications (Figure 3.10).

Test Your Knowledge

1. What determines the polarity (spectrum) of leprosy?
2. Which T-cell subtype is predominant in lepromatous leprosy?

3.3. Treatment and Management

Learning Outcome

1. Understand Standard Treatment Protocols for Cutaneous Tuberculosis;
2. Explain Standard Treatment Protocols for Leprosy;
3. Focus on Role of Antibiotics in Treatment;
4. Describe the Importance of Early Diagnosis and Intervention;
5. Learn Management of Complications and Co-morbidities;
6. Discuss Patient Education and Adherence to Treatment;
7. Know Role of Public Health Initiatives;
8. Understand Challenges in Treatment Accessibility.

Effective treatment and control of cutaneous tuberculosis and leprosy are required in alleviating the burden of these NTDs, particularly where the prevalence rates are high. For leprosy, multi-drug therapy (MDT) has immensely improved patient care, reducing disease morbidity and stigma (Momen-Heravi & Sharif, 2009). MDT consists of a course of antibiotics for a particular time, effectively killing *Mycobacterium leprae*. In Ethiopia, both the burden of leprosy and other NTDs remains high and the government's prioritization of an NTD Master Plan is aimed at increasing treatment and intervention activities (Deribe et al., 2012). In addition, public health initiative coordination and community campaigns will be essential towards the early detection of cases and treatment, with the overall aim of tackling not only the biological aspects of the disease but also the social effects of the disease states.

3.3.1. Standard Treatment Protocols for Cutaneous Tuberculosis

General therapeutic regimens for cutaneous TB are primarily antitubercular medications in agreement with standards set by the World Health Organization (WHO). The optimal regimen typically is a combination of isoniazid, rifampicin, pyrazinamide, and ethambutol administered during an initial two-month intensive phase, followed by continuation for four to six months. These protocols are essential for ensuring both the cure of skin lesions and the prevention of systemic dissemination of infection. Treatment, however, may be adjusted in response, and drug resistance is one of the complicating issues. Moreover, the experience of other mycobacterial infections, such as leprosy, highlights the permanent need for versatile protocols based on the response of individual patients and potential side effects of medicines, such as the problems discussed by Sarfo et al. (2011) and Lambert et al. (2016). Lastly, an individualized strategy is necessary to optimize therapeutic outcomes (Figure 3.11).

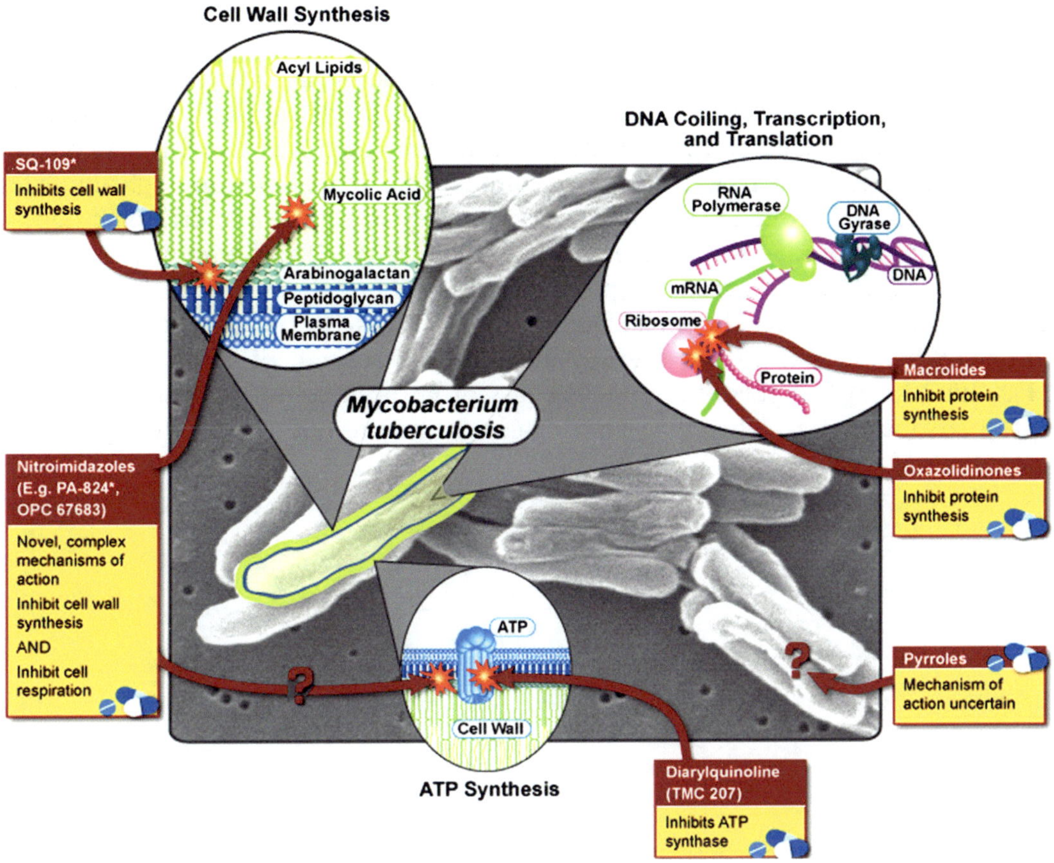

Figure 3.11. Standard treatment protocols for cutaneous tuberculosis (TB) primarily involve the use of antitubercular medications in accordance with guidelines established by the World Health Organization (WHO).

Source: https://upload.wikimedia.org/wikipedia/commons/0/08/Tuberculosis-drugs-and-actions.jpg.

3.3.2. Standard Treatment Protocols for Leprosy

Leprosy, being a *Mycobacterium leprae* infection, requires a combination-based strategy towards its control, relying heavily on standardized treatment protocols. The World Health Organization recommendations are a multidrug therapy (MDT) regimen, with rifampicin, clofazimine, and dapsone being the primary drugs, which have proven to eliminate the bacteria and prevent disability. The management of leprosy also includes managing immune-mediated sequelae, such as Type 1 reactions, that cause permanent nerve damage. Corticosteroids, like prednisolone, are the preferred treatment for Type 1 reactions, with immediate relief of symptoms. However, second-line agents such as ciclosporin have been introduced as effective second-line therapy for steroid non-responders or patients with adverse effects, bringing into perspective the need for more research on stronger leprosy drugs (Lambert et al., 2016). Thus, understanding these treatment regimens is key to minimizing long-term leprosy complications and improving patient quality of life.

3.3.3. Role of Antibiotics in Treatment

Antibiotics play a crucial role in the treatment of cutaneous tuberculosis and leprosy, primarily due to their efficacy in the eradication of the etiological bacterial infections by *Mycobacterium tuberculosis* and *Mycobacterium leprae*, respectively. Efficacy of the antibiotics in the treatment of these diseases is not only based on their efficacy in reducing bacterial load but also on the quality-of-life improvement of patients. In Ethiopia, for example, where the epidemiological burden of such neglected diseases as cutaneous leishmaniasis and leprosy is significant, strategic deployment of antibiotic therapy has witnessed achievements such as reaching leprosy elimination targets as early as 1999 (Deribe et al., 2012). Interestingly, research also reveals that effective antibiotic treatment can significantly decrease the level of mycolactone in patients with Buruli ulcer, demonstrating the complex interplay between antibiotic therapy and the progression of cutaneous infection (Sarfo et al., 2011). This finding supports the effectiveness of antibiotics not just in healing but even in preventing the advancement of disabling skin diseases like the one shown in Figure 3.12.

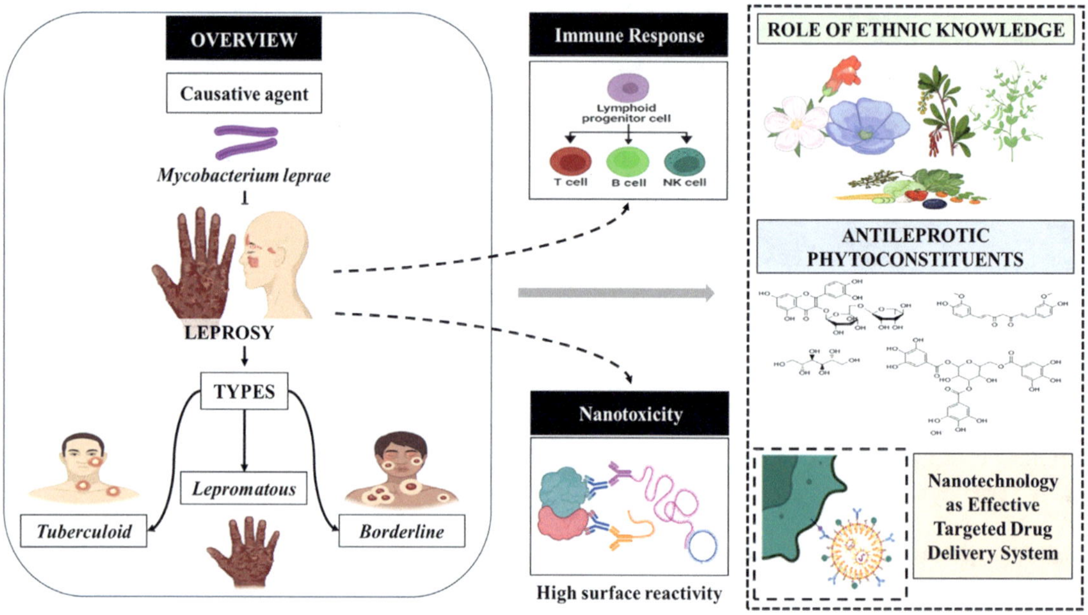

Figure 3.12. Antibiotics play a critical role in the treatment of cutaneous tuberculosis and leprosy.

Source: https://www.frontiersin.org/files/Articles/1361641/fphar-15-1361641-HTML-r1/image_m/FPHAR_fphar-2024-1361641_wc_abs.jpg.

3.3.4. Importance of Early Diagnosis and Intervention

The importance of early diagnosis and treatment of cutaneous tuberculosis and leprosy cannot be overestimated, as early treatment greatly alters patient prognosis. The early identification of skin lesions enables the initiation of immediate treatment protocols, which can prevent the advancement of the disease and the development of complications, such as erythema nodosum leprosum (ENL), a life-threatening and disabling condition that results from leprosy. Studies demonstrate that patients with ENL experience higher morbidity and mortality, and thus early management is warranted to avert these risks (Walker et al., 2014). In addition, the challenge presented by co-infections, which, in turn, complicates clinical presentation and leads to diagnostic misunderstandings, also indicates the need for quick diagnosis (Martínez et al., 2018). Consequently, the enhancement of diagnostic capabilities and implementation of prompt treatment processes is required in efficient management of such conditions and additionally concerning overall patient prognosis.

3.3.5. Management of Complications and Co-morbidities

Proper management of the complications and co-morbidities of cutaneous tuberculosis and leprosy patients is crucial in the enhancement of health outcomes. Erythema nodosum leprosum (ENL) is a severe complication of leprosy characterized by tender nodules, fever, and systemic manifestations, which can result in serious morbidity.

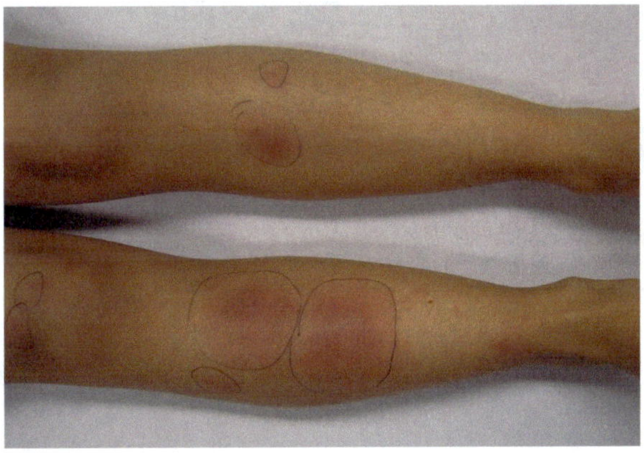

Figure 3.13. Erythema nodosum leprosum (ENL), a significant complication associated with leprosy, is characterized by painful nodules, fever, and systemic symptoms that may result in considerable morbidity.

Source: https://upload.wikimedia.org/wikipedia/commons/thumb/b/bb/ENlegs.JPG/1200px-ENlegs.JPG.

The need for prolonged treatment with high-doses of oral corticosteroids in the management of ENL may result in unwanted effects like increased mortality, as in one study where there was a higher rate of death among ENL patients compared to Type 1 reactions (Walker et al., 2014). In addition, co-infections such as tuberculosis impose additional complexities; new therapies such as delamanid, which selectively target various mycobacterial strains, are also vital in managing such complexities of cutaneous tuberculosis (Hazra, 2021). The treatment must encompass a holistic strategy for the treatment of multiple infections and their complexities (Figure 3.13).

3.3.6. Patient Education and Adherence to Treatment

Interventional patient education plays a very crucial role in enhancing adherence to treatment programs in cutaneous tuberculosis and leprosy, two diseases with direct impacts on public health in poor resource settings. Awareness of the conditions and their treatment strengthens patients' sense of control, which leads to better outcomes. Evidence highlights that patients who are provided with comprehensive education regarding their illness are more likely to adhere to prescribed regimens. Further, the necessity of addressing socio-demographic determinants, such as the place they reside in and drug availability, cannot be overstressed because such determinants also influence adherence rates (Perez et al., 2024). By utilizing methods such as patient counseling, educational materials, and community support, healthcare providers are able to bridge gaps in knowledge and empower patients. By a collaborative process that honors both biological and social barriers, patient adherence improvement leads to improved health and reduced disease transmission.

3.3.7. Role of Public Health Initiatives

Public health interventions play a critical role in the management of problems brought about by leprosy and cutaneous tuberculosis, particularly in resource-limited settings where these conditions prevail. In the Ethiopian context, where neglected tropical diseases (NTDs) are prevalent, inclusive public health planning will help in managing and preventing the disease. The Ethiopian government has recognized the necessity of these interventions by launching an NTD Master Plan to control the enormous burden of infection, with leprosy being among the leading public health concerns. Progress has been made, with achievement of the target of 1 case per 10,000 population leprosy elimination as early as 1999, but additional effort is necessary to consolidate and build on that progress (Deribe et al., 2012). Furthermore, bringing genomic methods into mainstream paradigms, as has been suggested in the NTDs debate, could improve treatment and intervention programs (Croft, 2016) (Figure 3.14).

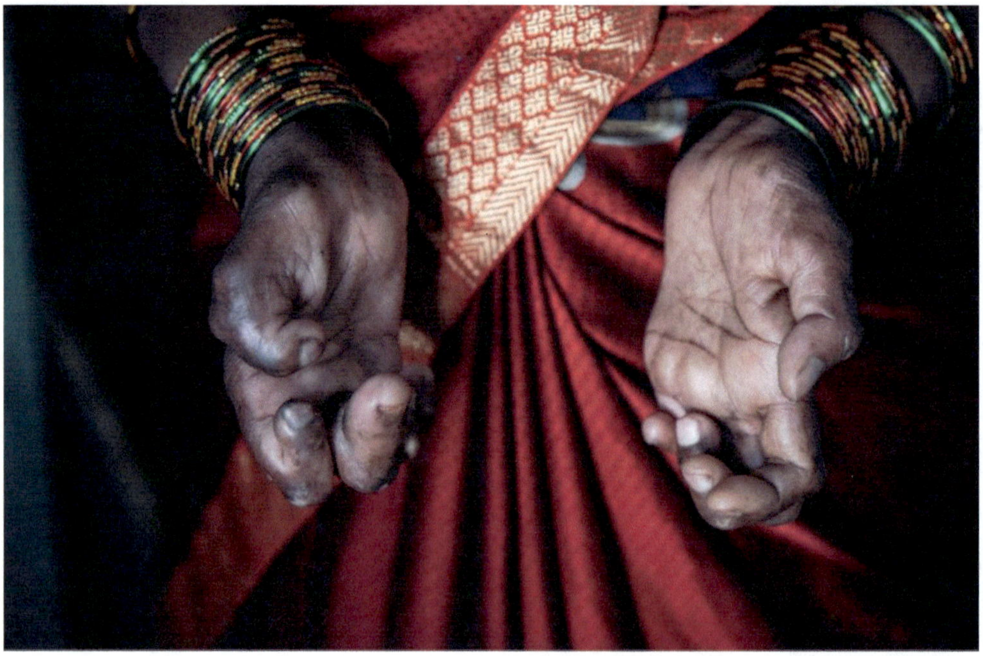

Figure 3.14. Public health initiatives play a crucial role in addressing the challenges posed by cutaneous tuberculosis and leprosy, particularly in resource-limited settings where these diseases flourish.

Source: https://static01.nyt.com/images/2019/04/23/science/00LEPROSY1/00LEPROSY1-superJumbo.jpg.

3.3.8. Challenges in Treatment Accessibility

Access to appropriate treatment for cutaneous tuberculosis and leprosy remains a significant challenge, particularly in low- and middle-income countries where the diseases are endemic. This impaired accessibility is also exacerbated by inadequate healthcare infrastructure, minimal numbers of qualified medical staff, and absent financing for disease control measures. Further, stigma against these conditions may deter individuals from accessing medical care, leading to underdiagnosis and continuing transmission. The shared biological and sociocultural roots of these diseases make the problem of meeting the accessibility of treatment one that needs to be addressed in a holistic manner. As emphasized by the VALIDATE Network, the burden of mycobacterial disease in poor-resource settings underscores the urgent need for new research and development approaches aimed at ensuring equitable access to therapeutics and diagnostics. An understanding of these shared challenges will assist in informing policy and supporting healthcare interventions, ultimately leading to better control of cutaneous tuberculosis and leprosy (Perez et al., 2024).

Test Your Knowledge

1. Which test is used to monitor treatment response in cutaneous TB?
2. Why is dapsone given in combination in leprosy?

3.4. Societal and Cultural Implications

Learning Outcome

1. Understand Historical Stigma associated with Both Diseases;
2. Explain Impact on Mental Health and Well-being;
3. Focus on Cultural Perceptions and Misconceptions;
4. Describe Role of Advocacy and Awareness Campaigns;
5. Learn Socioeconomic Factors Influencing Disease Spread;
6. Discuss Integration of Care into Community Health Systems;
7. Know Global Health Policies Addressing These Diseases;
8. Understand Future Challenges in Societal Acceptance.

The social and cultural impacts of cutaneous tuberculosis and leprosy extend way beyond individual health to encompass community structures and socioeconomic status. Both diseases have traditionally been linked with tremendous stigma, which has reinforced isolation and deprived the patient of essential social support networks. Stigmatization has the potential to perpetuate cycles of poverty since the diseased are discriminated against in securing employment and social associations, leading to reduced ability and life options.

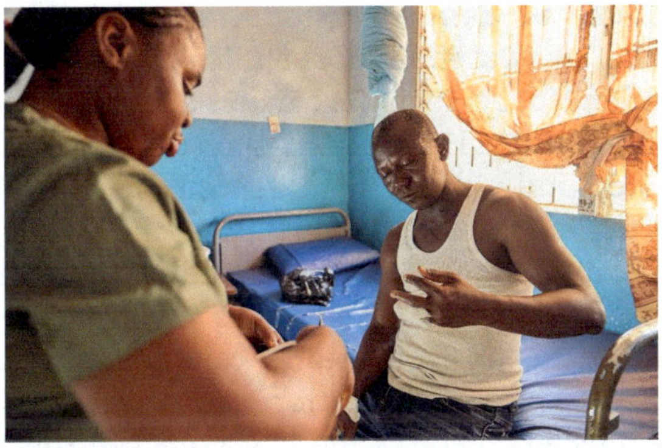

Figure 3.15. Stigmatization can perpetuate cycles of poverty, as affected individuals often face discrimination in employment and social settings, leading to reduced capabilities and life choices.

Source: https://www.who.int/images/default-source/departments/ntd-library/skin-ntds/activities-on-skin-related-ntds-in-sub-saharan-africa-3.jpg?sfvrsn=5c413ab4_5.

As the literature has indicated, such neglected tropical disease has its health cost worsened by societal attitudes and hence there is a dynamics of health and poverty as envisioned by Amartya Sen and Martha Nussbaum's capabilities approach (Wilsher,

2011). Aside from this, the existing antibiotic-resistant problem also calls for re-reading historical treatments of past pandemics to possibly discover advantages of going back to medicinal procedures of the past to aid current health policies (Harrison & Connelly, 2019). With this two-pronged focus, the spread of misinformation could be mitigated and public health efforts improved (Figure 3.15).

3.4.1. Historical Stigma Associated with Both Diseases

Both cutaneous tuberculosis and leprosy have throughout history been dominated by strong stigma, which has significantly influenced public perception and the treatment of victims. This stigmatization is typically the product of delusions about contagion and overall unawareness of such diseases, and this is followed by social exclusion and alienation of the victim. Historically, societies have also treated individuals with leprosy as morally tainted or cursed, in line with the broader pattern of stigmatization of individuals with neglected tropical diseases, as highlighted by their exclusion from health care systems and society. The stigmatization of these diseases not only exaggerates the psychological misery of the patients but also exacerbates their socioeconomic condition, thus trapping them in a vicious cycle of poverty and restricted life choices. These stigmas must be confronted, as observed in the discussion on the accompanying health burden, to make way for more humane and efficient public health intervention for both diseases (Wilsher, 2011; Deribe et al., 2012).

3.4.2. Impact on Mental Health and Well-being

The impact of cutaneous tuberculosis and leprosy extends beyond physical evidence, with a profound impact on mental well-being and overall health. Patients are typically confronted with psychological distress due to stigma, withdrawal from society, and the debilitating impact of prolonged disability. For instance, stigma of leprosy can lead to poor quality of life, with patients responding much lower on composite indicators of well-being, as in comparative studies where they also experience higher mental health morbidity and social isolation (Mousley et al., 2013). Moreover, the concurrent spread of poverty and access to healthcare exacerbates all these factors, as people residing in poverty-stricken settings may be deprived of adequate support structures for their mental well-being (Perez et al., 2024). Thus, any appropriate public health response for controlling cutaneous tuberculosis and leprosy needs to place top priority on mental healthcare to alleviate the psychological load of these conditions, which will be conducive to an empathetic and accepting community among affected populations (Figure 3.16).

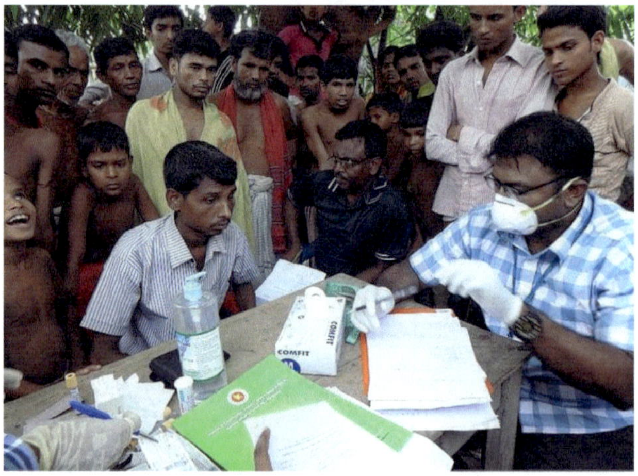

Figure 3.16. The impact of cutaneous tuberculosis and leprosy extends beyond physical manifestations, significantly affecting mental health and overall well-being.

Source: https://gumlet.assettype.com/down-to-earth%2Fimport%2Flibrary%2Flarge%2F2017-03-24%2F0.04931900_1490341666_tb-cdc-global.jpg?w=640&auto=format%2Ccompress.

3.4.3. Cultural Perceptions and Misconceptions

Cultural misconceptions and perceptions regarding cutaneous tuberculosis and leprosy have a significant impact on patient experience and treatment outcomes. The illnesses are usually highly stigmatized and are fueled by prehistoric thought patterns that blame them for danger and high contagious risk. For example, medical practitioners are common victims of patients who, driven by social fear, delay coming in for treatment and, as a result, prolong their conditions. These obstacles are based on ignorance on the part of both patients and providers about these diseases' transmission, as was evident in a study on Hansen's disease treatment-seeking experience, where there were misconceptions of its communicability (Kuhns, 2012). In the case of Cameroon, the history of leprosy elimination efforts by the country indicates how ignorance gets in the way of effective public health programs despite progress achieved after 2000 (Tabah, 2018). Education and advocacy are key to overcoming these cultural attitudes to enhance health outcomes as well as create an enabling environment for those infected.

3.4.4. Role of Advocacy and Awareness Campaigns

Advocacy and campaigns ensure awareness of diseases like cutaneous tuberculosis and leprosy, which have extensive implications for public health, particularly in communities where there are fewer resources. These efforts are meant to reverse the stigma surrounding NTDs since stigma can exacerbate health inequalities and undermine effective treatment programs, resulting in the trapping of individuals in poverty circles and exclusion. With heightened sensitization of symptoms, transmission, and management of cutaneous tuberculosis and leprosy, advocacy efforts may result in earlier detection and better access to care. In Ethiopia, for instance, where the incidence of NTDs is enormously high, advocacy efforts are needed to help stem the tide of misconceptions within society and foster an environment favorable to the affected (Deribe et al., 2012). Moreover, the integration of the capabilities approach in these advocacy endeavors highlights the mutual dependency of poverty and health, consequently advocating for a unified approach to the social determinants of health for NTDs (Wilsher, 2011) (Figure 3.17).

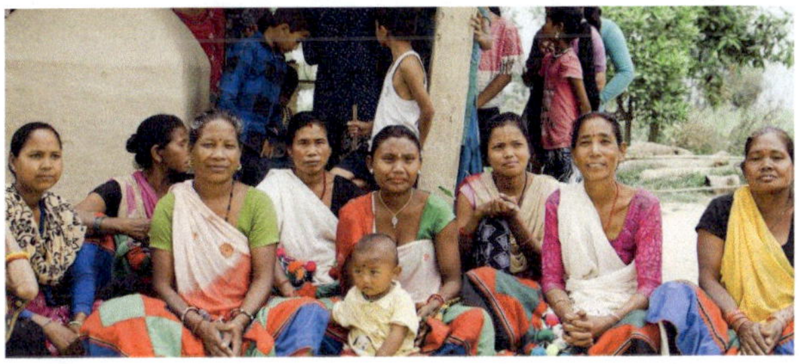

Figure 3.17. Advocacy and awareness campaigns play a pivotal role in addressing neglected tropical diseases (NTDs) like cutaneous tuberculosis and leprosy, which significantly affect public health, particularly in resource-limited settings.

Source: https://leprosymissioninternational.contentfiles.net/media/images/RS37670_RS9833__DSC6550.2e16d0ba.fill-900x400-c75.jpg.

3.4.5. Socioeconomic Factors Influencing Disease Spread

The link between socioeconomic determinants and cutaneous tuberculosis and leprosy disease transmission is considerable, particularly in low- and middle-income countries where the diseases are most prevalent. Economic constraints tend to limit access to healthcare resources, such as effective diagnosis and treatment, resulting in the continued disease transmission among populations. Socio-economic poor living conditions, coupled with a lack of education about such infections, exacerbate the situation because individuals may be unaware of symptoms or remedies. In addition to that, social stigmatization of leprosy leads to victims becoming more isolated, which complicates the efforts of public health campaigns to deliver their message and create a society that facilitates the spread of diseases. As highlighted by recent research, efforts at intervention have to target the shared biological and social determinants if they are to work against the infections (Perez et al., 2024). Despite advances through interventions such as multidrug therapy against leprosy, being careful about resistance draws attention to the complex interplay of socioeconomic determinants in the control and management of disease (Reibel et al., 2018).

3.4.6. Integration of Care into Community Health Systems

Integration of care into community health systems is essential in combating diseases such as cutaneous tuberculosis and leprosy, both of which disproportionately affect marginalized communities. Integration not only expands access to critical healthcare services but also maximizes coordination among a range of different healthcare providers, thereby boosting patient outcomes through improved coordination. As global health systems evolve, the impact of globalization allows for cross-border transfer of valuable health information and new treatment practices, but, in the process, poses problems like the transmission of communicable diseases (Murdan et al., 2014). The research on vaccines and disease management strategies, for example, for leprosy and tuberculosis, attests to the importance of healthcare models based on communities. The VALIDATE network is one demonstration of how collaborative vaccine development approaches are coming together with global health initiatives to ultimately benefit the health of vulnerable populations. Such integrated approaches are necessary to address these chronic public health problems sustainably (Figure 3.18).

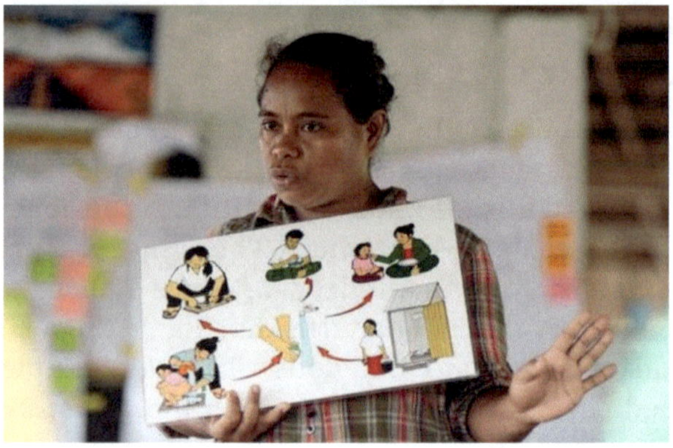

Figure 3.18. The integration of care into community health systems is pivotal for effectively addressing diseases such as cutaneous tuberculosis and leprosy, both of which disproportionately affect marginalized populations.

Source: https://www.who.int/images/default-source/departments/ntd-library/wash-ntd/wash-ntd-course.jpg?sfvrsn=a6034997_3.

3.4.7. Global Health Policies Addressing These Diseases

As part of comprehensive efforts towards effective public health interventions, global health policies have directed more attention towards the management of neglected tropical diseases like cutaneous tuberculosis and leprosy. These initiatives target better prevention, diagnosis, and treatment through cooperation on a worldwide basis. For example, the World Health Organization (WHO) determines that preventing seven tropical diseases in Africa will cost only 40 cents per person annually, a relatively low cost that could enhance health for millions of people with these illnesses (Molyneux et al., 2005). In addition, health innovations such as organ and stem cell transplantations are now faced with the spread of these underemphasized conditions, particularly in developing countries where the disease burden is high. Through the integration of holistic health models that prioritize observation and access to treatment, universal policies can readily mitigate the impact of cutaneous tuberculosis and leprosy, resulting in healthier populations worldwide.

3.4.8. Future Challenges in Societal Acceptance

With the medical fraternity improving awareness and treatment of Cutaneous Tuberculosis and Leprosy, future challenges regarding the acceptance of society are still a priority. Stigma has a large influence on how these neglected tropical diseases (NTDs) are viewed, usually discouraging people from receiving treatment and worsening their conditions. Stigma not only contributes to the low quality of life for the affected but also creates economic costs that ensnare families into poverty loops, which relates closely to the capabilities approach that has been contentious in the literature on NTDs (Wilsher, 2011). Moreover, new vaccine strategies and therapeutic technologies, outlined in recent NTD literature, will have to be complemented by efforts to diminish societal stigma associated with these diseases if equitable health outcomes are to be achieved. Sailing past social attitudes will be called for to fully involve patients with communities so that isolation and discrimination are avoided and the barriers to achievement of overall public health goals are dispelled.

Test Your Knowledge

1. What role does contact tracing play in public health management of leprosy?
2. What social determinant most strongly affects the prevalence of cutaneous TB?

SUMMARY

The two issues presented by cutaneous tuberculosis and leprosy are actual public health problems that need to be addressed by integrative intervention strategies. Such diseases, aside from compromising the health of individuals, impose a huge toll on the healthcare system, as is evident in nations such as Ethiopia, with one of the highest rates in the world of such neglected tropical diseases as leprosy, as noted in Deribe et al. (2012). Intervention against such diseases must be holistic, including early diagnosis and prevention and effective treatment, alongside education of communities to reduce stigma associated with such infection. Alongside, the immunological subtleties that come with it, as exemplified by the influence of immune reactions on systemic bacterial infections, demonstrate that knowledge regarding the underlying biological processes is critical to the development of effective therapeutic regimens, marking a need for continued research in this regard, as suggested by observations on immunity in studies like those presented in Moore et al. (2003).

While summarizing the key issues in the case of cutaneous tuberculosis and leprosy, it is evident that both conditions present with complex challenges in diagnosis and treatment since they share similar symptoms and are also susceptible to coinfection. For example, cutaneous leishmaniasis frequently occurs in concomitance with other pathogens, causing diagnostic difficulties and therapeutic problems, as evidenced by the frequency of coinfections within several populations, such as the high coinfection rates of *Trypanosoma cruzi* and helminthiasis among TL patients (Martínez et al., 2018). Furthermore, application of the bacillus Calmette-Guérin (BCG) vaccine extends beyond prevention against tuberculosis as it also exhibits efficacy in leprosy management, in spite of causing autoimmunity problems in some cases (Bernini et al., 2015). All such connections emphasize greater study of disease interaction for the aims of gaining an in-depth understanding of disease connectivity, enabling better correct diagnosis, and creating better treatment for affected populations.

KEY TERMS FROM THIS CHAPTER

- Leprosy
- Cutaneous tuberculosis
- Mycobacterium leprae
- Environmental niches
- Phagocyte activation
- Soft tissues
- Granuloma
- Immunosuppression
- Organisms
- Epidemiology
- Mycobacterium tuberculosis
- Mycobacterial species
- Innate immune system
- Respiratory tract
- Macrophages
- Malnutrition
- Coinfection
- T-lymphocytes

CRITICAL THINKING QUESTIONS

1. **The most common form of cutaneous tuberculosis in adults is:**
   a. *Lupus vulgaris*
   b. Scrofuloderma
   c. *Tuberculosis verrucosa* cutis
   d. *Miliary tuberculosis*
2. **Which of the following cutaneous TB forms occurs due to direct inoculation in a previously sensitized individual?**
   a. Scrofuloderma
   b. *Tuberculosis verrucosa* cutis
   c. *Lupus vulgaris*
   d. Tuberculid
3. **"Apple jelly nodules" seen on diascopy are characteristic of:**
   a. Leprosy
   b. Tinea corporis
   c. Lupus vulgaris
   d. Psoriasis
4. **The bacterium responsible for leprosy is:**
   a. *Mycobacterium tuberculosis*
   b. *Mycobacterium bovis*
   c. *Mycobacterium leprae*
   d. *Mycobacterium kansasii*
5. **The cardinal signs of leprosy include all EXCEPT:**
   a. Hypopigmented patch with sensory loss
   b. Thickened peripheral nerve
   c. Positive slit skin smear for AFB
   d. Elevated ESR

Short Answer Questions

1. What is the main immune mechanism involved in cutaneous tuberculosis?
2. Which type of hypersensitivity reaction underlies tuberculids?
3. What type of immune response predominates in tuberculoid leprosy?
4. Lepromatous leprosy is associated with which type of immunity?
5. What is the standard MDT (multidrug therapy) regimen for multibacillary leprosy?
6. Which drug in leprosy therapy is bactericidal?
7. What is the main reason patients delay seeking treatment for leprosy?
8. Which WHO program has been pivotal in reducing the global burden of leprosy?

Answers to Critical Thinking Questions

1. (a); 2. (b); 3. (c); 4. (c); 5. (d)

REFERENCES

1. Singh, N., Agrawal, S., & Rastogi, A. K. (1997). Infectious diseases and immunity: special reference to major histocompatibility complex. *Emerging infectious diseases*, *3*(1), 41–49. https://doi.org/10.3201/eid0301.970105(accessed on 23rd July 2025).

2. Reibel, F., Cambau, E., & Aubry, A. (2015). Update on the epidemiology, diagnosis, and treatment of leprosy. *Medecine et maladies infectieuses*, *45*(9), 383–393. https://doi.org/10.1016/j.medmal.2015.09.002(accessed on 23rd July 2025).

3. Murdan, S., Blum, N., Francis, S., Slater, E., Alem, N., Munday, M., Taylor, J. & Smith, F. (2014). *The Global Pharmacist*. Published by UCL School of Pharmacy and Development Education Research Centre, Institute of Education, University of London ISBN: 978-0-9574187-1-4. https://core.ac.uk/download/79499297.pdf (accessed on 23rd July 2025).

4. Lambert, S. M., Alembo, D. T., Nigusse, S. D., Yamuah, L. K., Walker, S. L., & Lockwood, D. N. (2016). A Randomized Controlled Double Blind Trial of Ciclosporin versus Prednisolone in the Management of Leprosy Patients with New Type 1 Reaction, in Ethiopia. *PLoS neglected tropical diseases*, *10*(4), e0004502. https://doi.org/10.1371/journal.pntd.0004502(accessed on 23rd July 2025).

5. Deribe, K., Meribo, K., Gebre, T., Hailu, A., Ali, A., Aseffa, A., & Davey, G. (2012). The burden of neglected tropical diseases in Ethiopia, and opportunities for integrated control and elimination. *Parasites & vectors*, *5*, 240. https://doi.org/10.1186/1756-3305-5-240(accessed on 23rd July 2025).

6. Bisht, M., Arya, A., & Choudhry, B. C. (2020). Histomorphological analysis and clinical correlation of neoplastic and non neoplastic skin lesions: a study in a tertiary care centre of Western Uttar Pradesh, India. *International Journal of Research in Medical Sciences*, *8*(8), 2820–2827. https://doi.org/10.18203/2320-6012.ijrms20203093(accessed on 23rd July 2025).

7. Martínez DY, Verdonck K, Kaye PM, et al. Tegumentary leishmaniasis and coinfections other than HIV. *PLoS Negl Trop Dis*. 2018;12(3):e0006125. Published 2018 Mar 1. doi:10.1371/journal.pntd.0006125(accessed on 23rd July 2025).

8. Gabriel, J. A., Weerasinghe, N., Balachandran, P., Salih, R., & Orchard, G. E. (2024). A Narrative Review of Molecular, Immunohistochemical and In-Situ Techniques in Dermatopathology. *British journal of biomedical science*, *81*, 13437. https://doi.org/10.3389/bjbs.2024.13437(accessed on 23rd July 2025).

9. Bernini, L., Manzini, C.U. and Ferri, C. (2015). BCG and Autoimmunity. In Vaccines and Autoimmunity (eds Y. Shoenfeld, N. Agmon-Levin and L. Tomljenovic). https://doi.org/10.1002/9781118663721.ch21 (accessed on 23rd July 2025).

10. Boffa, M. J., Farrugia, B., & DeGaetano, J. (2004). Lupus vulgaris in a Maltese patient. https://core.ac.uk/download/46601869.pdf (accessed on 23rd July 2025).

11. O'Brien, D. P., Leder, K., Matchett, E., Brown, G. V., & Torresi, J. (2006). Illness in returned travelers and immigrants/refugees: the 6-year experience of two Australian infectious diseases units. *Journal of travel medicine*, *13*(3), 145–152. https://doi.org/10.1111/j.1708-8305.2006.00033.x(accessed on 23rd July 2025).

12. Perez, R. L., Chase, J., & Tanner, R. (2024). Shared challenges to the control of complex intracellular neglected pathogens. *Frontiers in public health*, *12*, 1423420. https://doi.

org/10.3389/fpubh.2024.1423420(accessed on 23rd July 2025).

13. Sarfo, F. S., Le Chevalier, F., Aka, N., Phillips, R. O., Amoako, Y., Boneca, I. G., Lenormand, P., Dosso, M., Wansbrough-Jones, M., Veyron-Churlet, R., Guenin-Macé, L., & Demangel, C. (2011). Mycolactone diffuses into the peripheral blood of Buruli ulcer patients--implications for diagnosis and disease monitoring. *PLoS neglected tropical diseases*, *5*(7), e1237. https://doi.org/10.1371/journal.pntd.0001237(accessed on 23rd July 2025).

14. Pate, M. B., Smith, J. K., Chi, D. S., & Krishnaswamy, G. (2010). Regulation and dysregulation of immunoglobulin E: a molecular and clinical perspective. *Clinical and molecular allergy : CMA*, *8*, 3. https://doi.org/10.1186/1476-7961-8-3(accessed on 23rd July 2025).

15. Moore, T. A., Lau, H. Y., Cogen, A. L., Monteleon, C. L., & Standiford, T. J. (2003). Anti-tumor necrosis factor-alpha therapy during murine Klebsiella pneumoniae bacteremia: increased mortality in the absence of liver injury. *Shock (Augusta, Ga.)*, *20*(4), 309–315. https://doi.org/10.1097/01.shk.0000087203.34916.45Harrison, F., & Connelly, E. (2019). Could medieval medicine help the fight against antimicrobial resistance? https://core.ac.uk/download/266992301.pdf (accessed on 23rd July 2025).

16. Croft, S. L. (2016). Neglected tropical diseases in the genomics era: Re-evaluating the impact of new drugs and mass drug administration. https://core.ac.uk/download/42635798.pdf (accessed on 23rd July 2025).

17. Mousley, E., Deribe, K., Tamiru, A., & Davey, G. (2013). The impact of podoconiosis on quality of life in Northern Ethiopia. *Health and quality of life outcomes*, *11*, 122. https://doi.org/10.1186/1477-7525-11-122 (accessed on 23rd July 2025).

18. Dinçer Rota, D., & Emeksiz, M. C. (2020). Granulomatous skin infections. Turkderm-Turkish Archives of Dermatology and Venereology, 55(1), 1-8.. https://core.ac.uk/download/539818597.pdf (accessed on 23rd July 2025).

19. Walker, S. L., Lebas, E., Doni, S. N., Lockwood, D. N., & Lambert, S. M. (2014). The mortality associated with erythema nodosum leprosum in Ethiopia: a retrospective hospital-based study. *PLoS neglected tropical diseases*, *8*(3), e2690. https://doi.org/10.1371/journal.pntd.0002690(accessed on 23rd July 2025).

20. Molyneux, D. H., Hotez, P. J., & Fenwick, A. (2005). "Rapid-impact interventions": how a policy of integrated control for Africa's neglected tropical diseases could benefit the poor. *PLoS medicine*, *2*(11), e336. https://doi.org/10.1371/journal.pmed.0020336(accessed on 23rd July 2025).

21. Fiqnasyani, S. E., Mudigdo, A., Novriana, D. E., et al. (2023). Lucio phenomenon in pregnancy: A histopathology review. https://core.ac.uk/download/639385429.pdf (accessed on 23rd July 2025).

22. Franco-Paredes, C., Marcos, L. A., Henao-Martínez, A. F., Rodríguez-Morales, A. J., Villamil-Gómez, W. E., Gotuzzo, E., & Bonifáz, A. (2018). Cutaneous mycobacterial infections. *Clinical Microbiology Reviews, 32*. https://doi.org/10.1128/cmr.00069-18 (accessed on 23rd July 2025).

23. Hazra, M. (2021). A rational pharmacotherapeutic study of the prevalent prescription patterns of delamanid, ofloxacin, levofloxacin, and bedaquiline among the multi-drug-resistant tuberculosis patients in global multi-center tertiary care hospitals. https://core.ac.uk/download/539896183.pdf (accessed on 23rd July 2025).

24. Jayaraman, R. (2012). A study on diagnostic significance of nerve conduction studies in early detection of pure neurotic Hansen's disease. https://core.ac.uk/download/287236524.pdf (accessed on 23rd July 2025).

25. Kevadiya, G. V., & Shah, P. H. (2024). Histopathological analysis of granulomatous lesions of skin and its correlation with clinical diagnosis at a tertiary care hospital, Bhavnagar. *Annals of Pathology and Laboratory Medicine.* https://www.semanticscholar.org/paper/68bea1710b458b49f858da18caf63443682498ff (accessed on 23rd July 2025).

26. Kodnani, A., & Shah, J. M. (2016). A comparative overview of histopathology of granulomatous lesions of skin. *International Journal of Clinical and Biomedical Research, 2*(1), 6–9. Retrieved from https://sumathipublications.com/index.php/ijcbr/article/view/7(accessed on 23rd July 2025).

27. Kuhns, K. E. (2012). What's to know? Navigating knowledge gaps of Hansen's disease in the U.S. https://core.ac.uk/download/71423600.pdf (accessed on 23rd July 2025).

28. Padmavathy, L., Lakshmana Rao, L., et al. (2005). Mycobacterial antigen in tissues in diagnosis of cutaneous tuberculosis. https://core.ac.uk/download/83048882.pdf (accessed on 23rd July 2025).

29. Martinez, A. N., Phetsuksiri, B., Plikaytis, B. B., Boehme, C. C., Cardoso, C. C., et al. (2011). Evaluation of qPCR-based assays for leprosy diagnosis directly in clinical specimens. https://core.ac.uk/download/pdf/8627235.pdf (accessed on 23rd July 2025).

30. Momen-Heravi, M., & Sharif, A. (2009). Leprosy of the larynx: A case report. Acta medica Iranica 47(6):485-487. https://core.ac.uk/download/143838177.pdf (accessed on 23rd July 2025).

31. Murray, C. J. L., Ikuta, K. S., Sharara, F., Swetschinski, L. R., Robles Aguilar, G., Gray, A. P., Han, C., et al. (2022). Global burden of bacterial antimicrobial resistance in 2019: A systematic analysis. *The Lancet, 399*, 629–655. https://doi.org/10.1016/s0140-6736(21)02724-0 (accessed on 23rd July 2025).

32. Phillips, R. O., Sarfo, F. S., Landier, J., Oldenburg, R., Frimpong, M., Wansbrough-Jones, M., Abass, K., Thompson, W., Forson, M., Fontanet, A., Niang, F., & Demangel, C. (2014). Combined inflammatory and metabolic defects reflected by reduced serum protein levels in patients with Buruli ulcer disease. *PLoS neglected tropical diseases, 8*(4), e2786. https://doi.org/10.1371/journal.pntd.0002786(accessed on 23rd July 2025).

33. Ramanathan, V. D. (1998). Studies on the immunopathology of tuberculosis. https://core.ac.uk/download/48015688.pdf (accessed on 23rd July 2025).

34. Richens, J. (2004). Genital manifestations of tropical diseases. https://core.ac.uk/download/1669842.pdf (accessed on 23rd July 2025).

35. Tabah, E. N. (2018). Skin neglected tropical diseases in Cameroon: The need for integrated control and elimination. https://core.ac.uk/download/211690333.pdf (accessed on 23rd July 2025).

36. Wilsher, E. J. (2011). The impact of neglected tropical diseases, and their associated stigma, on people's basic capabilities. https://core.ac.uk/download/176851.pdf (accessed on 23rd July 2025).

HYPERPIGMENTATION DISORDERS

4

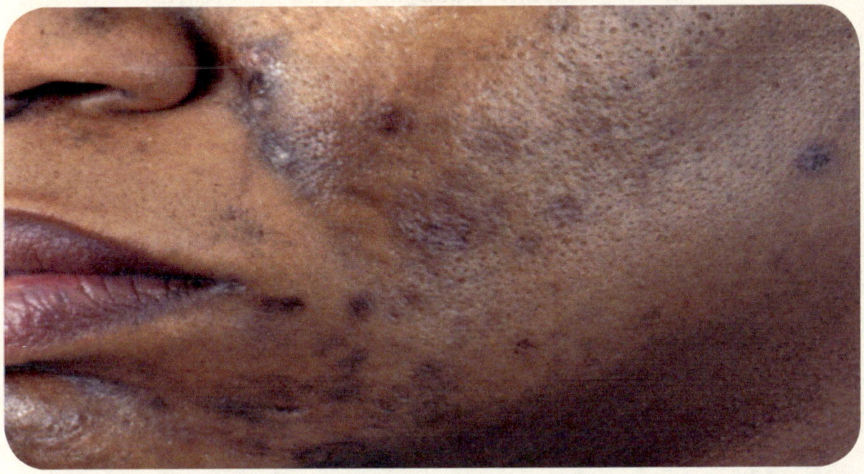

LEARNING OBJECTIVES

After studying this chapter, you will be able to:

1. Understand Hyperpigmentation;
2. Explain Melasma;
3. Describe Post-Inflammatory Hyperpigmentation (PIH);
4. Focus on Other Hyperpigmentation Disorders.

Introduction

Hyperpigmentation disorders, including conditions such as melasma and post-inflammatory hyperpigmentation (PIH), represent a critically difficult entity within the dermatology specialty, with varied populations of patients worldwide. They are characterized by augmented melanin production secondary to a diverse array of intrinsic and extrinsic factors, specifically UV light and environmental pollutants. As highlighted by literature, hyperpigmentation occurs most frequently in patients with darker skin types, and for them, it exerts a profound psychosocial impact, affecting self-esteem and overall quality of life (Edpuganti et al., 2025). Respecting the intricate nature of these conditions is particularly critical, as they constitute a wide clinical spectrum and accompanying pathophysiological mechanisms (Maymone, 2016). Additionally, the prevalence of hyperpigmentation coupled with a relative dearth of comprehensive dermatological studies requires an active investigation of the treatment modalities in use, their availability, and their efficiency in enhancing the quality of life of the afflicted.

4.1. Understanding Hyperpigmentation

Learning Outcome

1. Understand Definition and Mechanisms of Hyperpigmentation;
2. Explain Types of Hyperpigmentation Disorders;
3. Focus on Role of Melanin in Skin Pigmentation;
4. Describe Genetic Factors Influencing Hyperpigmentation;
5. Learn Environmental Triggers (Sun Exposure, Pollution);
6. Discuss Hormonal Influences (Pregnancy, Contraceptives);
7. Know Skin Types and their Susceptibility;
8. Understand Psychological Effects of Hyperpigmentation;
9. Explain the Importance of Skin Care in Prevention.

Disorders of hyperpigmentation are an important dermatology problem, which includes abnormal hypersecretion of melanin in the form of darkened spots on the skin. Melasma and post-inflammatory hyperpigmentation (PIH) are two of the most common types, which affect an individual's self-esteem and overall quality of life. Evidence points out that the impact of such disorders can be colossal, with patient studies indicating that patients who are diagnosed with PIH also demonstrate a mean Dermatology Life Quality Index (DLQI) score of 7.89, which indicates a substantial decrease in health-related quality of life (Maymone, 2016).

Moreover, environmental factors such as sun exposure are also the cause of the exacerbation of hyperpigmentation, and ultraviolet radiation (UVR) is a major reason behind such changes (Rodríguez-Luna et al., 2023). Hence, it becomes important to learn about the multifactorial etiology of hyperpigmentation in order to create proper treatment and management strategies (Figure 4.1).

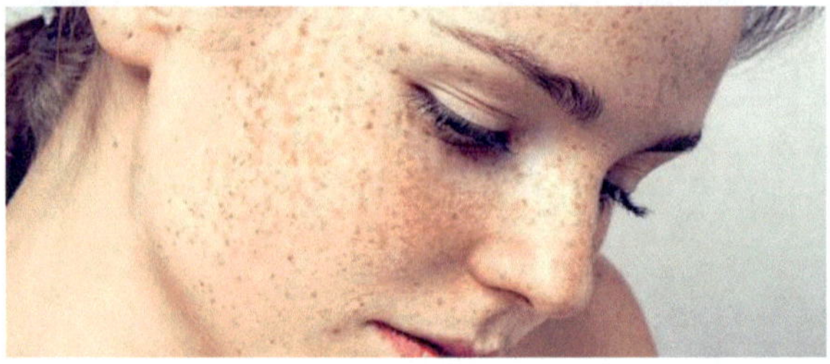

Figure 4.1. Hyperpigmentation disorders.

Source: https://lh3.googleusercontent.com/proxy/rjlzeSxt85OsL_GkM7rv31yYMQjKDtpshdHtxdIXjcyLSm9rY3S1Iu8clSG0mqn_VrubXT_1AWFNsKqDJfEyU0M8z1MTGWz3zDUoDhEWZ9ySLh28ptQM-PwCuBhjIj0T.

4.1.1. Definition and Mechanisms of Hyperpigmentation

Hyperpigmentation is a condition where there is an increase in melanin production resulting in localized skin darkening and is prevalent in other dermatoses such as melasma and post-inflammatory hyperpigmentation (PIH). Based on detailed descriptions in existing literature, hyperpigmentation arises from various mechanisms, including increased melanin synthesis, enhanced melanocyte density, and aberrant distribution of both endogenous and exogenous pigments in the skin (Maymone, 2016).

These processes are triggered by key factors such as ultraviolet (UV) light exposure, inflammation, and endocrine alteration, resulting in a noticeably altered skin appearance (Maymone, 2016). The consequences of hyperpigmentation extend beyond the cosmetic problem because individuals allegedly have a moderate to severe impact on their well-being, particularly in conditions like melasma and PIH, where the psychological profile is affected (Damodaran & Nair, 2022). It is crucial to comprehend these mechanisms to develop helpful therapeutic interventions and improve patient outcomes.

4.1.2. Types of Hyperpigmentation Disorders

Hyperpigmentation diseases are classified into several categories, primarily melasma and post-inflammatory hyperpigmentation (PIH), among others. Melasma often develops as bilateral facial pigmentation, usually brought about by hormonal changes, sun, and hereditary factors, predominantly affecting people with darker skin types. In contrast, PIH develops after trauma or inflammation of the skin, where additional melanin is deposited following injury, acne, or irritants. The nature and severity of these disorders can significantly influence the quality of life of patients who have them. Studies have reported lower health-related quality of life (HRQoL) scores among melasma and PIH patients compared to those with other types of hyperpigmentation disorders, reflecting the psychosocial consequence of these dermatological disorders (Maymone, 2016; Edpuganti et al., 2025). Understanding these differences is vital to the planning of personalized treatment programs aimed at both the aesthetic and emotional concerns that face patients (Figure 4.2).

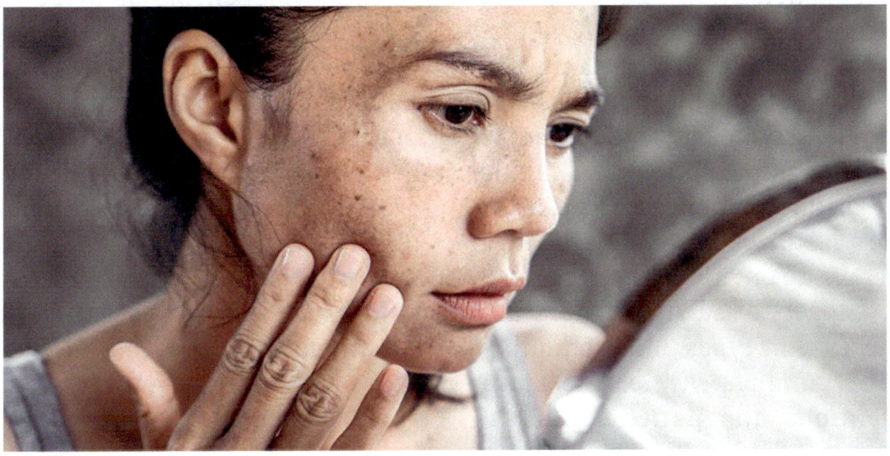

Figure 4.2. Melasma.

Source: https://gennev.com/wp-content/uploads/2025/05/6604d100de80def7d028f2ab_Hormones-and-Melasma_-How-to-Manage-the-Dark-Spots-On-Your-Skin.jpg.

4.1.3. Role of Melanin in Skin Pigmentation

Melanin plays a significant role in determining the pigmentation of the skin, acting as an innate protective barrier against harmful ultraviolet (UV) radiation. It is synthesized by highly specialized epidermal cells, the melanocytes, which, on exposure to a variety of stimuli, such as UV radiation, synthesize melanin. It plays an important role in preventing damage to the skin, though overproduction leads to hyperpigmentation disorders such as melasma and post-inflammatory hyperpigmentation (PIH). Studies demonstrate that hyperpigmentation is prevalent in individuals with darker shades of skin, demonstrating a high correlation between the production of melanin and a state of well-being of the skin. Moreover, their psychosocial impact is wide in the sense that they have been proven to be detrimental to the quality of life of an individual, particularly for post-inflammatory hyperpigmentation and melasma, whose health-related quality of life scores are lower (Maymone, 2016; Edpuganti et al., 2025). Understanding the intricate function of melanin not only illuminates its protective function but also illuminates the routes to common skin diseases related to its dysregulation.

4.1.4. Genetic Factors Influencing Hyperpigmentation

Genetic determinants of hyperpigmentation are an intricate interaction among genetic determinants and environmental precipitants that significantly influence the formation of such skin disorders as melasma and post-inflammatory hyperpigmentation (PIH). Genetic susceptibilities, particularly in individuals with Fitzpatrick skin types III-VI, are also key players in controlling the skin's reaction to environmental aggressors like UV radiation, the most vital initiator of hyperpigmentation (Edpuganti et al., 2025). Genetic differences can also affect the formation and dissemination of melanin and raise the risk for hyperpigmentation diseases (Maymone, 2016). Genes specific to melanocyte function and inflammation are implicated in this susceptibility, with implications that patients with these family histories are likely to have more severe reactions to environmental triggers. As psychosocial impacts of such disorders are significant in darker skin types, understanding their genetic underpinnings will lead to more directed interventions and patient gains in dermatology (Figure 4.3).

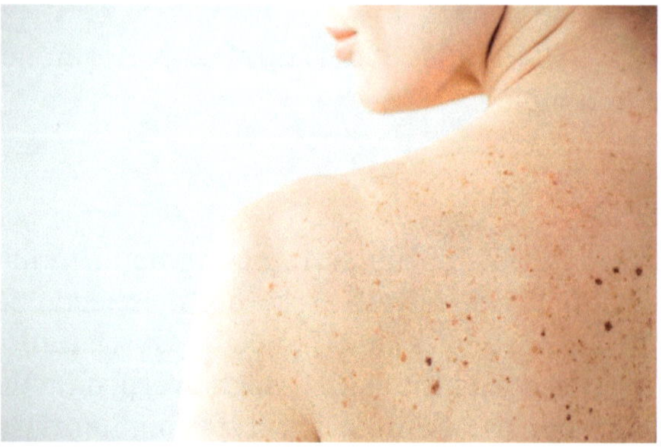

Figure 4.3. Genetic factors influencing hyperpigmentation.

Source: https://www.ripponmedicalservices.co.uk/images/easyblog_articles/156/b2ap3_large_woman-with-skin-pigmentation-issues.jpg.

4.1.5. Environmental Triggers (Sun Exposure and Pollution)

The role of environmental triggers, especially sun exposure and pollution, is immense in the pathogenesis of hyperpigmentation disorders like melasma and post-inflammatory hyperpigmentation (PIH). Hyperpigmentation is caused primarily by Ultraviolet (UV) radiation, causing not only intensified pigmentation but also skin damage, which can lead to conditions such as skin cancer. Recent studies emphasize that exposure to visible and UV light is involved in the pathogenesis of these conditions, with DNA damage many years after sun exposure has ceased (Rodríguez-Luna et al., 2023). Environmentally, cigarette smoke and particulate matter have also been shown to be involved in the induction of hyperpigmentation via the creation of oxidative stress and inflammation in the skin (Edpuganti et al., 2025). Thus, comprehension of these environmental factors is critical when designing prevention and treatment strategies in individuals, particularly those with darker complexion who are at higher risk for such conditions.

4.1.6. Hormonal Influences (Pregnancy and Contraceptives)

Hormonal influences, particularly during pregnancy and due to the use of contraceptives, are key causes of hyperpigmentation disorders such as melasma and post-inflammatory hyperpigmentation (PIH). Pregnant females have such dramatic fluctuations in estrogen and progesterone levels, resulting in the excessive production of melanin that leads to brown patches characteristic of melasma. Similarly, hormonal contraceptives that also interfere with systemic levels of hormones can precipitate or exacerbate these pigmentation disorders in susceptible individuals. It is necessary to grasp these hormonal balances, for they not only contribute to the incidence of dermatologic disorders, but also to the psychological status of the affected. Research has shown that pregnant women with melasma have a significant impact on quality of life, just like individuals with other conditions of hyperpigmentation, emphasizing the significance of having to tackle both the dermatological and psychosocial aspects of these diseases (Maymone, 2016; Edpuganti et al., 2025) (Figure 4.4).

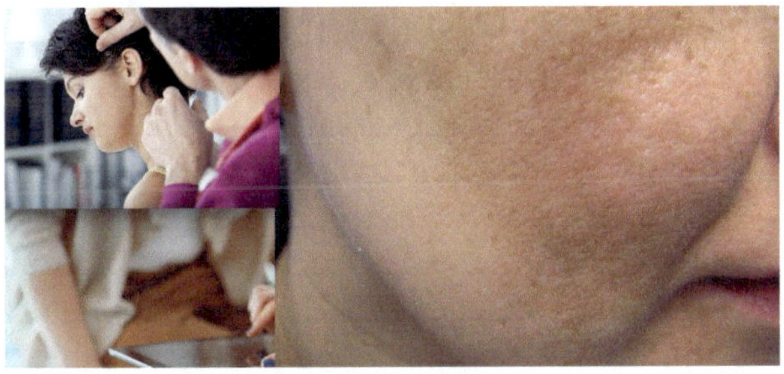

Figure 4.4. Hormonal influences, particularly those occurring during pregnancy and due to contraceptive use, play a substantial role in the manifestation of hyperpigmentation disorders such as melasma and post-inflammatory hyperpigmentation (PIH).

Source: https://www.skintherapyletter.com/wp-content/uploads/2016/01/melasma-post-inflammatory-hyperpigmentation.jpg.

4.1.7. Skin Types and their Susceptibility

The susceptibility of skin types to hyperpigmentation disorders such as melasma and post-inflammatory hyperpigmentation (PIH) holds important differences among different population groups. Skin types, particularly those classified based on Fitzpatrick's scale, have a high disparity in melanin production and responsiveness to stimuli, with individuals with darker skin types being more affected by hyperpigmentation disorders. Research determines that melasma is prevalent in women of color and is connected to UV, genetics, and hormonal function (Lawson et al., 2017). Furthermore, the impact of hyperpigmentation disorders also goes beyond physical appearance, seriously affecting a person's quality of life. In a study, PIH and melasma patients rated their health-related quality of life lower, which indicates a high emotional burden of these illnesses (Maymone, 2016). Hence, awareness about skin types and their susceptibility is required in formulating effective treatment plans in dermatologic treatment.

4.1.8. Psychological Effects of Hyperpigmentation

Psychological effects of hyperpigmentation, such as disorders like melasma and post-inflammatory hyperpigmentation (PIH), are often severe and multifaceted. Patients frequently complain of a reduction in body image and self-esteem from societal pressures that often stigmatize skin flaws.

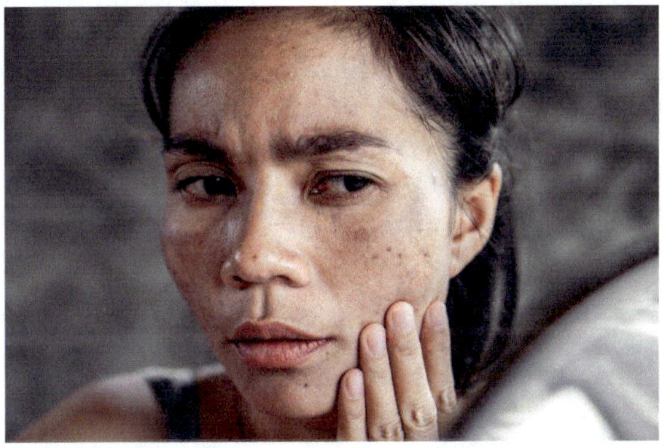

Figure 4.5. Individuals frequently report a decline in self-esteem and body image, stemming from societal beauty standards that often stigmatize skin imperfections.

Source: https://www.drhealthclinic.com/wp-content/uploads/2023/12/PigmentationTreatment.jpg.

This can result in social withdrawal, depression, and anxiety, further increasing the emotional cost of visible skin disease. Research has demonstrated that such psychological impacts are particularly prominent in the scenario of individuals with darker complexion, who, apart from the private concerns, suffer from more general social pressures and discrimination about their appearance (Edpuganti et al., 2025). Moreover, the efficacy of treatment interventions, i.e., non-ablative lasers, has been questioned, creating desperation among individuals in search of effective treatments. Overall, the connection between mental well-being and hyperpigmentation stresses the significance of comprehensive prevention measures that address both the physical and emotional signs of such illnesses (Figure 4.5).

4.1.9. Importance of Skin Care in Prevention

Correct skincare is crucial in the prevention of hyperpigmentation disorders such as melasma and post-inflammatory hyperpigmentation (PIH), which have a significant impact on people, particularly those with darker skin. The direct cause of the said diseases is ultraviolet (UV) radiation, further highlighting the need for continuous use of broad-spectrum sunscreen in reducing the harmful impacts of the sun and risk of skin injury (Rodríguez-Luna et al., 2023). Furthermore, exposure to environmental pollutants like air pollution and cigarette smoke necessitates protective skin precautions with antioxidant-containing products to reverse oxidative stress, a proven cause of hyperpigmentation (Edpuganti et al., 2025). By employing a conscientious skincare regimen directed against such environmental aggressors, not only does one enhance the look of their skin but also safeguards their skin's health and minimizes the psychological effect more classically encountered with hyperpigmentation disorders, thereby improving overall quality of life.

Test Your Knowledge

1. What role does inflammation play in triggering pigment changes?
2. Which vitamin deficiency can lead to generalized hyperpigmentation?

4.2. Melasma

Learning Outcome

1. Understand the Definition and Characteristics of Melasma;
2. Explain Common Causes and Risk Factors;
3. Focus on Diagnosis and Clinical Evaluation;
4. Describe Treatment Options (Topical, Procedural);
5. Learn the Role of Sun Protection in Management;
6. Discuss Recurrence Rates and Long-term Management;
7. Know Differences between Melasma and Other Disorders;
8. Understand the Impact of Melasma on Self-esteem.

Melasma is a prevalent hyperpigmentary condition that disproportionately impacts individuals with darker skin types, particularly women, as reported in recent research. This acquired condition is typified by dark brown irregular facial patches, primarily triggered by causes such as ultraviolet (UV) light, hormonal changes, and genetic predisposition (Lawson et al., 2017). Psychosocial effects of melasma are extremely significant and quite commonly bring about distress and diminished quality of life in patients, even more so in women of color who could be under societal judgment of their looks in the first place (Edpuganti et al., 2025). While it has a high prevalence rate, melasma has been poorly represented in dermatology studies, resulting in an inadequate number of well-rounded treatment strategies appropriate for individuals with darker skin types. Management can only be optimal if its characteristic pathophysiology and risk factors are well understood, further highlighting the necessity for proper public awareness of both prevention and affordable treatment options for the multifactorial nature of this condition.

4.2.1. Definition and Characteristics of Melasma

Melasma is a common skin condition where there is a presence of brown or gray-brown color patches, primarily on sun-exposed regions of the body, such as the face. Melasma is a form of hyperpigmentation that arises because of excessive melanin production, the pigment responsible for the color of the skin, by the dysregulation of melanocytes, the specialized cells responsible for pigment production.

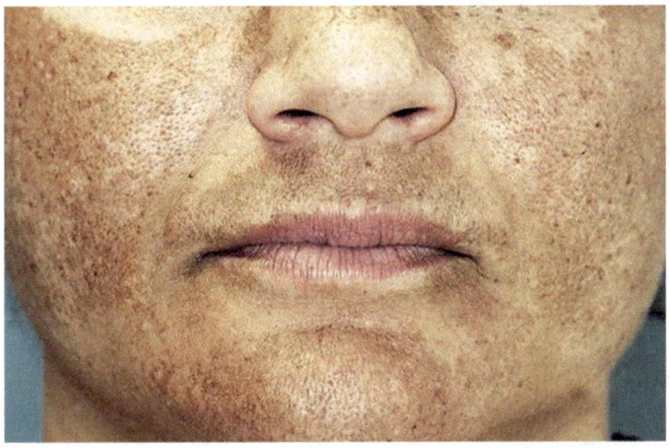

Figure 4.6. Melasma is defined as a common skin condition characterized by the development of brown or gray-brown patches, primarily on sun-exposed areas such as the face.

Source: https://www.athena-skin-hair-dental.com/wp-content/uploads/2023/11/Melasma.jpg.

A number of causes are accountable for the formation of melasma, including hormonal changes, particularly during pregnancy or with oral contraceptives, genetic predisposition, and repeated exposure to sunlight. Notably, research indicates that the patient's health-related quality of life is significantly impacted by melasma, and the patients report moderate to severe distress linked with their condition, as observed in Dermatology Life Quality Index (DLQI) scores among such patients (Maymone, 2016). It is crucial to identify the mechanisms of melanogenesis to come up with effective treatments and therapies for the management of melasma (Maddaleno et al., 2021) (Figure 4.6).

4.2.2. Common Causes and Risk Factors

Melasma and post-inflammatory hyperpigmentation (PIH) are hyperpigmentation disorders that are caused by a number of interconnected causes and risk factors. Particularly, ultraviolet (UV) radiation is a significant catalyst, particularly for patients with Fitzpatrick skin types III-VI, as it causes excess melanin release that has been found to cause these conditions (Edpuganti et al., 2025). Tobacco smoking and atmospheric pollution have also been found to contribute to the progression of hyperpigmentation, suggesting lifestyle takes center stage in dictating skin wellness (Edpuganti et al., 2025). Furthermore, the psychosocial consequence of these disorders is substantial; patients have diminished quality of life, especially those with melasma and PIH, who report more health-related quality of life problems. Understanding these common causes and risk factors is significant for preventive and curative strategies aimed at both the physical and psychological impacts observed with hyperpigmentation diseases.

4.2.3. Diagnosis and Clinical Evaluation

Effective diagnosis and clinical evaluation of hyperpigmentation disorders like melasma and post-inflammatory hyperpigmentation (PIH) necessitate an entire understanding of the characteristic features that accompany these disorders. Clinicians must consider numerous factors, including demographics of the patient, disease duration, and specific skin type, particularly when dealing with patients of color, who have the risk for dyschromias. Accurate assessment usually involves the use of prevalidated scales of measurement, such as the Melasma Area Severity Index (MASI), to quantify disease severity, combined with patient self-assessment quantified using questionnaires such as the Dermatology Life Quality Index (DLQI) to determine quality-of-life impact (Maymone, 2016). Studies indicate that knowledge of one's own diagnosis is strongly associated with level of education and current skin care routines (Maymone, 2016). Additionally, recognition of the nuances of clinical presentation among racially and ethnically diverse populations is significant because it can have a profound effect on treatment regimen and patient outcomes (Figure 4.7).

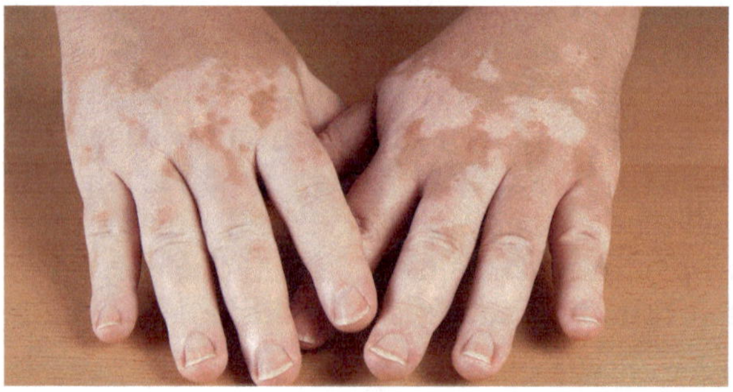

Figure 4.7. Dyschromias.

Source: https://m3.healio.com/~/media/images/news/print/healio-psoriatic-disease/2021/02_february/adobestock_224739107_og.jpg.

4.2.4. Treatment Options (Topical and Procedural)

Management of hyperpigmentation disorders, such as melasma and post-inflammatory hyperpigmentation (PIH), demands insight into the treatment options, topical or procedural. Topical treatments comprise agents such as hydroquinone, tretinoin, and corticosteroids, which inhibit the formation of melanin and promote the regeneration of skin.

The efficacy of such treatments can be unpredictable, necessitating an individualized approach in the clinical setting. Procedural treatments, particularly laser therapies such as the Q-switched Nd:YAG laser, have been in demand due to their ability to penetrate deeper layers of the skin and create remarkable improvement in hyperpigmented lesions. However, post-inflammatory hyperpigmentation issues raised by these procedures highlight the need for effective prophylactic practices, as evidenced by studies which demonstrate that topical clobetasol and brimonidine did not significantly reduce PIH incidence, although enhancing patient satisfaction after treatment. Furthermore, the use of procedural modalities demands that patient education and counseling be heavily taken into account because these parameters are crucial in successful results from the treatment, especially in disorders such as acne, which has the ability to cause hyperpigmentation (Kandhari et al., 2022).

4.2.5. Role of Sun Protection in Management

In the management of hyperpigmentation disorders such as melasma and post-inflammatory hyperpigmentation (PIH), the role of sun protection comes forth as a critical factor in successful management strategies. Exposure to ultraviolet (UV) radiation is the most important cause of hyperpigmentation and thus, in those at risk, it is highly important to adopt universal sun protection measures like frequent use of broad-spectrum sunscreens, protective clothing, and seeking shade during the peak sun hours. Evidence indicates that UV radiation not only increases existing pigmentation but also causes its cause in susceptible groups, such as Fitzpatrick skin types III-VI (Edpuganti et al., 2025). Ongoing exposure has long-term implications for quality of life and is linked to psychosocial morbidity in the form of frustration and low self-esteem, indicating preventive treatment is vital (Parveen et al., 2019). Therefore, daily sun protection strategies are required to manage hyperpigmentation best and minimize its psychosocial effect (Figure 4.8).

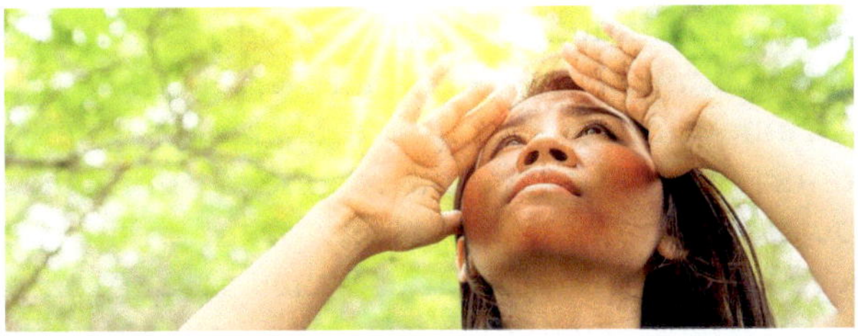

Figure 4.8. Exposure to ultraviolet (UV) radiation is a primary trigger for hyperpigmentation, making it imperative for individuals at risk to adopt comprehensive sun protection measures, including the regular use of broad-spectrum sunscreens, protective clothing, and seeking shade during peak sunlight hours.

Source: https://www.hopkinsmedicine.org/-/media/images/health/1_-conditions/skin/ultraviolet-radiation-hero-image.jpg?h=500&iar=0&mh=500&mw=1300&w=1295&hash=27B5FE1F9C1C74AB1637C0105FEAB793.

4.2.6. Recurrence Rates and Long-term Management

Hyperpigmentation disorders like melasma require a multidisciplinary approach when it comes to managing them, and this involves a thorough insight into recurrence rates and long-term management. Melasma is well known for being chronic and recurrent and may often require a multimodal treatment to manage effectively. Recurrence is triggered by continuous sun exposure, hormonal instability, and personal skin types, especially among individuals of Middle Eastern, Asian, or Hispanic origin (Philipp-Dormston, 2024). Clinically, treatment modalities such as meticulous photoprotection, the use of topical agents such as tranexamic acid, and chemical peels have been helpful, but perhaps would not completely eliminate relapse risk (Philipp-Dormston, 2024). Notably, research indicates that the use of diluted concentrations of tranexamic acid can be high in terms of providing pigmentation improvements while at the same time decreasing recurrence rates (Rangapriya, 2017). Thus, continuous education and individualized treatment plans are essential to the patient, emphasizing the necessity for continuous care to avoid relapse and enhance cosmetic outcomes.

4.2.7. Differences between Melasma and Other Disorders

It should be known that melasma is different from other hyperpigmentation conditions, such as post-inflammatory hyperpigmentation (PIH), which requires accurate diagnosis and management. Melasma typically manifests as symmetrical brown macules on sun-damaged areas of the face in darker-skinned women and is strongly associated with ultraviolet (UV) exposure, hormonal changes, and genetic predisposition (Lawson et al., 2017).

PIH typically develops after skin injury or inflammation, leading to discoloration at the injured site or lesions of acne. Interestingly, in one study, patients with melasma were also shown to have an identical health-related quality of life (HRQoL) impact as PIH patients, referring to the psychological impact of the condition (Maymone, 2016). Notwithstanding the fact that they are similar, the pathophysiologies of such forms of hyperpigmentation are rather diverse, necessitating specialized treatment modalities responsible for both cosmetic and psychological implications (Figure 4.9).

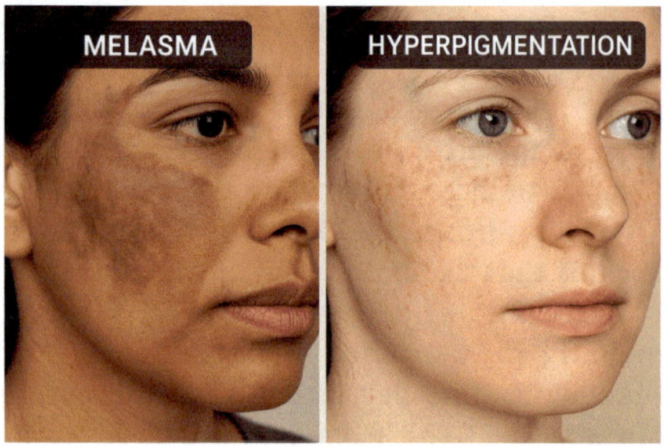

Figure 4.9. Understanding the differences between melasma and other hyperpigmentation disorders, such as post-inflammatory hyperpigmentation (PIH), is crucial for effective diagnosis and treatment.

Source: https://www.cliqueclinic.com/wp-content/uploads/2025/05/melasma_vs_hyperpigmentation__understanding_the_difference__treatment_approaches-2-768x512.png.

4.2.8. Impact of Melasma on Self-esteem

The impact of melasma on self-esteem is profound and multifaceted, particularly for individuals with this skin condition. Melasma, characterized by symmetrical patches of hyperpigmentation in sun-exposed areas, can significantly alter one's appearance as well as evoke emotional distress. Studies have indicated that the prevalence of melasma has been significantly correlated with compromised quality of life, especially among females, as it tends to bring about self-consciousness and feelings of inadequacy. This affective burden is also compounded by cultural beauty standards, underlining blemish-free and clear skin. The aforementioned example thus makes people suffering from melasma manifest diminished social functioning and work productivity via perceived flaws. Besides, the psychosocial influence is particularly sensational in dark-skinned people, highlighting the necessity to know more and explore how hyperpigmentation disorders impact psychological well-being (Said, 2016; Edpuganti et al., 2025). By treating these factors, interventions can be developed to limit the negative impact on self-esteem that melasma produces.

Test Your Knowledge

1. How does hydroquinone work in melasma treatment?
2. What is the most common histological type of melasma?

4.3. Post-Inflammatory Hyperpigmentation (PIH)

Learning Outcome

1. Understand Definition and Causes of PIH;
2. Explain Common Conditions Leading to PIH;
3. Focus on Mechanism of PIH Development;
4. Describe Diagnosis and Differentiation from Other Disorders;
5. Learn Treatment Strategies for PIH;
6. Discuss the Role of Skin Care in Prevention;
7. Know the Psychological Impact of PIH;
8. Understand the Importance of Patient Education;
9. Explain Emerging Therapies and Research.

PIH is an extremely common skin condition that develops following inflammation or injury to the skin, which results in localized darkening due to melanin overproduction.

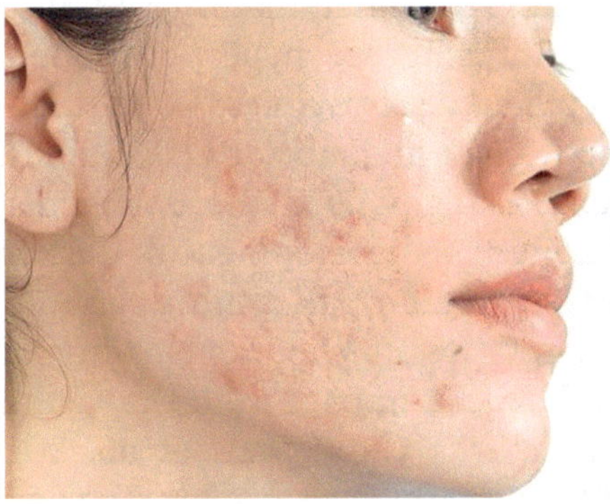

Figure 4.10. Post-inflammatory hyperpigmentation (PIH).

Source: https://images-1.eucerin.com/~/media/eucerin/international/about-skin/indications/postinflammatory-hyperpigmentation/pih-update2018/euc-int_about-skin_pih_00_teaser.jpg.

It is extremely prevalent among individuals with darker skin types, which actually increases the psychosocial impact among them, e.g., lower quality of life and self-esteem issues regarding appearance (Edpuganti et al., 2025). The pathophysiology of PIH involves complex biological responses, in which inflammatory mediators initiate melanocyte stimulation due to skin injury, e.g., acne, eczema, or surgery. Significantly, one recent case demonstrated the occurrence of PIH after breast augmentation by the periareolar incision, which brings about the conditions correlated with both surgical and nonsurgical inflammatory events. Awareness of the precipitants and management plan for PIH is useful in dermatological practice, as effective management can significantly improve patient outcomes and satisfaction (Figure 4.10).

4.3.1. Definition and Causes of Post-Inflammatory Hyperpigmentation (PIH)

PIH is a common skin condition comprising darkened patches caused by increased melanin production following skin damage or inflammation. It happens when skin damage, say acne, eczema, or chemical burns, elicits an inflammatory local reaction, which subsequently results in hyperactivity of melanocytes, the pigment cells (Damodaran & Nair, 2022). The excess melanin thus created may form deep dark spots that tend to be long-lasting, long after the injury has healed, hence greatly impacting an individual's appearance and, in turn, quality of life (Maymone, 2016).

The intensity of PIH may differ based on, among other things, skin type, the level of inflammation, and how the individual reacts to injury. In addition, other factors like sun exposure can worsen PIH, and prevention and management become important for the affected individuals. It is important to comprehend these mechanisms in order to treat the conditions effectively and enhance patient outcomes in post-inflammatory hyperpigmentation disorders.

4.3.2. Common Conditions Leading to Post-Inflammatory Hyperpigmentation (PIH)

PIH usually occurs due to an array of skin disorders that cause inflammation, thereby leading to an excess production of melanin. The common etiologies of PIH involve acne, eczema, psoriasis, and other inflammatory dermatoses, which have the ability to break down the skin barrier and result in hyperactivity of melanocytes through injury (Maymone, 2016).

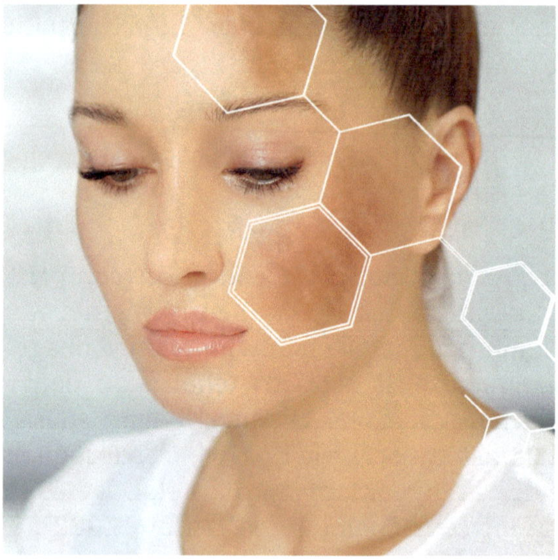

Figure 4.11. Common conditions leading to post-inflammatory hyperpigmentation (PIH) include acne, eczema, psoriasis, and other inflammatory dermatoses, all of which can damage the skin barrier and result in increased melanocyte activity in response to injury.

Source: https://www.clinikally.com/cdn/shop/articles/DAILY_BLOG_BANNER_-_IMAGE_vaishnavi_7_93dbdd9c-f243-4ea9-b591-ef494187c131_1200x1200_crop_center.png?v=1688709828.

Also, precipitating causes such as ultraviolet light exposure, tobacco smoking, and atmospheric pollution increase the risk of onset of hyperpigmentation, notably in individuals with Fitzpatrick skin types III-VI, who are categorically more susceptible to such changes (Edpuganti et al., 2025). Psychosocial impact is considerable; PIH patients have been known to portray diminished health-related quality of life, with studies indicating significant emotional distress linked with apparent cutaneous change. This interaction of these variables is the essence of the difficulty in treating PIH and the necessity for integrative treatment approaches that address both the dermatologic and psychological components of the disease (Figure 4.11).

4.3.3. Mechanism of Post-Inflammatory Hyperpigmentation (PIH) Development

PIH development is a multicausal process that is triggered by various inflammatory cutaneous conditions, which induce increased melanin production in melanocytes. Following inflammation, acne spots or eczema, the skin reacts by initiating the inflammatory cascade and subsequently inducing the hyperproduction of melanin as a shield to ultraviolet (UV) radiation. This hyperactivity of melanocytes results in the deposit of excess pigment in the epidermis or dermis and hence the development of darkened spots on the skin. Notably, PIH is more common in Fitzpatrick skin types III-VI patients, who suffer a higher psychosocial impact from the visibility of these dark marks (Edpuganti et al., 2025). Treatment modalities such as brightening agents and chemical peels have experienced variable success in reducing pigmentation, and so there is a need for certain therapeutic interventions based on skin type and individual skin characteristics, as well as the nature of the hyperpigmentation (Khoo & Halim, 2016).

4.3.4. Diagnosis and Differentiation from Other Disorders

Diagnosis of disorders of hyperpigmentation, such as melasma and post-inflammatory hyperpigmentation (PIH), relies on careful clinical evaluation and differentiation from other dermatologic disorders. Accurate diagnosis is important because various factors, like the duration of the condition, symptoms associated with it, and patient history, can influence clinical presentations. As a case in point, melasma and PIH are often mistaken for each other since they present comparable characteristics; however, some tests, such as the Melasma Area Severity Index (MASI), assist in distinguishing between these conditions and other conditions, such as solar lentigo or peri-orbital hyperpigmentation, that may have different etiologies and treatment results (Maymone, 2016). Moreover, consideration must be given to underlying factors such as skin type and prior skin trauma, since both may increase hyperpigmentation and complicate diagnosis (Damodaran & Nair, 2022). Lastly, an enlightened understanding of these differences not only enables effective management but also optimizes patient outcome in both health and quality of life (Figure 4.12).

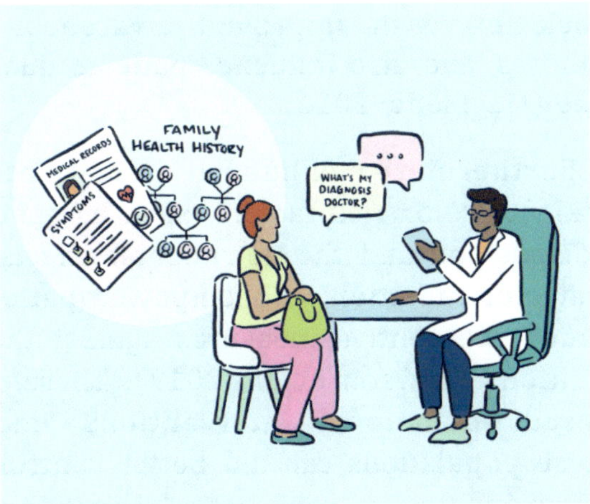

Figure 4.12. Accurate diagnosis is essential, as various factors like duration of the condition, associated symptoms, and patient history can influence clinical presentations.

Source: https://framerusercontent.com/images/iWI4Di5mBAurC3n0ByITVbFfSA.png.

4.3.5. Treatment Strategies for Post-Inflammatory Hyperpigmentation (PIH)

PIH can be treated through a multidisciplinary approach, as the condition can significantly interfere with the quality of life and psychosocial status of a person. Pharmacological and non-pharmacological modalities are effective treatment options that are based on patient's skin type and concern. Of the several options available, topical formulations such as hydroquinone, retinoids, and ascorbic acid are commonly utilized to manage the diminution of melanin synthesis and skin regeneration. Procedural therapies like chemical peeling, laser therapy, and dermabrasion have also been more frequently employed clinically but can be predisposed to side effects and differing efficacies (Parveen et al., 2019). Because of the complexity of PIH, physicians are increasingly employing natural treatments and plant extracts for incorporation into treatment regimens that are supposed to be less likely to cause side effects, responding to patient expectations of less damaging and less invasive treatments (Edpuganti et al., 2025).

4.3.6. Role of Skin Care in Prevention

The prevention role of skin care for melasma and post-inflammatory hyperpigmentation (PIH) disorders cannot be overemphasized. Effective skin care routines for protection from the sun and use of topical treatments can go a long way in avoiding the occurrence of such conditions. Ultraviolet (UV) radiation is the main stimulant for hyperpigmentation and therefore proper sun protection is essential; default in this leads not only to pigmentation but also to the development of skin cancer, as determined by recent studies (Edpuganti et al., 2025). Besides traditional photoprotection, more recent natural products like Fernblock® have the promise to limit UV-induced injury and enhance simultaneous pigmentary issues, suggesting a two-pronged approach to skin health (Rodríguez-Luna et al., 2023). Therefore, it is important to adopt prudent skin care practices, not merely for aesthetic purposes, but in an effort to promote overall integrity of skin and combat psychosocial morbidity associated with hyperpigmentation disorders (Figure 4.13).

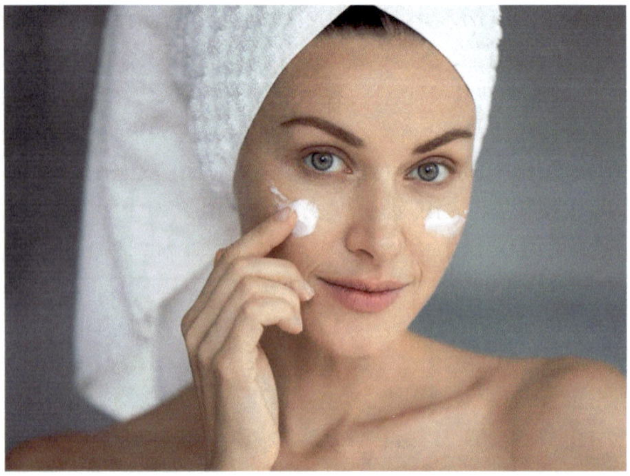

Figure 4.13. Effective skin care routines that focus on sun protection and the use of topical agents can significantly mitigate the risk of developing these conditions.

Source: https://cdn.shopify.com/s/files/1/0039/6073/3763/files/banner_8a596792-686e-4263-b106-a8d7a1bc4fb4_1024x1024.webp?v=1688124547.

4.3.7. Psychological Impact of Post-Inflammatory Hyperpigmentation (PIH)

The psychological impact of PIH extends beyond physical appearance, having a significant psychological impact on mental health and quality of life. PIH patients are more likely to develop anxiety and depression, typically due to the sociocultural demands on skin appearance, particularly in societies with great emphasis placed on the smooth, unblemished color of the skin. In darker populations, such conditions are likely to be sources of social distress as well as decreased self-esteem, which is indicative of the psychosocial nature of disorders of pigmentation. Findings indicate that while PIH is prevalent, it remains underreported in dermatologic studies, where solely clinical findings prevail over psychological impacts (Edpuganti et al., 2025). As people with these populations continue through their day-to-day lives, how visible their condition becomes exacerbates feelings of loneliness and distress, necessitating a broader treatment model that addresses both physical and psychological aspects (Fung et al., 2010).

4.3.8. Importance of Patient Education

Adequate patient education is paramount in the treatment of hyperpigmentary conditions such as melasma and post-inflammatory hyperpigmentation (PIH) because it enables patients to gain the proper information about their condition and treatment. A study finds that higher levels of education have a significant association with improved awareness of diagnoses, and also influence patients quality of life (Maymone, 2016).

Furthermore, enhanced sensitization of skin of color risk factors, such as genetic predisposition and the detrimental effects of ultraviolet radiation, can empower patients to adopt preventive measures against these conditions (Lawson et al., 2017). Therefore, focused educational interventions among diverse populations can aid better control of hyperpigmentation, consequently resulting in better health-related quality of life. By putting patient education as the top priority, healthcare professionals can induce active participation, allowing patients to make informed choices about their skin care and their treatment regimen, thereby improving overall results in hyperpigmentation treatment (Figure 4.14).

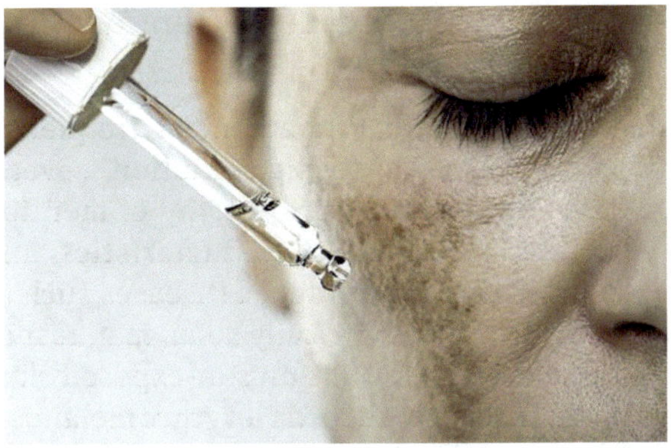

Figure 4.14. Effective patient education is paramount in managing hyperpigmentation disorders such as melasma and post-inflammatory hyperpigmentation (PIH), as it equips individuals with the essential knowledge to understand their conditions and treatment options.

Source: https://content.health.harvard.edu/wp-content/uploads/2024/03/b7f72e1d-9140-458c-8c6f-db079648757b.jpg.

4.3.9. Emerging Therapies and Research

The current advances in the treatment of hyperpigmentation disorders such as melasma and post-inflammatory hyperpigmentation (PIH) indicate the shift towards more efficient and targeted treatments. New studies indicate the application of new laser technology, the Q-switched 1064/532-nanometer laser, which has produced encouraging results in the treatment of benign hypermelanosis, particularly among the Asian population. This picosecond laser has been found to provide improved aesthetic outcomes compared to traditional treatments, with a high rate of satisfaction among patients after treatment (Cannarozzo et al., 2023). Furthermore, the multifactorial etiology of hyperpigmentation conditions calls for an integrative solution that, besides embracing the latest technological treatments, also includes lifestyle modifications and increased public awareness of risk factors, as suggested in studies focusing on psychosocial impacts and trigger factors such as UV radiation and pollution (Edpuganti et al., 2025). As science continues to advance, the future of treatments for hyperpigmentation seems increasingly promising.

Test Your Knowledge

1. What role do chemical peels play in PIH?
2. Which topical agent used in acne can worsen PIH if used improperly?

4.4. Other Hyperpigmentation Disorders

Learning Outcome

1. Understand Overview of Less Common Hyperpigmentation Disorders;
2. Explain Lentigines and Their Characteristics;
3. Focus on Nevus of Ota and its Implications;
4. Describe Drug-induced Hyperpigmentation;
5. Learn the Role of Systemic Diseases in Hyperpigmentation;
6. Discuss Diagnosis and Management of Rare Disorders;
7. Know the Importance of Differential Diagnosis;
8. Understand Patient Support and Resources.

Though post-inflammatory hyperpigmentation (PIH) and melasma are usually the most highlighted in describing disorders of hyperpigmentation, numerous other disorders are also worth mentioning owing to their distinctive nature and clinical significance. Lentigines, café-au-lait macules, and solar lentigines result from a wide range of etiologic factors, ranging from genetic susceptibility to sunlight. Treatment modalities for the conditions vary and can include topical depigmenting agents and laser therapy specifically designed to treat specific pigmentation (Khoo & Halim, 2016). Interestingly, it has been demonstrated that persons with varied hyperpigmentation disorders differently impact their health-related quality of life, such that PIH and melasma have a profound psychological effect compared to other types of hyperpigmentation (Maymone, 2016). Management of these diverse disorders not only accumulates information on their clinical management but also highlights the need for a tailored therapeutic approach that considers patient-specific experience and response to treatments.

4.4.1. Overview of Less Common Hyperpigmentation Disorders

While melasma and PIH are most frequently reported forms of hyperpigmentation, several less common disorders are worthy of mention due to their distinctive characteristics and impact on affected individuals. Diseases such as lentigines, which are typically solar, manifest as flat, tiny, dark skin lesions on sun-exposed skin. Similarly, diseases such as erythromelanosis follicularis manifest a combination of follicular erythema and pigmentation with challenges in diagnosis and treatment. Besides, the prevalence of hyperpigmentation in individuals with darker skin types indicates heightened sensitivity to dyschromias caused by conditions like acne, and therefore the management of such diseases is crucial towards improving quality of life, especially in women of color (Lawson et al., 2017). The implication of hyperpigmentation extends beyond the aesthetic, as some studies indicate that disorders can create enormous psychological distress, again emphasizing the importance of prolonged patient education and targeted therapeutic interventions (Maymone, 2016) (Figure 4.15).

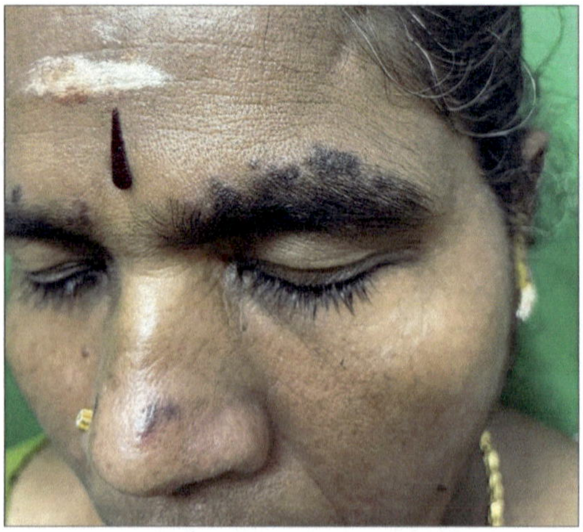

Figure 4.15. Facial dyschromias.

Source: https://cosmoderma.org/content/130/2024/4/1/img/CSDM-4-130-g006.png.

4.4.2. Lentigines and Their Characteristics

Lentigines, otherwise referred to as age spots or liver spots, constitute a distinct form of hyperpigmentation in the form of flat, small, brown lesions observed predominantly on sun-exposed skin regions. The cause lies in localized overproduction of melanin, which may be triggered by repeated ultraviolet (UV) radiation over time, and therefore, they are prevalent in subjects with Fitzpatrick skin types III-VI with a high tendency for the development of hyperpigmentation disorders. The development of lentigines is an important marker for sun damage as their formation has been shown to be linked with a higher risk of skin cancer and highlights the need for photoprotection (Maymone, 2016). While usually innocuous, lentigines can be psychologically disconcerting due to cosmetic issues and may also contribute to the overall severity of hyperpigmentation disorders such as melasma and post-inflammatory hyperpigmentation, thus influencing patients' health-related quality of life (Maymone, 2016).

4.4.3. Nevus of Ota and Its Implications

Nevus of Ota is an asymptomatic condition of hyperpigmentation that primarily manifests as hyperpigmented macules on the eyelid and facial skin because of melanin accumulation in the dermal layer. The condition, usually encountered in patients of Asian origin, is also associated with increased perceptions concerning cosmetic defects, and thus, the majority of individuals prefer dermatological treatment. Laser has emerged as a preferred modality to treat Nevus of Ota since it is capable of targeting melanin selectively with minimal damage to the adjacent tissues. More importantly, Q-switched lasers have gained immense popularity because of their ability to reduce pigmented lesions without much potential for scarring, thus placing them within the total treatment modalities for hyperpigmentation disorders like melasma and post-inflammatory hyperpigmentation (PIH) (Žužul, 2014). An appreciation of the importance of Nevus of Ota is crucial, alongside its effect not only upon cosmetic appearance but also its link with other ocular and systemic manifestations (Figure 4.16).

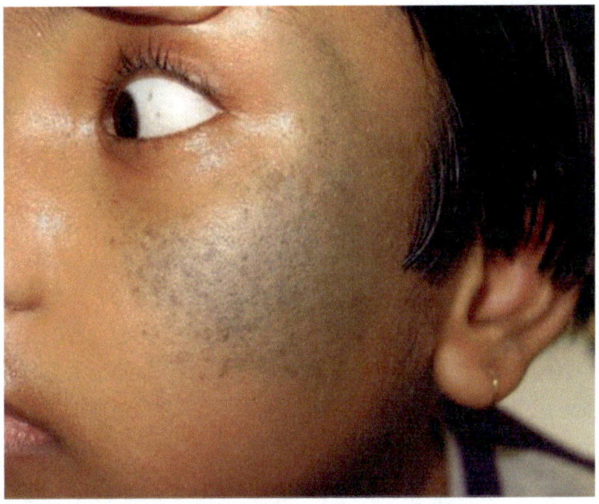

Figure 4.16. Nevus of Ota.

Source: https://www.indianpediatrics.net/june2014/images/im3-1.jpg.

4.4.4. Drug-induced Hyperpigmentation

A drug-induced hyperpigmentation is a significant category of hyperpigmentation disorders, which is characterized by the skin's adverse response to several drugs. The condition occurs in patients on therapy with drugs such as antimalarials, certain chemotherapeutic agents, and even certain antibiotics and may lead to an undesirable darkening of the skin. The resulting hyperpigmentation has serious psychosocial effects, particularly among darker-skinned individuals, deteriorating the perception of stigma and affecting quality of life (Edpuganti et al., 2025). Proper management of drug-induced hyperpigmentation is not just the identification and removal of causative drugs but also the application of interventions such as depigmenting agents and laser therapy to prevent the pigmentation (Khoo & Halim, 2016). The inconsistent response of different individuals to therapy creates a challenge to achieve the best outcome. Therefore, more attention to drug-induced hyperpigmentation mechanisms and their treatment is necessary in order to improve care in patients.

4.4.5. Role of Systemic Diseases in Hyperpigmentation

Systemic illness may be significantly involved in the pattern and progression of hyperpigmentation diseases, such as melasma and post-inflammatory hyperpigmentation (PIH). Endocrine illnesses and diabetes mellitus have been reported to influence melanin production, worsening the pigmentation in susceptible individuals.

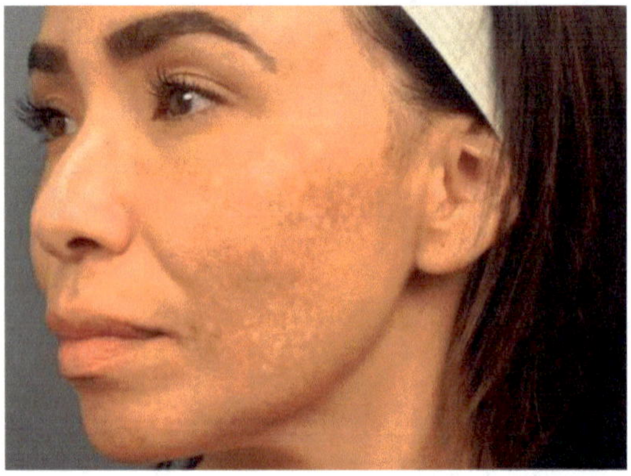

Figure 4.17. Conditions like diabetes and endocrine disorders are known to impact melanin production, often exacerbating pigmentation issues in susceptible individuals.

Source: https://www.skintherapyletter.com/wp-content/uploads/2016/01/fig-1a.jpg.

The complex interplay between such systemic disease and hyperpigmentation may lead to an atypical clinical presentation, which must be managed efficiently. In practice, assessment of hyperpigmentation often extends beyond alterations on local skin, where careful evaluation of underlying systemic disorders likely to be the cause of abnormal melanin distribution and function is required. Moreover, quality of life implications of such diseases continue to be of relevance, as evidenced by research proving a direct correlation between the degree of hyperpigmentation and decreased health-related quality of life (HRQoL) (Maymone, 2016). Overall, it is important to recognize the role of systemic diseases in the formation of effective treatment methods for patients with hyperpigmentation disorders (Khoo & Halim, 2016) (Figure 4.17).

4.4.6. Diagnosis and Management of Rare Disorders

The treatment and clinical diagnosis of melasma and post-inflammatory hyperpigmentation (PIH) necessitate a complex understanding of both clinical presentation and the psychological impact of the conditions. The patients have multifactorial cases according to skin type and disease pathologies, which are extremely variable, particularly among darker phototypes.

There is a requirement to measure the severity of these disorders through the use of tools like the Melasma Area Severity Index (MASI), which is crucial for drawing up treatment plans that include chemical, physical, and pharmaceutical treatments. Also, awareness of the effect of hyperpigmentation on quality of life related to health is essential; evidence in the literature indicates that diseases like PIH and melasma significantly interfere with patients' well-being, making it important that they are managed effectively (Maymone, 2016). Therefore, early diagnosis and tailored treatment approaches are essential in optimizing outcomes for patients presenting with these frequently-stigmatized conditions (Maymone, 2016).

4.4.7. Importance of Differential Diagnosis

In dermatology, particularly in the case of pigmentary disorders such as melasma and post-inflammatory hyperpigmentation (PIH), the importance of differential diagnosis cannot be overstated. Differential diagnosis between them is absolutely critical since their presentation clinically overlaps, thus posing the risk of misdiagnosis and inappropriate therapy. For instance, while melasma is most commonly associated with UV exposure and hormonal effects, PIH is typically the outcome of irritation or inflammation of the skin, which may be commonly observed in patients with darker skin types who are prone to dyschromias, as documented in the literature (Lawson et al., 2017). Moreover, the understanding of the specific mechanisms that cause these disorders, such as melanin production and external factors' impact, contributes to making diagnosis more effective and efficient and effective treatment feasible (Damodaran & Nair, 2022). Last but not least, a correct differential diagnosis is necessary to tailor treatments according to the individual needs of patients with these hyperpigmentation disorders.

4.4.8. Patient Support and Resources

Access to resources and patient support are necessary for patients with hyperpigmentation disorders such as post-inflammatory hyperpigmentation (PIH) and melasma. Apart from physically changing how a person looks, these conditions interfere with quality of life to a significant extent, as the studies have indicated that nearly 22% of people who have them have had severe life disruptions due to their condition (Maymone, 2016). Good management practices, including education on the significance of sun protection, are imperative, considering the fact that individuals with skin of color are more likely to be at higher risk due to variation in photoprotection behaviors (Krutmann et al., 2023). Health professionals are also mandated to enhance patient activation by improving communication about the treatment process and resources available, i.e., support groups and educational materials. By creating a comprehensive system of support, patients can better deal with their condition, eventually improving their health-related quality of life and compliance rates with recommended treatments (Figure 4.18).

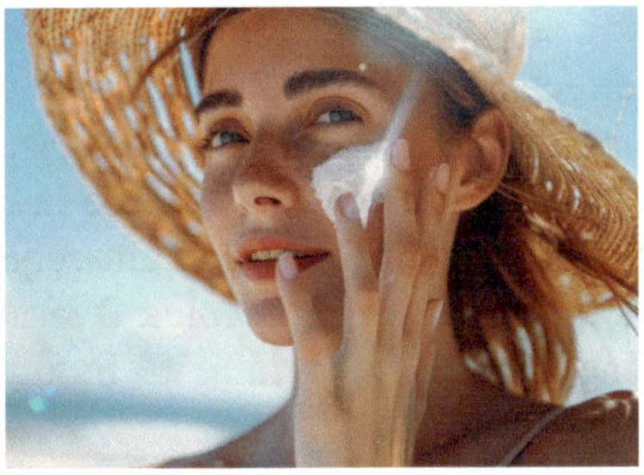

Figure 4.18. Effective management strategies, including education on the importance of sun protection, are essential, particularly since individuals with skin of color are often at a heightened risk due to disparities in photoprotection practices.

Source: https://drrashmisharma.in/wp-content/uploads/2024/05/Importance-of-Sun-Protection-Dr.-Rashmi-Sharma-.png.

Test Your Knowledge

1. What is the pigment responsible for bluish-gray dermal discoloration in ochronosis?
2. What is a distinguishing feature of café-au-lait spots in neurofibromatosis type I?

SUMMARY

Hyperpigmentation diseases, like melasma and post-inflammatory hyperpigmentation (PIH), are multifactorial diseases that need careful understanding and effective management. Their multifactorial pathogenesis stresses the demand for customized treatment programs for specific skin types and environmental exposures. As noted, UV light is an important causative agent of such disorders, with the need for good photoprotection emphasizing preventive measures (Khoo & Halim, 2016). Furthermore, treatments such as brightening creams, chemical peels, and laser treatments have been noted as effective interventions, with patient response differing widely. Of particular concern is their psychosocial effect, since they directly affect the quality of life of patients with such a condition, most particularly those with darker skin types (Edpuganti et al., 2025). Therefore, raising awareness and promoting access to effective treatment remain key in stemming this prevalent condition.

The disease process of hyperpigmentation disorders, particularly melasma and post-inflammatory hyperpigmentation (PIH), brings to the fore some pertinent factors towards their etiology and management. Melasma, an irreversible facial pigmentation condition that occurs predominantly in women, is controlled by genetic susceptibility and solar exposure, among others, such that control is complicated by the fact that it is multifactorial. Most of the treatments at hand, from topically to procedurally based treatments, are of limited therapeutic effectiveness and necessitate relapses or side effects. The application of nanotechnology in topical therapy is accompanied by promising developments, improving drug delivery and therapeutic efficiency. It is also important to understand the depigmentation paradox, where individuals with some diseases like vitiligo receive treatment for a light color, while others might request depigmentation for cosmetic reasons, which shows the complex approach towards color. Overall, the therapeutic setting for hyperpigmentation disorders is evolving, but much remains to be done (Khoo & Halim, 2016).

KEY TERMS FROM THIS CHAPTER

- Melasma
- Dermatology
- Hyperpigmentation
- Self-esteem
- Colossal
- Ultraviolet radiation (UVR)
- Melanocyte density
- Endogenous
- Inflammation
- Post-inflammatory hyperpigmentation (PIH)
- Extrinsic factors
- Psychosocial impact
- Quality of life
- Sun exposure
- Melanin synthesis
- Aberrant distribution
- Exogenous pigments
- Cosmetic problem

CRITICAL THINKING QUESTIONS

1. **Which of the following is the most common cause of hyperpigmentation?**
   a. Addison's disease
   b. Melasma
   c. Acanthosis nigricans
   d. Post-inflammatory hyperpigmentation (PIH)
2. **Which condition shows a "mask-like" distribution of pigmentation on the face?**
   a. Lichen planus
   b. Melasma
   c. Freckles
   d. Café-au-lait spots
3. **Which of the following drugs can cause hyperpigmentation?**
   a. Minocycline
   b. Isotretinoin
   c. Acetaminophen
   d. Omeprazole
4. **Acanthosis nigricans is most commonly associated with which underlying condition?**
   a. Hypothyroidism
   b. Addison's disease
   c. Insulin resistance
   d. Anemia
5. **Which of the following is a dermal cause of hyperpigmentation?**
   a. Freckles
   b. Lentigines
   c. Dermal melanocytosis
   d. Post-acne macules

Short Answer Questions

1. Which enzyme is central to melanin biosynthesis in the skin?
2. Which type of UV radiation is most responsible for stimulating melanogenesis?
3. What is the most common precipitating factor for melasma?
4. Which gender is more commonly affected by melasma?
5. What is the most common cause of post-inflammatory hyperpigmentation?
6. Which skin types are at greater risk of PIH?
7. Which genetic disorder features hyperpigmented macules on the lips and oral mucosa?
8. What is the pigment responsible for bluish-gray dermal discoloration in ochronosis?

Answers to Critical Thinking Questions

1. (d); 2. (b); 3. (a); 4. (c); 5. (c)

REFERENCES

1. Parveen, N., S. Ali, A., & A. Ali, S. (2019). On the Intricacies of Facial Hyperpigmentation and the Use of Herbal Ingredients as a Boon for Its Treatment: Cosmeceutical Significance, Current Challenges and Future Perspectives. IntechOpen. doi: 10.5772/intechopen.84257(accessed on 23rd July 2025).
2. Cannarozzo, G., Del Re, C., Negosanti, F., Bennardo, S., Amoruso, G. F., Nisticò, S. P., & Bennardo, L. (2023). Q-Switched Nd:YAG Laser to Manage Hyperpigmentation in Asians: A Multicenter Study. *Cosmetics*, *10*(2), 44. https://doi.org/10.3390/cosmetics10020044(accessed on 23rd July 2025).
3. Kandhari, S., Girdhar, M., Kulkarni, D. S., Arsiwala, S., Sakhiya, J., Karthikeyan, K., Murthy, S., Dhawan, S., Mallela, V. B., & Rathi, S. (2022). Expert consensus on the management of acne in India. *International Journal of Research in Medical Sciences*, *10*(4), 980–990. https://doi.org/10.18203/2320-6012.ijrms20220998(accessed on 23rd July 2025).
4. Buainain de Castro Maymone, M. (2016). Skin hyperpigmentation disorders: Associations and impact on health-related quality of life. https://open.bu.edu/bitstream/2144/19513/1/BuainaindeCastroMaymone_bu_0017E_12224.pdf (accessed on 23rd July 2025).
5. Lawson, C. N., Hollinger, J., Sethi, S., Rodney, I., Sarkar, R., Dlova, N., & Callender, V. D. (2017). Updates in the understanding and treatments of skin & hair disorders in women of color. *International journal of women's dermatology*, *3*(1 Suppl), S21–S37. https://doi.org/10.1016/j.ijwd.2017.02.006(accessed on 23rd July 2025).
6. Maddaleno, A. S., Camargo, J., Mitjans, M., & Vinardell, M. P. (2021). Melanogenesis and Melasma Treatment. *Cosmetics*, *8*(3), 82. https://doi.org/10.3390/cosmetics8030082 (accessed on 23rd July 2025).
7. Damodaran, A., & Nair, N. (2023). Skin Pigmentation and Cosmetic Considerations for Even Skin Tone. IntechOpen. doi: 10.5772/intechopen.108693(accessed on 23rd July 2025).
8. Edpuganti, S., Subhash, S., Siras, S., Sajeev, S., mesineni, S., Devakumar, D., & shahinsha, M. (2025). Prevalence of Hyperpigmentation Disorders in Fitzpatrick skin types. *International Journal of Progressive Sciences and Technologies, 50*(1), 499-513. doi:http://dx.doi.org/10.52155/ijpsat.v50.1.7148(accessed on 23rd July 2025).
9. Fung, T. K., Leung, A. Y. H., & Liang, R. H. S. (2010). Functional characterization of a novel nucleoporin gene *NUP98* in zebrafish embryo. https://core.ac.uk/download/38032875.pdf (accessed on 23rd July 2025).
10. Rodríguez-Luna, A., Zamarrón, A., Juarranz, Á., & González, S. (2023). Clinical Applications of *Polypodium leucotomos* (Fernblock®): An Update. *Life (Basel, Switzerland)*, *13*(7), 1513. https://doi.org/10.3390/life13071513(accessed on 23rd July 2025).
11. Krutmann, J., Piquero-Casals, J., Morgado-Carrasco, D., Granger, C., Trullàs, C., Passeron, T., & Lim, H. W. (2023). Photoprotection for people with skin of colour: needs and strategies. *The British journal of dermatology*, *188*(2), 168–175. https://doi.org/10.1093/bjd/ljac046(accessed on 23rd July 2025).
12. Khoo, Y.T., & Halim, A.S. (2016). Treatment modalities for hyperpigmented skin lesions: A brief overview. *Journal of Surgical Dermatology*. https://core.ac.uk/download/132566787.pdf (accessed on 23rd July 2025).

13. Ly, F. (2023). Pigmentary disorders in Black skin: From pathophysiology to treatment. https://core.ac.uk/download/560378319.pdf (accessed on 23rd July 2025).

14. Mokhtarzadegan, M., Kiafar, M. R., Ghasemiyeh, P., Fazlinejad, R., Rasekh, S., & Mohammadi-Samani, S. (2024). Different therapeutic approaches in melasma: Advances and limitations. https://core.ac.uk/download/614681802.pdf (accessed on 23rd July 2025).

15. Philipp-Dormston, W. G. (2024). Melasma: A step-by-step approach towards a multimodal combination therapy. https://core.ac.uk/download/615297566.pdf (accessed on 23rd July 2025).

16. Rangapriya, M. (2017). Efficacy, safety and tolerability of oral tranexamic acid vs modified Kligman formula in moderate to severe melasma. https://core.ac.uk/download/327695968.pdf (accessed on 23rd July 2025).

17. Said, R. N. (2016). Hubungan melasma dengan tingkat kualitas hidup pada wanita. https://core.ac.uk/download/148610287.pdf (accessed on 23rd July 2025).

18. Žužul, K. (2014). The use of lasers in dermatology. https://core.ac.uk/download/197824559.pdf (accessed on 23rd July 2025).

HYPOPIGMENTATION AND DEPIGMENTATION DISORDERS

5

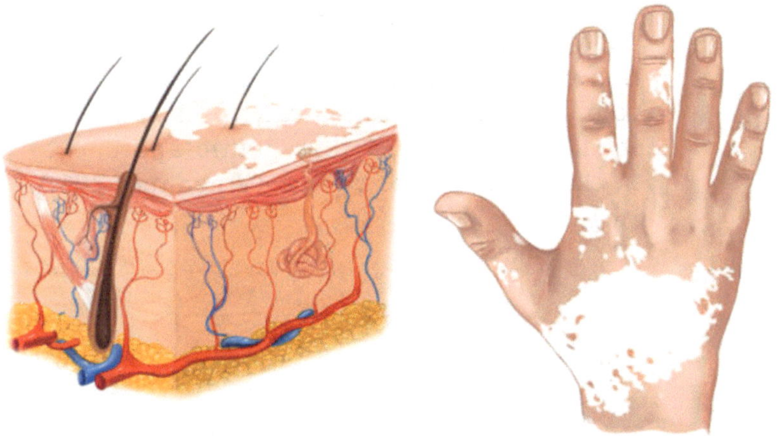

LEARNING OBJECTIVES

After studying this chapter, you will be able to:

1. Understand Vitiligo;
2. Explain Albinism;
3. Describe Societal and Cultural Perspectives.

Introduction

The study of depigmentation and hypopigmentation disorders, especially albinism and vitiligo, is a critical aspect of dermatological and psychological health. Vitiligo, caused by the selective destruction of melanocytes, leads to distinct patches of depigmented skin, affecting an individual's physical attractiveness and psychological quality of life. The disease, often accompanied by social embarrassment and emotional distress, is a classic example of the profound impact of skin diseases on quality of life. Likewise, albinism, which is a genetic disorder that leads to lowered melanin production, has its own set of challenges in that it is visible and lends itself to risks such as sun sensitivity and eye issues. In treating these disorders, it is necessary to comprehend the complex interplay of genetic, autoimmune, and environmental influences that lead to their development and exacerbation. Introduction of newer management strategies also warrants exploration, hopefully leading to better patient management and greater understanding of these multifactorial diseases (Witek et al., 2025).

5.1. Vitiligo

Learning Outcome

1. Understand Definition and Classification of Vitiligo;
2. Explain Causes and Risk Factors;
3. Focus on Symptoms and Clinical Presentation;
4. Describe Diagnosis and Differential Diagnosis;
5. Learn the Psychological Impact on Patients;
6. Discuss the Role of Lifestyle and Home Remedies.

Vitiligo is a common hypopigmentation condition characterized by the progressive loss of melanocytes, leading to well-defined, depigmented patches of skin. Common in around 0.5%–1% of the world's population, Vitiligo has been said to impose considerable disruption on an individual's quality of life, with attendant psychological distress, especially among patients of dark skin color who are subjected to stigmatization from society (Baldini et al., 2017). The aetiology of Vitiligo remains multifactorial, with the autoimmune hypothesis gaining momentum, comparing the illness to other autoimmune illnesses such as thyroid diseases. Further, Vitiligo's classic description in historic healthcare traditions, such as Ayurveda, places it under Shwitra, underlining its age-old position as a skin disorder. This multi-faceted approach to Vitiligo highlights the need for holistic therapeutic interventions addressing not just physical symptoms but also the psychological impacts of the condition (Baldini et al., 2017).

5.1.1. Definition and Classification of Vitiligo

Vitiligo is a multifaceted acquired skin disease involving the depigmentation of the skin due to the loss of functional melanocytes. This disorder is classified into several types, predominantly localized vitiligo, which is restricted to specific locations on the body, and generalized vitiligo, which is diffuse. Each of these subtypes has specific depigmentation patterns and has the potential to significantly impact a patient's psychological well-being since it is so outwardly apparent. Current studies have characterized an autoimmune etiology in vitiligo, which is attested by the presence of circulating autoantibodies to melanocyte antigens and further detailing its pathogenetics (Waterman, 2002). Classification is further extended to a more severe type of vitiligo, including segmental vitiligo that mainly occurs asymmetrically and is possibly less amenable to treatment. It is essential to comprehend these classifications in an attempt to develop targeted therapeutic approaches in the treatment of vitiligo (Vinodhini, 2018) (Figure 5.1).

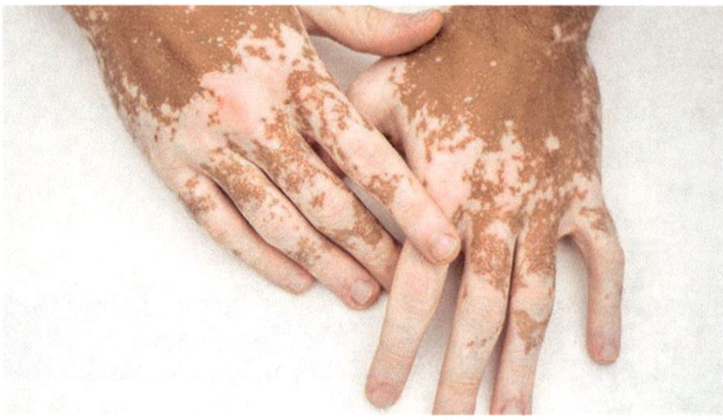

Figure 5.1. Vitiligo is a complex acquired skin disorder characterized by the loss of functional melanocytes, leading to the development of depigmented patches on the skin.

Source: https://my.clevelandclinic.org/-/scassets/images/org/health/articles/12419-vitiligo.

5.1.2. Causes and Risk Factors

Depigmentation and hypopigmentation disorders such as albinism and vitiligo could be caused by an interaction of gene, immunological, and environmental factors. Genetic inheritance plays a significant role in this regard, as demonstrated by the recurrence pattern in individuals suffering from these conditions. Environmental stimuli, for example, exposure to specific chemicals or skin injury, can also induce or exacerbate these conditions, again highlighting the need for awareness of one's surroundings and lifestyle. Increased emphasis on the immunological aspect is needed, given the fact that diseases like leucoderma are defined by loss of melanocytes via their autoimmune destruction (Kaur & Kaur, 2012). Besides, while depigmentation in some populations can be considered to be largely a cosmetic issue, it is a cause of significant concern in darker skin color groups and could impact the psychological status. Overall, all these factors bring home the complexity of how hypopigmentation and depigmentation disorders look.

5.1.3. Symptoms and Clinical Presentation

The clinical presentation of depigmentation and hypopigmentation conditions, such as vitiligo and albinism, is attended by well-defined symptoms that significantly affect the quality of life. In vitiligo, patients typically present with patches of colored loss of skin that lead to contrast with surrounding skin and also cause emotional and social embarrassment. In contrast to albinism, more comprehensive issues arise with patients who have albinism, such as visual abnormalities in the forms of reduced acuity of vision and hypoplasia of the fovea, both of which appear within both oculocutaneous albinism and ocular albinism (Neveu et al., 2022). Both of these vision issues normally co-occur with hair and skin hypopigmentation, indicating the shared influence of genetic factors within the condition. Also, pigmentation disorders can be accompanied by systemic symptoms, like in Vici syndrome, where hypopigmentation is accompanied by worsening neurodevelopmental issues (Byrne et al., 2016). The identification of such symptoms is crucial for appropriate diagnosis and management (Figure 5.2).

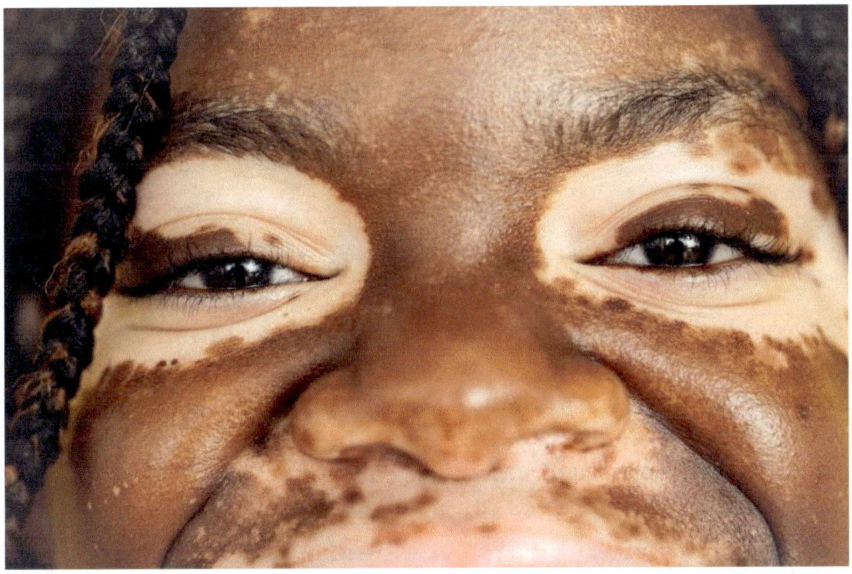

Figure 5.2. In vitiligo, patients typically exhibit patches of skin that lose pigment, leading to a contrast with surrounding areas, which can also result in emotional distress and social stigma.

Source: https://news.northwestern.edu/assets/Stories/2025/01/vitiligo1940__FitMaxWzk3MCw2NTBd.jpg.

5.1.4. Diagnosis and Differential Diagnosis

Diagnosis of hypopigmentation and depigmentation conditions such as vitiligo and albinism is typically complex, involving extensive knowledge of the clinical presentation along with the pathogenic mechanisms. These conditions can be classified under a variety of different types of pigmentation disorders, characterized by either decreased (hypopigmentation) or completely absent (depigmentation) melanin production. Dermatologists thus have to navigate through a wide variety of differential diagnoses that could produce comparable presentations, such as post-inflammatory hypopigmentation or other skin diseases, possibly resulting in comparable appearances (Jusuf, 2017). The challenge is not only in determining clinical features but also in incorporating patient history and response to treatment, which will vary tremendously from individual to individual. As stressed in recent studies, the identification of the genetic determinants that regulate these conditions is important for the purpose of offering accurate diagnosis and for developing personalized therapeutic regimens, ultimately improving the quality of life in these affected patients (Albretsen, 2022).

5.1.5. Psychological Impact on Patients

Psychological impacts of hypopigmentation and depigmentation disorders, such as vitiligo and albinism, can be extreme and impact patients' self-esteem and interpersonal relationships. Patients often feel stigmatized and discriminated against due to the visible appearance of their disorders, tending to result in anxiety, depression, and compromised quality of life. According to research, while depigmentation is a cosmetic goal for some, especially for patients with vitiligo who need therapeutic interventions, it is also characterized by complex emotional responses, which include jealousy and feelings of inadequacy when compared to other people who have perfect skin. Furthermore, social pressure to conform to beauty standards exacerbates such psychological issues, resulting in out-of-pocket payments for expensive cosmetic procedures, which, incidentally, are insufficient (Witek et al., 2025). Thus, provision for the psychological implications is key in developing holistic care plans addressing the physical and emotional needs of the affected patients (Figure 5.3).

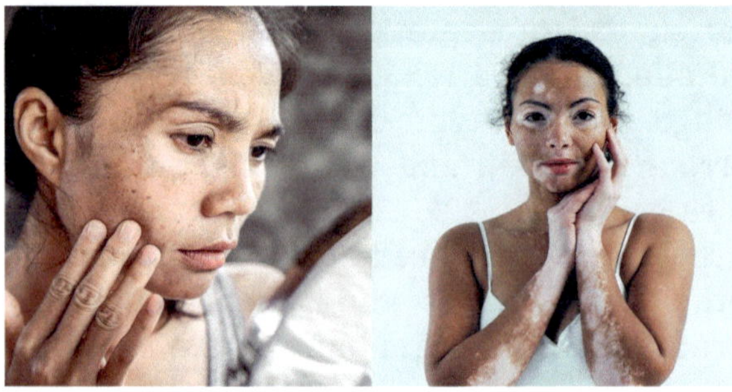

Figure 5.3. Individuals often experience stigma and discrimination due to the visible nature of their conditions, which can lead to anxiety, depression, and a diminished quality of life.

Source: https://skinnfit.in/wp-content/uploads/2024/07/Hypopigmentation-vs-Vitiligo.jpg.

5.1.6. Treatment Options and Management Strategies

For the therapy of depigmentation and hypopigmentation disorders such as vitiligo and albinism, treatment and management are very diverse, a demonstration of the complexity of these conditions. Effective therapies usually have elements involving combined topical treatments, phototherapy, and surgery for the purposes of re-pigmentation or improvement of skin appearance. Topical corticosteroids and calcineurin inhibitors are usually first-line treatments for localized vitiligo, with broader cases responding to light treatments, including narrowband ultraviolet B (NB-UVB) phototherapy. Aesthetic solutions may also be pursued through depigmentation treatments, with variable results, as studies report both treatment expectations and social impacts of skin appearance. In addition, therapies such as melanocyte transplantation can be reassuring for patients with stable vitiligo (Witek et al., 2025). Ultimately, treatment should be according to the individual's unique circumstances, and considerate care in regard to the potential of side effects and psychological impacts.

5.1.7. Role of Lifestyle and Home Remedies

Management of hypopigmentation and depigmentation disorders such as vitiligo and albinism may extend beyond the clinic to encompass lifestyle modification and home remedies, which are a vital component of patient care. These patients are instructed to adopt a sun-protective lifestyle, employing broad-spectrum sunscreens to minimize UV damage effects as well as prevent subsequent skin issues. Apart from this, certain home remedies, such as the use of supportive topical medications, can even make the skin look better; their effectiveness is largely dependent on variation among individuals. Systematic review of clinical trials suggests that the use of topical agents in combination with phototherapy can be effective, as reported in a funded pilot study on home hand-held phototherapy for vitiligo (Eleftheriadou, 2025). While lifestyle modification and home use provide a supplementary measure, professional treatment must be combined with these to provide optimal results in managing these conditions (Figure 5.4).

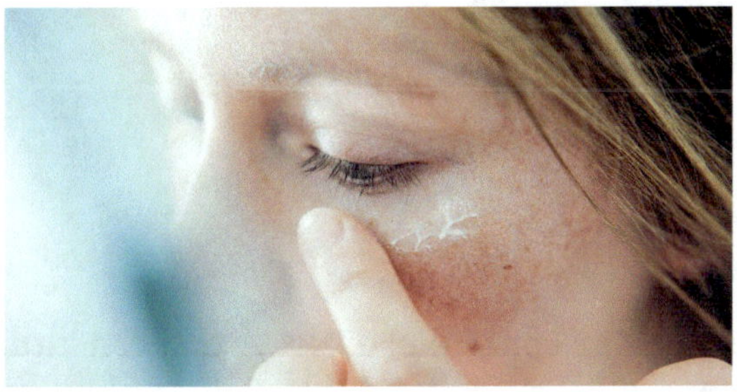

Figure 5.4. Certain home remedies, such as the application of supportive topical agents, may help enhance skin appearance; however, their effectiveness varies widely among individuals.

Source: https://media.post.rvohealth.io/wp-content/uploads/2022/01/female-face-eye-cream-1200-628-facebook-1200x628.jpg.

Test Your Knowledge

1. Which test is useful to assess the extent of depigmentation under ultraviolet light?
2. What is the mainstay of treatment for localized vitiligo?

5.2. Albinism

Learning Outcome

1. Understand Definition and Types of Albinism;
2. Explain Genetic Basis and Inheritance Patterns;
3. Focus on Physical Characteristics and Symptoms;
4. Describe Associated Health Issues (e.g., Vision Problems);
5. Learn Social and Cultural Implications;
6. Discuss Diagnosis and Screening Methods;
7. Know Treatment and Management of Symptoms;
8. Understand Advocacy and Support for Individuals with Albinism.

Albinism is a congenital disorder that constitutes a complete or partial deficiency of skin, hair, and eye pigmentation that is secondary to a lack of functional melanocytes. The ensuing hypopigmentation may cause profound visual impairment and a high risk of skin cancer due to increased vulnerability to ultraviolet light.

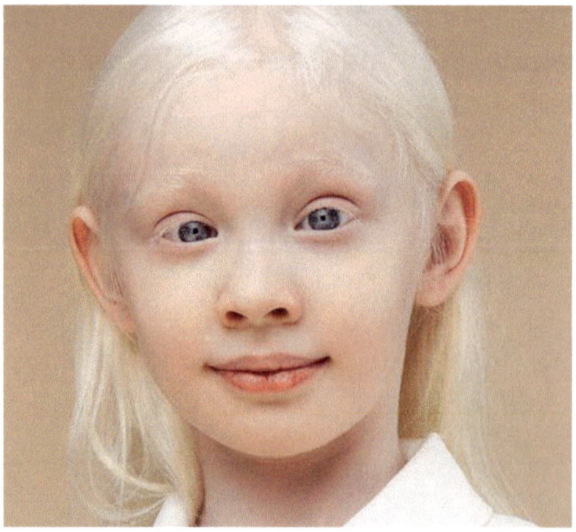

Figure 5.5. Albinism is a genetic condition characterized by a complete or partial absence of pigment in the skin, hair, and eyes due to the lack of functional melanocytes.

Source: https://www.ambrosiaclinic.com/wp-content/uploads/2023/09/Albinism-ambrosia.jpg.

Albinism patients often have social stigmatization and psychological issues that have adverse effects on their self-concept and quality of life. Besides, the different presentations of albinism complicate diagnosis and treatment since symptoms may be highly variable among affected persons.

According to quotes in literature, studies on key enzymes involved in pigmentary processes can inform us regarding the genetic mechanisms of this condition and hence enable us to devise appropriate diagnostic methods and therapy, improving the lives of affected individuals (Albretsen, 2022). Current advances in therapeutic approaches, including the use of plant-based remedies, also offer hopeful avenues for managing the influence of albinism (Kaur & Kaur, 2012) (Figure 5.5).

5.2.1. Definition and Types of Albinism

Albinism is a genetic disease caused by an absence of melanin production, resulting in partial or full hypopigmentation of the skin, hair, and eyes. The illness is mainly classified into a number of classes, of which Oculocutaneous Albinism (OCA) and Ocular Albinism (OA) are the most common. OCA affects both the skin and eyes, resulting in severe visual disabilities, while OA is mostly eye-related, with the skin and hair least affected.

The genes responsible for albinism are mutations in genes involved in producing melanin, such as TYR, OCA2, and TYRP1. Also, albinos are more likely to develop skin cancer due to the lack of protective melanin. This understanding is crucial in further developing the care and management methods of the affected patients, underlining the need for higher awareness and research into the effective treatments for this often misunderstood disorder (Witek et al., 2025; Waterman, 2002).

5.2.2. Genetic Basis and Inheritance Patterns

The genetic cause of hypopigmentation and depigmentation disorders such as vitiligo and albinism is complex with a number of patterns of inheritance that eventually influence pigment production. In albinism, genetic mutations in genes responsible for melanin production lead to a significant reduction or complete absence of pigment from the skin, hair, and eyes, a classic instance of autosomal recessive inheritance. Studies have shown that mutations in specific pigmentation genes are under the influence of genetic and environmental factors, a classic example of a multifactorial model of inheritance in which gene-environment interactions are of utmost relevance (Sturm & Duffy, 2012).

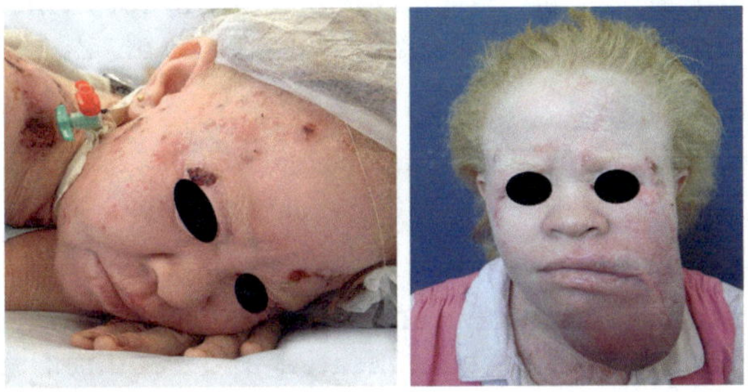

Figure 5.6. In albinism, for instance, mutations in genes responsible for melanin synthesis lead to a significant reduction or complete absence of pigment in the skin, hair, and eyes, demonstrating a classic example of autosomal recessive inheritance.

Source: https://static.elsevier.es/multimedia/03650596/0000009400000005/v9_201912130752/S0365059619300583/v9_201912130752/en/main.assets/gr6.jpeg.

Similarly, the gray morphism of Southern right whales is another example of the genetic etiology of pigmentation abnormalities. It has been revealed through research that both fewer melanocytes and smaller melanosomes are present in the gray morphs, ultimately implying that pigmentation differences can be brought about by intricate genetic mechanisms that influence cell formation and pigment production (Eroh et al., 2017) (Figure 5.6).

5.2.3. Physical Characteristics and Symptoms

Physical features and symptoms of hypopigmentation and depigmentation disorders, such as vitiligo and albinism, occur mainly by means of clear-cut alteration of the color of the skin. Vitiligo patients usually have patches of depigmented skin that vary in size and amount, forming a stark color contrast to their normal skin color; these also tend to extend to hair and mucous membranes, thus affecting the overall look substantially. Albinism, however, is a systemic lack of melanin production, resulting in uniformly pale skin, hair, and eye color in the patient. This color loss not only impacts beauty but also has important implications on psychological health and social functioning in accordance with societal definitions of beauty and normality. Furthermore, even though local depigmentation within fair skin may be less apparent, it is particularly potent within pigmented skin, thereby making therapeutic approaches more targeted in such populations (Kala, 2013).

5.2.4. Associated Health Issues (e.g., Vision Problems)

Patients suffering from hypopigmentation and depigmentation conditions such as vitiligo and albinism are afflicted with a myriad of associated health issues, particularly involving vision. Albinism, which is the absence of melanin production, often results in ocular findings such as photophobia, nystagmus, and poor visual acuity primarily due to the lack of pigment within the retina required for optimal light absorption and image sharpness. These individuals have been found to substantially struggle with visual impairment caused by albinism, with some of them requiring low-vision rehabilitation services. Individuals with vitiligo may also experience psychosocial problems, but eye complications of these illnesses can be debilitating. Both culture and clinical practice have realized the medicinal value of herbal drugs, such as *Parangipattai chooranam*, in curing these disorders, which reflects the importance of holistic care as uncovered by some research (Vadivelan, 2013; Vinodhini, 2018) (Figure 5.7).

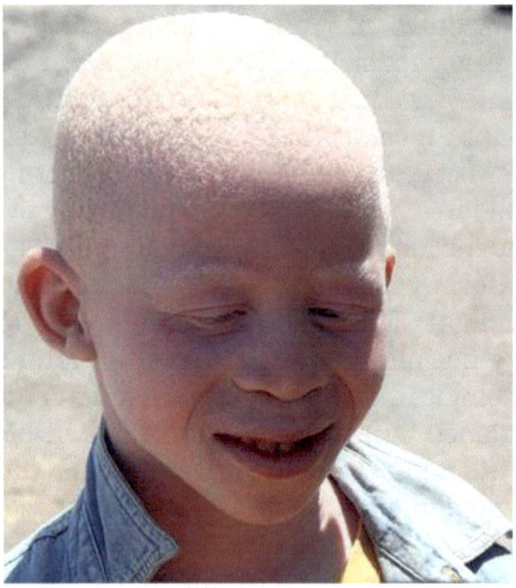

Figure 5.7. Albinism, characterized by a deficiency in melanin production, often results in ocular complications, including photophobia, nystagmus, and reduced visual acuity, primarily due to the lack of pigment in the retina that is essential for optimal light absorption and image clarity.

Source: https://www.physio-pedia.com/images/thumb/9/9a/Albinisitic_man_portrait.jpg/300px-Albinisitic_man_portrait.jpg.

5.2.5. Social and Cultural Implications

Social and cultural consequences of depigmentation and hypopigmentation disorders, primarily vitiligo and albinism, are enormous and multifaceted. Patients undergo enormous stigmatization and discrimination, particularly in societies where lighter skin is desirable. Sight of depigmented areas causes psychological burden, e.g., anxiety and depression, which in turn reinforces inadequacy and social isolation. As noted, although depigmentation may be sought for cosmetic purposes in some groups, this is an expression of a broader societal preoccupation with skin color and beauty standards that can create envy on the part of those with vitiligo who have accessed treatments for depigmentation to present a homogeneous appearance. Further, the prevalence of diseases like oculocutaneous albinism in specific geographic regions underscores the need for culturally suitable awareness and education of these conditions, with extensive psychosocial effects, for which there is little information (Manga et al., 2013).

5.2.6. Diagnosis and Screening Methods

Diagnosis of depigmentation and hypopigmentation conditions, such as vitiligo and albinism, is complicated and requires an integrative method. Clinicians will typically be faced with the diversity of presentation and the potential overlap with other dermatological entities, making it confusing to diagnose. Identification of critical enzymes and genetic determinants of pigmentation can aid in establishing a more accurate diagnosis. Techniques such as genomic sequencing and gene expression analysis become essential in determining the causative factors of depigmentation, particularly in determining the local versus systemic nature of the process. Moreover, understanding the importance of depigmentation across various skin types is essential; while some people may not find depigmented lesions to be bothersome, pigmented individuals may experience devastating psychosocial effects like low self-esteem and social stigmatization (Albretsen,

2022). Hence, goal-oriented diagnoses can enhance treatment protocols and patient outcomes (Figure 5.8).

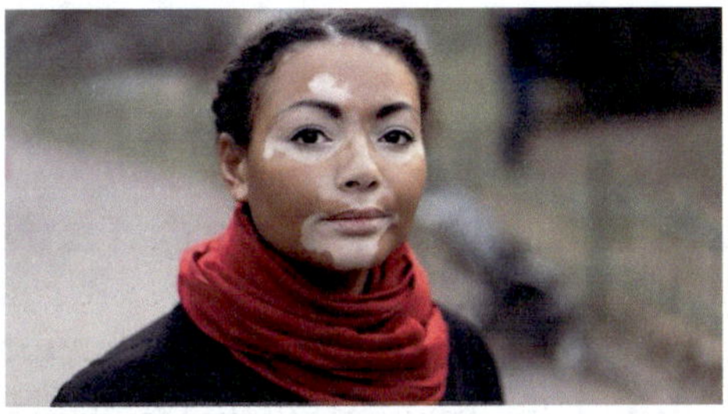

Figure 5.8. The identification of key enzymes and genetic factors involved in pigmentation can aid in establishing a more accurate diagnosis.

Source: https://i0.wp.com/post.medicalnewstoday.com/wp-content/uploads/sites/3/2022/05/GettyImages-1142517253_slide-1.jpg?w=1155.

5.2.7. Treatment and Management of Symptoms

Treatment of hypopigmentation and depigmentation disorders, particularly vitiligo and albinism, involves an integrative treatment protocol for alleviating symptoms as well as the quality of life in patients afflicted with these disorders. Topical agents such as corticosteroids and calcineurin inhibitors are typically employed to suppress patches of skin and induce repigmentation. As well, patients will often pursue many various cosmetic treatments, including chemical and laser peeling, to address visible discrepancies in skin color. Recent research has shown that some herbal formulations, such as Parangipattai chooranam and Annabedhi chenduram, were seen to lower depigmentation by a great extent and improve the appearance of the skin in clinical trials of patients undergoing treatment for ailments such as Venpulli, in which half of the cases showed moderate improvement (Vinodhini, 2018). Thus, an interdisciplinary approach using medical, herbal, and cosmetic interventions is critical to effectively deal with the disorders.

5.2.8. Advocacy and Support for Individuals with Albinism

Protection and advocacy for persons with albinism persons are necessary to ensure the elimination of the stigma and violence that otherwise accompany the condition. There have been cases of sickening abuse of individuals with albinism, particularly in KwaZulu-Natal, where cultural beliefs contribute to their vulnerability (Shabalala, 2023). These misconceptions sometimes create destructive beliefs that the body organs of individuals with albinism possess magical powers, which increase violence and discrimination (Mbatha, 2021). Effective advocacy initiatives must try to raise awareness and educate policymakers as well as the general public regarding the unique challenges this stigmatized group encounters. Support mechanisms, like educational interventions conducted by social workers, play a central role in fostering resilience in individuals with albinism. Through the creation of safe spaces and promoting acceptance, advocacy fuels the empowerment of individuals with albinism, ultimately working to dismantle harmful stereotypes and protect their rights (Figure 5.9).

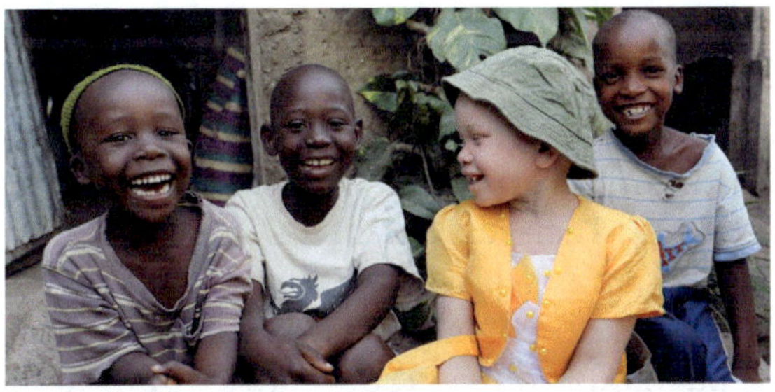

Figure 5.9. The advocacy and support for individuals with albinism are critical in combating the stigma and violence often associated with this condition.

Source: https://images.theconversation.com/files/173343/original/file-20170612-10242-14n6vqy.jpg?ixlib=rb-4.1.0&rect=0%2C224%2C5760%2C2793&q=45&auto=format&w=1356&h=668&fit=crop.

Test Your Knowledge

1. What is the role of tyrosinase in melanin production?
2. What preventive advice is crucial for patients with albinism?

5.3. Societal and Cultural Perspectives

Learning Outcome

1. Understand Historical Views on Skin Color and Beauty;
2. Explain Media Representation of Hypopigmentation Disorders;
3. Focus on Cultural Beliefs and Myths Surrounding Vitiligo and Albinism;
4. Describe Impact of Social Media on Awareness and Acceptance;
5. Learn Role of Advocacy Groups and Organizations;
6. Discuss Education and Outreach Programs;
7. Know Legal Protections and Discrimination Issues;
8. Understand Global Perspectives on Skin Disorders;
9. Explain Future Trends in Societal Attitudes.

The social and cultural perception of depigmentation and hypopigmentation disorders, such as albinism and vitiligo, is complex and typically marred with issues. Patients with such disorders are typically stigmatized, ostracized, and sometimes physically abused, particularly in regions where cultural beliefs breed myths about their conditions. For instance, research indicates a high level of abuse of albinos because of myths that their body parts are believed to possess magical healing properties, and this leads to rampant infringement of their rights and security (Shabalala, 2023). Moreover, people's awareness is often low, and this aggravates the discrimination and social exclusion of the affected persons (Téot et al., 2021). It is the task of managing these social attitudes; it requires an interdisciplinary approach incorporating education and public engagement for dismantling harmful assumptions and fostering an inclusive view of hypopigmentation disorders, ultimately leading to a more accommodating environment for individuals afflicted with such disorders.

5.3.1. Historical Views on Skin Color and Beauty

In the past, attitudes regarding skin color and beauty have played a major role in bringing about social norms, particularly regarding skin illnesses like albinism and vitiligo. In different cultures and throughout different centuries, light skin has been equated with beauty, privilege, and status, while dark skin has been stigmatized. This has been compounded by media and colonialist representations favoring Eurocentric aesthetics. In addition, individuals with hypopigmented disorders like vitiligo and albinism have historically been stigmatized, configured as other and discriminated against. As our medical understanding of the disorders deepens, it is important to resist and subvert the skin color bias.

The challenge lies in reconciling generally accepted standards of attractiveness with a more inclusive acceptance of variation. A comprehensive strategy combining both historical view and modern observation is necessary to embrace acceptance and reduce stigma regarding differences in skin color, particularly with disorders like vitiligo and albinism (Téot et al., 2021) (Figure 5.10).

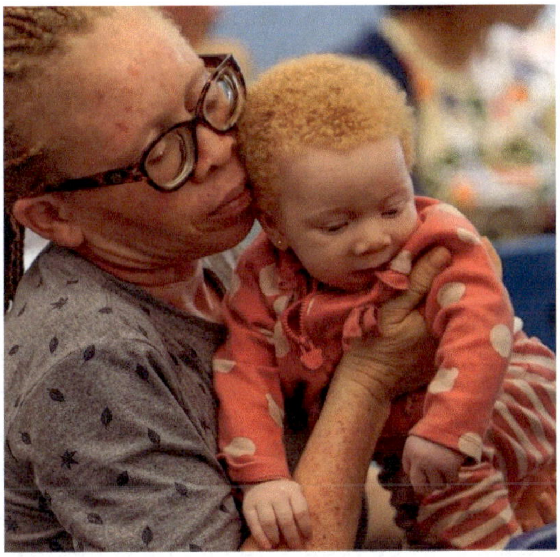

Figure 5.10. Individuals with hypopigmented conditions like vitiligo and albinism have historically been marginalized, viewed as other and often subjected to discrimination.

Source: https://media.licdn.com/dms/image/sync/v2/D4D27AQF_saZhLQE5WA/articleshare-shrink_800/articleshare-shrink_800/0/1731768215943?e=2147483647&v=beta&t=rj4UvTDs91YhcYPCUv3_60c6IMB4zHAoPSI--H13K2s.

5.3.2. Media Representation of Hypopigmentation Disorders

The media portrayal of hypopigmentation conditions such as vitiligo and albinism also affects public attitude and self-concept of the individuals. They are often reduced to stereotypical depictions based on otherness in most instances. The portrayals serve to perpetuate stigma and disinformation. For instance, actors or models used in commercial scripts or movies may be depicted as exotic or broken, reinforcing negative stereotypes overruling the multifaceted experiences of the affected individuals. Therefore, vitiligo patients, whose loss of functional melanocytes (Waterman, 2002) may cause them perhaps to feel less than lovely in a society that prizes conventional conceptions of beauty, may find it difficult to accept themselves. Alternatively, evolving media landscapes are beginning to depict more authentic, varied narratives, with the intention of inducing empathy and acceptance. For instance, advances in skin equivalent research project the biological underpinnings of pigmentation disorders, implying a future potential for better-educated portrayals in media (Mead, 2022). Such changes are critical toward eliciting empathy and debunking stigma surrounding hypopigmentation disorders.

5.3.3. Cultural Beliefs and Myths Surrounding Vitiligo and Albinism

Myths and beliefs regarding vitiligo and albinism strongly shape social attitudes as well as the control of persons affected by these hypopigmentation conditions. Individuals afflicted with albinism in the majority of cultures are highly discriminated against due to the lack of accurate information regarding their condition, including the myth that their body parts are magical or bring prosperity and wealth.

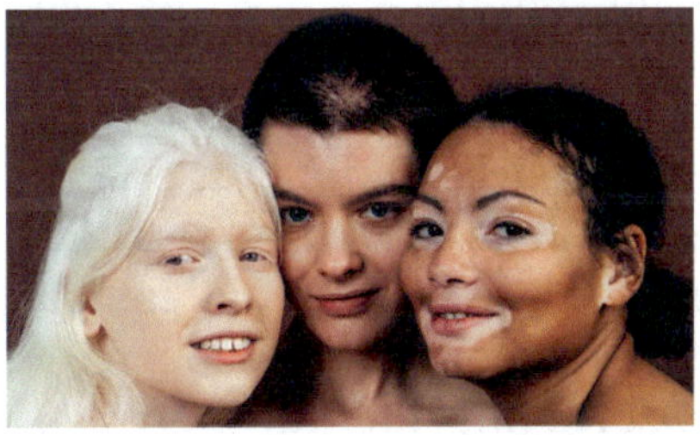

Figure 5.11. Cultural beliefs and myths surrounding vitiligo and albinism significantly inform societal attitudes and treatment of individuals affected by these hypopigmentation disorders.

Source: https://www.kayakalpglobal.com/health/wp-content/uploads/2023/05/Famous-people-with-vitilig.webp.

These myths have gruesome repercussions, including violence and homicide, as illustrated by the research, which claims that individuals with albinism live in terror of abuse or lethal attacks on grounds of cultural superstition about their affliction (Shabalala, 2023). Vitiligo, similarly often seen through a lens of stigma and ignorance, can result in social exclusion and psychic trauma among its victims. Therefore, countering these cultural myths is crucial in raising awareness and attaining a tolerant society where the humanity and dignity of all individuals are respected irrespective of their complexion (Mbatha, 2021) (Figure 5.11).

5.3.4. Impact of Social Media on Awareness and Acceptance

The role played by social media in the development of public awareness and knowledge of hypopigmentation and depigmentation disorders, such as vitiligo and albinism, cannot be overstated. Social media sites like Twitter and Instagram have provided avenues for sharing patients' personal stories and experiences that build solidarity and a community sense among patients with the conditions. In providing images and descriptions of their experiences, they are contributing to a growing visibility that transcends societal constructions of beauty and color. Not only does this greater representation encourage self-acceptance, but it also educates the broader public about the facts of living with these disorders. Social media campaigns also frequently provide resources for treatment and advocacy, bridging the gap between medical knowledge and patient life. Lastly, these digital interactions are pivotal to demolishing stigmas surrounding hypopigmentation illnesses, as evident in recent research on skin wellness and social attitudes (Marie, 2013; Téot et al., 2021).

5.3.5. Role of Advocacy Groups and Organizations

Advocacy groups and organizations play a core role in raising awareness and providing support to patients affected by hypopigmentation and depigmentation conditions such as vitiligo and albinism. These groups not only foster a sense of community among patients but also serve as bridge intermediaries between impacted individuals and the medical establishment, offering access to information, resources, and accessible treatments. Through the mobilization of efforts to educate the public and medical professionals, advocacy organizations underscore the benefits of learning about these disorders, combat stigma, and promote acceptance. Moreover, they usually collaborate with clinicians and researchers in developing improved treatment approaches and best practices, as discussed in materials on scar and wound care (Téot et al., 2021). The collaboration ensures that new innovations and therapies are properly disseminated to practitioners and patients as well, ultimately improving the level of care for those afflicted with these conditions (Figure 5.12).

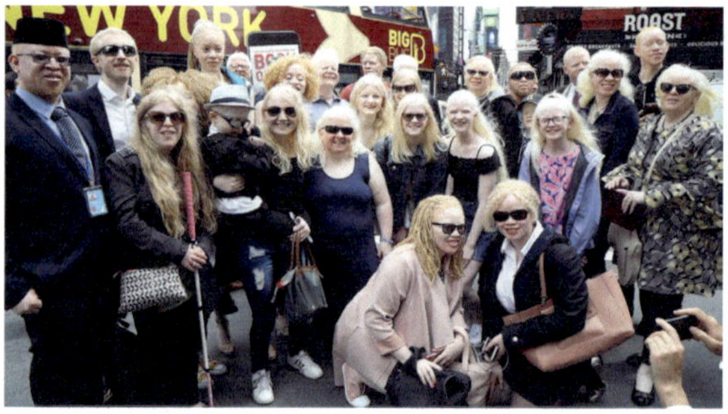

Figure 5.12. Advocacy groups and organizations play a critical role in raising awareness and providing support for individuals affected by hypopigmentation and depigmentation disorders, such as vitiligo and albinism.

Source: https://untoday.org/wp-content/uploads/2024/05/05_GLOBAL-AFFAIRS-12.jpg.

5.3.6. Education and Outreach Programs

Good education and outreach programs play a significant role in problem-solving related to patients suffering from hypopigmentation and depigmentation disorders, i.e., albinism and vitiligo. They aim to develop an awareness of the biological, social, and psychological status of such conditions and thereby work towards a more tolerant society. By providing proper information about genetic and evolutionary reasons behind skin pigmentation, as discussed in recent research literature, these measures can deter social stigma commonly associated with differential skin color (Mosca & Morrone, 2023). Further, outreach programs invite medical professionals for efforts to advance policies favoring the affected, raising the visibility of their rights and needs among medical professionals (Mikhly & Ruiz, 2015). Through extensive education about the medical as well as social consequences of hypopigmentation disorders, these programs can significantly facilitate the affected individuals, resulting in enhanced health status and quality of life.

5.3.7. Legal Protections and Discrimination Issues

With reference to hypopigmentation and depigmentation diseases such as albinism and vitiligo, the protection against discrimination by law is still acutely needed by individuals with these conditions. They often lead to physical stigmatization and social ostracization, even by ignorance and unawareness on the part of society. Legislation, such as the Americans with Disabilities Act (ADA) and the Rehabilitation Act, offers protections against employment discrimination and enables citizens to seek redress when they are not provided with equal treatment in the workforce or public places. Sadly, the enforcement and application of such legislations fall short because a large number of individuals who are affected do not have information about their rights or the proof needed to prove discrimination. Hence, it is important to push for increased legal protection and enlightenment of the people to the facts of these disorders to make the realization of an environment that is inclusive, where individuals are not discriminated against because of their skin conditions, a reality (Donkor et al., 2022) (Figure 5.13).

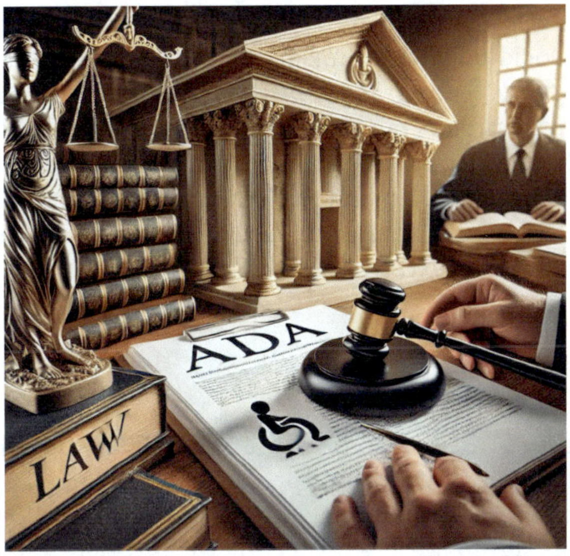

Figure 5.13. Legal frameworks, such as the Americans with Disabilities Act (ADA) and the Rehabilitation Act, offer safeguards against employment discrimination and enable individuals to seek recourse in cases of unequal treatment in the workplace or public spaces.

Source: https://know-the-ada.com/wp-content/uploads/2024/06/The-Legal-Framework-of-the-ADA.webp.

5.3.8. Global Perspectives on Skin Disorders

The world perspective of skin disorders, particularly hypopigmentation and depigmentation disorders like albinism and vitiligo, is characterized by interaction between medical awareness and cultural perception. In most areas, traditional remedies based on local flora are at the forefront of treatment for such disorders, such as in South African research where indigenous medicine plants are employed to rejuvenate skin condition and tone (Mahachi, 2013). Moreover, identification of genetic factors in isolates offers a clear conceptualization of the disorders and makes it possible for effective healthcare intervention. For instance, research among such populations as the Amish and Pakistani groups has advanced what is known about hereditary eye disease associated with albinism, necessitating accurate genetic testing as well as subsequent clinical implications (Lin, 2021). This coming together of traditional wisdom and contemporary scholarship necessitates the importance of an integrative strategy toward skin health in the global context.

5.3.9. Future Trends in Societal Attitudes

Future attitudes of society towards people afflicted with hypopigmentation and depigmentation disorders, such as vitiligo and albinism, are expected to undergo a sea change. Increased awareness of vitiligo being an autoimmune disorder, brought forth by recent research, is increasing sensitivity towards the disorder and its psycho-emotional implications, as ignorance more than knowledge lies at the basis of misconceptions and stigma (Kadhim et al., 2023). Consequently, educational programs can fight negative stereotypes and promote broader acceptance in society, leading to a more tolerant environment for individuals suffering from such conditions. Second, the impact of social media as the primary source of information is transforming public perception, as the sites provide avenues for the sharing of personal experiences and ensure visibility (Kadhim et al., 2023). As knowledge advances, it can be hoped that stigma regarding these disorders will decrease, and it will pave the way for a future in which there is more understanding and more acceptance of variations in individual skin health and colour (Figure 5.14).

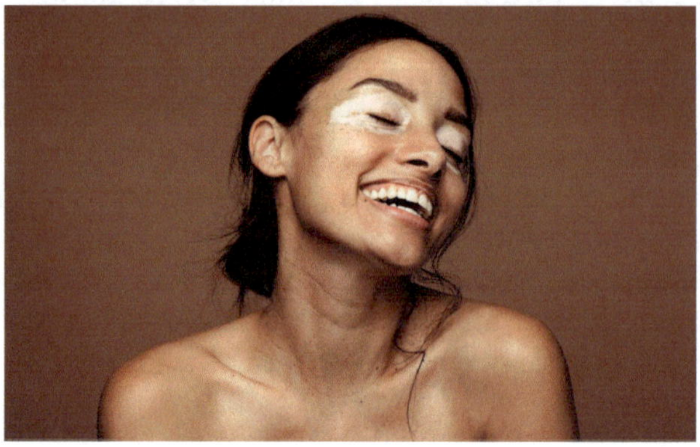

Figure 5.14. Increased awareness of the autoimmune nature of vitiligo is fostering a more empathetic understanding of the condition and its psychological implications, as misconceptions and stigma often stem from a lack of knowledge.

Source: https://drmaggieyu.com/wp-content/uploads/2023/05/iStock-1332337830-1184x755.jpg.

Test Your Knowledge

1. What role do patient support groups play in managing vitiligo?
2. How can education reduce misconceptions about albinism?

SUMMARY

It is not only crucial to have knowledge about hypopigmentation and depigmentation disorders such as vitiligo and albinism for appropriate clinical management, but also to confront their psychological and social implications by patients. These diseases recognize the complexity of the biology of melanocytes and highlight the importance of more research in clinical and basic dermatology. New findings in the field have indicated promising avenues for treatment and more insight into the mechanisms of these conditions, as indicated in new frontiers regarding vitiligo and albinism (Filipp et al., 2018). One needs, however, to realize the reality that depigmentation can be an issue and an aesthetic wish, shaping individuality and wider definitions of beauty. By supporting inclusive approaches that pursue education and compassion, we can better serve individuals who are going through the profound impacts of these disorders.

In summarizing the matters addressed in this chapter regarding hypopigmentation and depigmentation disorders, particularly vitiligo and albinism, it is crucial to cite the complexity of such conditions. Vitiligo, which is the depigmentation of skin by autoimmune mechanisms, has the potential to inflict severe psychological trauma on the victims if consideration is taken for cosmetic appearance and social perception. The therapeutic aspect of depigmentation also seems to be double-edged in that, although it has remedies for cosmetic treatment, including chemical peels, it has the potential to induce jealousy among others who are opting for such therapy. However, conditions like albinism result in an insufficiency of melanin production, with special protection against environmental harm due to increased sensitivity to sunlight (Dnyane, 2023). Knowledge of the causative factors and physiological responses involved in such conditions, along with the influence of environmental agents as demonstrated in experimental studies using animal models like the Smyth line chickens, further proves the complexity involved in controlling and studying such conditions (Dong, 2012).

KEY TERMS FROM THIS CHAPTER

Depigmentation
Albinism
Psychological health
Social embarrassment
Sun sensitivity
Genetic
Exacerbation
Aetiology
Autoimmune illnesses
Hypopigmentation disorders
Vitiligo
Depigmented skin
Genetic disorder
Eye issues
Autoimmune
Patient management
Autoimmune hypothesis
Thyroid diseases

CRITICAL THINKING QUESTIONS

1. **Which of the following is a true depigmenting disorder (complete loss of melanin)?**
   a. Pityriasis alba
   b. Tinea versicolor
   c. Vitiligo
   d. Nevus depigmentosus
2. **Which condition is associated with "chalk-white" macules with well-defined borders?**
   a. Tinea versicolor
   b. Vitiligo
   c. Pityriasis alba
   d. Idiopathic guttate hypomelanosis
3. **What is the most likely diagnosis in a child with hypopigmented, ill-defined facial patches and fine scaling?**
   a. Vitiligo
   b. Pityriasis alba
   c. Tinea corporis
   d. Psoriasis
4. **The most common cause of hypopigmented patches in adolescents in tropical countries is:**
   a. Vitiligo
   b. Pityriasis versicolor
   c. Albinism
   d. Psoriasis
5. **Which stain is most helpful in diagnosing tinea versicolor?**
   a. Gram stain
   b. Ziehl-Neelsen stain
   c. KOH mount
   d. PAS stain

Short Answer Questions

1. What is the primary pathophysiological mechanism in vitiligo?
2. Which of the following is the most common clinical presentation of vitiligo?
3. Which enzyme defect causes oculocutaneous albinism type 1?
4. What are the common ocular manifestations in albinism?
5. What are common social stigmas faced by patients with vitiligo?
6. Which cultural beliefs may affect treatment-seeking behavior in albinism?

Answers to Critical Thinking Questions

1. (c); 2. (b); 3. (b); 4. (b); 5. (c)

REFERENCES

1. Albretsen, A. S. M. (2022). Depigmentation–Possible causes of change in phenotype, potential genetic mechanisms, and methods for investigating the cause of depigmentation. https://core.ac.uk/download/646165086.pdf (accessed on 23rd July 2025).
2. Baldini, E., Carbotta, G., Catania, A., et al. (2017). Vitiligo and autoimmune thyroid disorders. https://core.ac.uk/download/127588138.pdf (accessed on 23rd July 2025).
3. Witek, A., Parys, J., Mikosińska, A., Kaźmierczak, M., Mossakowski, M., Kałuziak, P., ... Bieś, R. (2025). Vitiligo Review: etiopathogenesis, diagnosis and treatment. *Quality in Sport, 37*, 57367. https://doi.org/10.12775/QS.2025.37.57367(accessed on 23rd July 2025).
4. Filipp, F. V., Birlea, S., Bosenberg, M. W., Brash, D., Cassidy, P. B., Chen, S., D'Orazio, J. A., Fujita, M., Goh, B. K., Herlyn, M., Indra, A. K., Larue, L., Leachman, S. A., Le Poole, C., Liu-Smith, F., Manga, P., Montoliu, L., Norris, D. A., Shellman, Y., Smalley, K. S. M., ... Box, N. F. (2018). Frontiers in pigment cell and melanoma research. *Pigment cell & melanoma research*, *31*(6), 728–735. https://doi.org/10.1111/pcmr.12728(accessed on 23rd July 2025).
5. Eroh, G. D., Clayton, F. C., Florell, S. R., Cassidy, P. B., Chirife, A., Marón, C. F., Valenzuela, L. O., Campbell, M. S., Seger, J., Rowntree, V. J., & Leachman, S. A. (2017). Cellular and ultrastructural characterization of the grey-morph phenotype in southern right whales (Eubalaena australis). *PloS one*, *12*(2), e0171449. https://doi.org/10.1371/journal.pone.0171449(accessed on 23rd July 2025).
6. Neveu, M. M., Padhy, S. K., Ramamurthy, S., Takkar, B., Jalali, S., Cp, D., Padhi, T. R., & Robson, A. G. (2022). Ophthalmological Manifestations of Oculocutaneous and Ocular Albinism: Current Perspectives. *Clinical ophthalmology (Auckland, N.Z.)*, *16*, 1569–1587. https://doi.org/10.2147/OPTH.S329282(accessed on 23rd July 2025).
7. Dnyane, P. (2023). Towards the development of a systems pharmacology model for vitiligo. http://dspace.ncl.res.in:8080/xmlui/bitstream/handle/20.500.12252/6281/Thesis_Pooja_Dnyane_10BB18A26028_Final_Copy.pdf?sequence=1 (accessed on 23rd July 2025).
8. Dong, L. (2012). A role of environmental components in autoimmune vitiligo of Smyth Line chickens. https://core.ac.uk/download/84119000.pdf (accessed on 23rd July 2025).
9. Donkor, C. M. Y. A., Aryee-Boi, J., Osazuwa, I. R., Afflu, F. K., & Alexis, A. F. (2022). *Atlas of dermatological conditions in populations of African ancestry*. Springer. https://books.google.com/books?id=uHI3zwEACAAJ (accessed on 23rd July 2025).
10. Sturm, R. A., & Duffy, D. L. (2012). Human pigmentation genes under environmental selection. *Genome biology*, *13*(9), 248. https://doi.org/10.1186/gb-2012-13-9-248(accessed on 23rd July 2025).
11. Eleftheriadou, V. (2025). Setting priorities and reducing uncertainties for the treatment of vitiligo. https://core.ac.uk/download/33566258.pdf (accessed on 23rd July 2025).
12. Téot L, Mustoe TA, Middelkoop E, et al., editors. Textbook on Scar Management: State of the Art Management and Emerging Technologies [Internet]. Cham (CH): Springer; 2020. Available from: https://www.ncbi.nlm.nih.gov/books/NBK586066/ doi: 10.1007/978-3-030-44766-3 (accessed on 23rd July 2025).
13. Byrne, S., Jansen, L., U-King-Im, J. M., Siddiqui, A., Lidov, H. G., Bodi, I., Smith, L., Mein, R., Cullup, T., Dionisi-Vici, C., Al-Gazali, L., Al-Owain, M., Bruwer, Z., Al Thihli, K., El-Garhy, R.,

Flanigan, K. M., Manickam, K., Zmuda, E., Banks, W., Gershoni-Baruch, R., ... Jungbluth, H. (2016). EPG5-related Vici syndrome: a paradigm of neurodevelopmental disorders with defective autophagy. *Brain : a journal of neurology, 139*(Pt 3), 765–781. https://doi.org/10.1093/brain/awv393(accessed on 23rd July 2025).

14. Jusuf, N. K. (2017). Pattern of pigmentation disorder in Cosmetic Dermatology Clinic H. Adam Malik General Hospital, Medan, 2012–2015. https://core.ac.uk/download/639382319.pdf (accessed on 23rd July 2025).

15. Kadhim, S. E., Kareem, S. S., & Mohammed, Z. H. (2023). Knowledge of nursing students and their attitude towards vitiligo. https://cdnx.uobabylon.edu.iq/undergrad_projs/7daJryH0TUy315kjzAJLHw.pdf (accessed on 23rd July 2025).

16. Kala, G. (2013). A study on Swetha Kuttam. https://core.ac.uk/download/235666191.pdf (accessed on 23rd July 2025).

17. Kaur, N., & Kaur, S. (2012). A REVIEW ON LEUCODERMA AND REPORTED HERBS FOR ITS TREATMENT. *Journal of Drug Delivery and Therapeutics, 2*(3). https://doi.org/10.22270/jddt.v2i3.157(accessed on 23rd July 2025).

18. Manga, P., Kerr, R., Ramsay, M., & Kromberg, J. G. (2013). Biology and genetics of oculocutaneous albinism and vitiligo - common pigmentation disorders in southern Africa. *South African medical journal = Suid-Afrikaanse tydskrif vir geneeskunde, 103*(12 Suppl 1), 984–988. https://doi.org/10.7196/samj.7046(accessed on 23rd July 2025).

19. Lin, S. (2021). Defining the clinical and molecular spectrum of inherited eye diseases in community settings. https://core.ac.uk/download/479013070.pdf (accessed on 23rd July 2025).

20. Mahachi, J. (2013). Medicinal properties of some plants used for the treatment of skin disorders in the O. R. Tambo and Amathole municipalities of the Eastern Cape Province, South Africa. https://core.ac.uk/download/327305548.pdf (accessed on 23rd July 2025).

21. Marie, K. L. (2013). Chemical and genetic control of melanocyte development, proliferation and regeneration in zebrafish. https://core.ac.uk/download/429736645.pdf (accessed on 23rd July 2025).

22. Mbatha, S. M. (2021). Trafficking in persons living with albinism in South Africa. https://core.ac.uk/download/481484899.pdf (accessed on 23rd July 2025).

23. Mead, H. D. (2022). Incorporation of pigment-producing cells into novel 3D skin equivalents to study the role of the dermal compartment upon pigmentation in skin equivalents. https://core.ac.uk/download/533445235.pdf (accessed on 23rd July 2025).

24. Mikhly, M., & Ruiz, A. (2015). The role of the medical profession in swaying public policy: Exploring physician responsibility and advocacy. *The Einstein Journal of Biology and Medicine, 30*(1–2), 2–5. https://www.einstein.yu.edu/ejbm (accessed on 23rd July 2025).

25. Mosca, S., & Morrone, A. (2023). Human skin pigmentation: From a biological feature to a social determinant. *Healthcare, 11*, 2091. https://doi.org/10.3390/healthcare11142091 (accessed on 23rd July 2025).

26. Shabalala, M. M. (2023). Development of intervention strategies to address the abuse and brutal killing of people with albinism in KwaZulu-Natal. https://core.ac.uk/download/639419075.pdf (accessed on 23rd July 2025).

27. Vadivelan, S. (2013). A study on Venpulli. https://core.ac.uk/download/235669973.pdf (accessed on 23rd July 2025).

28. Vinodhini, R. (2018). Clinical evaluation of *Parangipattai Chooranam* (internal) and *Annabedhi Chenduram* (external) for Venpulli (vitiligo) in children. https://core.ac.uk/download/235669873.pdf (accessed on 23rd July 2025).

29. Waterman, E. A. (2002). An investigation into the role of autoimmunity in vitiligo. https://core.ac.uk/download/14343331.pdf (accessed on 23rd July 2025).

VESICULOBULLOUS DISEASES

6

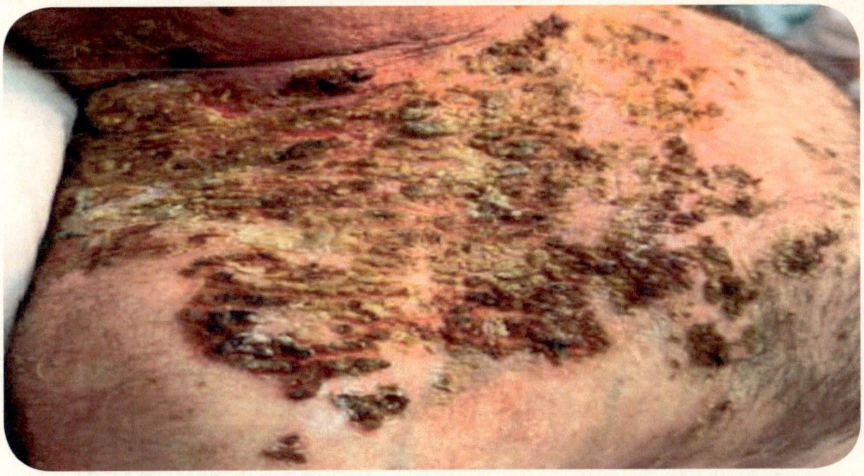

LEARNING OBJECTIVES

After studying this chapter, you will be able to:

1. Understand Pemphigus;
2. Explain Bullous Pemphigoid;
3. Describe Diagnosis and Differential Diagnosis;
4. Focus on Treatment and Management Strategies.

Introduction

Vesiculobullous disorders comprise a heterogeneous group of conditions that are characterized by the formation of bullae and blisters on the skin due to disruption of epidermal adhesion caused by various stimuli. Among the vesiculobullous diseases, pemphigus and bullous pemphigoid are two classic autoimmune diseases. Pemphigus is defined by intraepidermal blistering, expressed primarily in the form of pemphigus vulgaris and pemphigus foliaceous, with several other less common forms having specific clinical and immunopathological features (Porro et al., 2014). Comparatively, bullous pemphigoid is defined by subepidermal splitting, and hence clinically disparate but pathophysiologically allied. Understanding of the underlying mechanisms, including the immune response against structural components of the skin, is necessary for proper diagnosis and management of these diseases (Taş Aygar & Gönül, 2023). With advancing science, the nomenclature and understanding of such diseases improve, and hence there is a need for ongoing academic research and clinical perception.

6.1. Pemphigus: An Overview

Learning Outcome

1. Understand Definition and Classification of Pemphigus;
2. Explain Types of Pemphigus;
3. Focus on Etiology and Risk Factors;
4. Describe Pathophysiology of Pemphigus;
5. Learn Clinical Manifestations and Symptoms;
6. Discuss Diagnostic Methods and Criteria;
7. Know Treatment Options and Management Strategies;
8. Understand Prognosis and Potential Complications.

The pemphigus disease group is a spectrum of autoimmune skin disorders comprising the development of blisters in the epidermis due to disruption of cell adhesion. This disruption is primarily a result of the development of autoantibodies against desmogleins, which are integral structural elements of desmosomes that maintain cellular integrity.

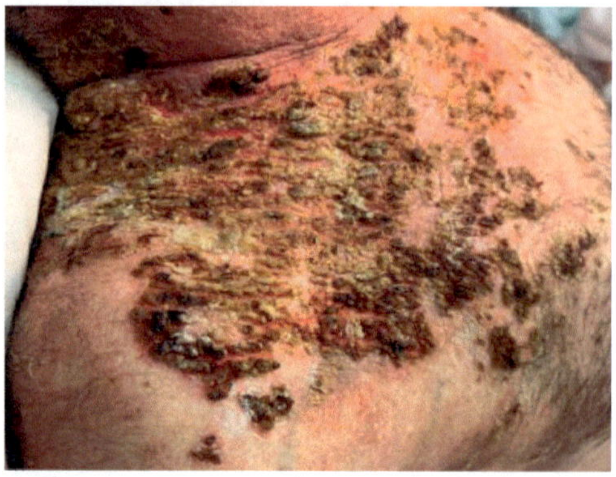

Figure 6.1. The pemphigus group of diseases represents a spectrum of autoimmune skin disorders characterized by the development of blisters in the epidermis due to the disruption of cell adhesion.

Source: https://www.mdpi.com/dermato/dermato-04-00007/article_deploy/html/images/dermato-04-00007-g015-550.jpg.

Pemphigus vulgaris, the most frequent form, typically presents with painful ulcers and cutaneous blisters in the mouth and usually follows an early diagnosis and treatment to prevent severe consequences. Differentiation of pemphigus from other vesiculobullous diseases, such as cicatricial pemphigoid, is particularly important for management. Cicatricial pemphigoid is differentiated by erosive mucosal lesions and their potential to lead to the development of serious complications, including blindness and airway obstruction (Ayvaz et al., 2018). Moreover, overall familiarity with ulcerative lesions in these diseases can enable clinicians to cope with the diagnostic challenges and utilize appropriate interventional strategies (Mortazavi et al., 2016) (Figure 6.1).

6.1.1. Definition and Classification of Pemphigus

Pemphigus is a group of autoimmune vesiculobullous disorders characterized by the development of blisters on the skin and mucous membranes due to disruption of intercellular adhesion in the epidermis. It is primarily segregated into two general categories: pemphigus vulgaris, tending to start with painful mucosal lesions followed by skin involvement, and pemphigus foliaceous, with the dominance of skin lesions with minimal mucosal involvement.

There are also rare variants like pemphigus herpetiformis and IgA pemphigus that present in distinctive clinical and histopathological ways, making pemphigus classification more complex (Porro et al., 2014). The realization of these classifications is essential since they inform clinical practice and therapy, with an emphasis on correct diagnosis using immunofluorescence analysis and clinical evaluation, particularly in differentiating pemphigus from other autoimmune dermatological diseases (Leuci et al., 2019).

6.1.2. Types of Pemphigus (e.g., Pemphigus Vulgaris, Pemphigus Foliaceus)

Pemphigus is a group of autoimmune illnesses characterized by the formation of vesicles and bullae and is predominantly targeted against the skin and mucous membranes. Of the most prevalent forms, pemphigus vulgaris and pemphigus foliaceus are noted due to their varying clinical presentation and pathophysiologic underpinnings from the others. Pemphigus vulgaris, the more severe condition, typically presents with painful mucosal ulcers and promptly fragile bullae with resulting severe morbidity and impaired quality of life (Kumar et al., 2019). Pemphigus foliaceus presents with superficial skin lesions that do not have a tendency for involvement of mucosal membranes and is a milder disease form (Ates, 2018). Correct diagnosis relies on clinical evaluation, histopathological examination, and direct immunofluorescence in order to ascertain the localization of the split in the epidermis, which allows for correct discrimination between these types of pemphigus and other vesiculobullous disorders (Figure 6.2).

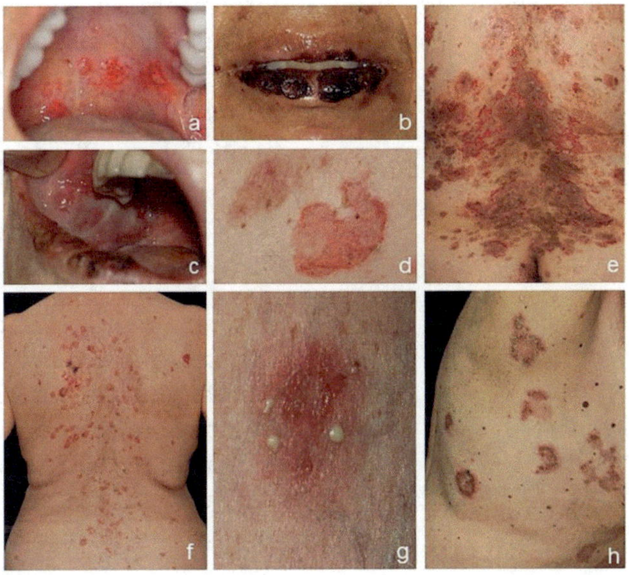

Figure 6.2. Pemphigus is a group of autoimmune disorders characterized by the formation of vesicles and bullae, primarily affecting the skin and mucous membranes.

Source: https://images-provider.frontiersin.org/api/ipx/w=1200&f=png/https://www.frontiersin.org/files/Articles/1363032/fimmu-15-1363032-HTML/image_m/fimmu-15-1363032-g001.jpg.

6.1.3. Etiology and Risk Factors

The pathogenesis and etiologic factors in vesiculobullous disorders such as pemphigus and bullous pemphigoid are highly associated with autoimmune dysfunction of the integrity of the skin. These conditions are induced by the formation of blisters because of the disruption of epidermal cell adhesion or at the dermo-epidermal junction. Pemphigus, for instance, results when autoantibodies target desmosomal proteins, leading to epidermal cell loss of cohesion, while bullous pemphigoid results from antibodies against hemidesmosomal proteins BP180 and BP230, which anchor the epidermis to the dermis (Yayla et al., 2018). Risk factors include old age, since bullous pemphigoid occurs predominantly in the elderly, and genetic susceptibility, which suggests an intrinsic defect in immune regulation (Raghuwanshi et al., 2023). Environmental influences such as drugs and infection can activate these diseases, testifying to the multicentric nature of their etiology.

6.1.4. Pathophysiology of Pemphigus

The pathophysiology of pemphigus, an autoimmune blistering disease group, is characterized predominantly by the production of autoantibodies against desmosomal antigens, which destroy keratinocyte adhesion.

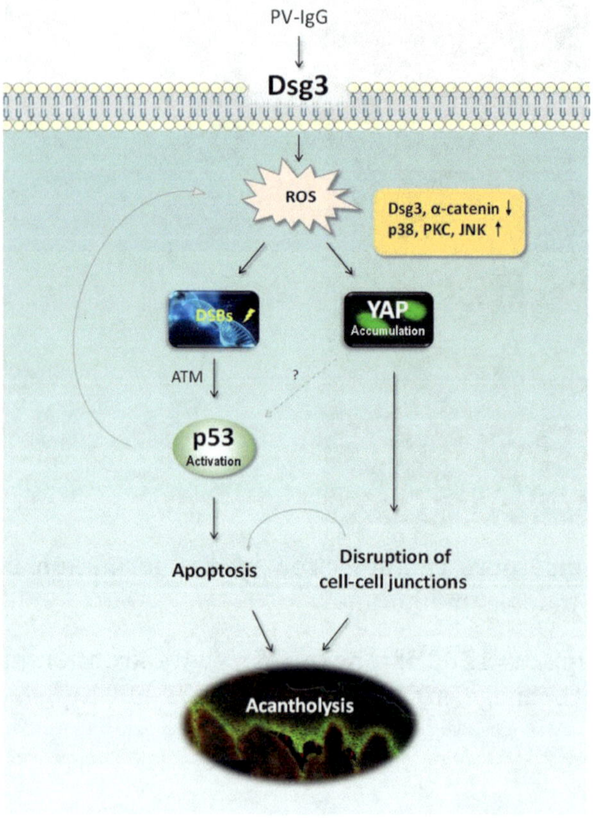

Figure 6.3. The pathophysiology of pemphigus.

Source: https://www.mdpi.com/life/life-11-00621/article_deploy/html/images/life-11-00621-g001.png.

The autoimmune response compromises the integrity of the epidermis and forms intraepithelial blisters. Pemphigus vulgaris, the most common variant, is associated with anti-desmoglein 3 antibodies, and pemphigus foliaceus with desmoglein 1. The antibodies interfere with intercellular adhesion such that the involved keratinocytes go through acantholysis, which clinically manifests as painful erosions and vesicles over the skin and mucous membranes. Accurate diagnosis is crucial because treatment is vastly different; thus, comprehensive evaluation through clinical assessment and direct immunofluorescence is required in disease establishment and determination of appropriate management options. An understanding of these mechanisms is crucial to improve the therapeutic plan and patient outcome in pemphigus (Yayla et al., 2018; Mohanapriya, 2020) (Figure 6.3).

6.1.5. Clinical Manifestations and Symptoms

Clinical manifestations of vesiculobullous diseases, particularly pemphigus and bullous pemphigoid, are a serious challenge since they are not homogeneous. Pemphigus vulgaris, for instance, presents with painful, superficial vesicles and bullae that have a tendency to affect mucus membranes, but most often the oral cavity, which may precede the cutaneous lesions in some individuals by weeks (Jayasri, 2012). In contrast to bullous pemphigoid, which also tends to begin with tense bullae on erythematous or uninvolved skin and has less likelihood of oral mucosa involvement than pemphigus (Mohanapriya, 2020), both conditions can lead to severe morbidity due to pain, dysphagia, and secondary infection of the ruptured vesicles. Besides, an early diagnosis by careful clinical examination coupled with histopathological assessment and direct immunofluorescence is also essential in effectively managing these diseases and promoting improved patient outcomes.

6.1.6. Diagnostic Methods and Criteria

Accurate diagnosis is a major factor in the treatment of vesiculobullous diseases such as pemphigus and bullous pemphigoid because it straightforwardly informs treatment regimens and prognostic outcomes. Traditional diagnostic methods, like clinical tests and histopathological analysis, prove to be insufficient in light of the heterogeneous presentation. This necessitates the addition of complex procedures, e.g., direct immunofluorescence (DIF), which, as proven, renders diagnosis far more precise. Literature is assertive that combined clinical features, histopathological findings, and DIF yield the best result even in the event of indefinite histopathological findings (Mohanapriya, 2020). Besides, early diagnosis of oral manifestations is important due to the fact that the involvement of the oral cavity is frequent in autoimmune bullous diseases and can precede the occurrence of cutaneous lesions (Jayasri, 2012). Hence, an interdisciplinary approach through these techniques is required in order to provide effective control and improved patient outcomes for vesiculobullous diseases (Figure 6.4).

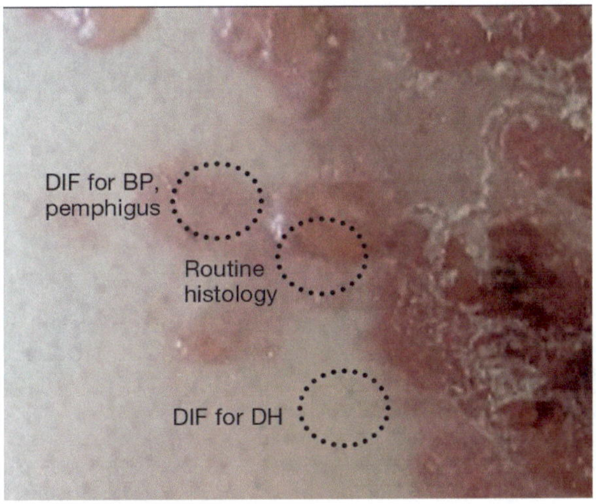

Figure 6.4. Direct immunofluorescence (DIF).

Source: https://cdn.mdedge.com/files/s3fs-public/CT108005023_e_Fig.JPG.

6.1.7. Treatment Options and Management Strategies

The treatment of vesiculobullous disorders, especially pemphigus and bullous pemphigoid, requires a holistic approach specific to the unique needs of each patient. In pemphigus, systemic corticosteroids remain the cornerstone of treatment, administered in 86.9% of the patients to avert the disease's potentially severe outcomes; however, it is necessary to add steroid-sparing drugs to prevent long-term side effects, such as mycophenolate mofetil and azathioprine, utilized in 58.3% of the patients (Budianti et al., 2021). Conversely, the treatment of bullous pemphigoid emphasizes both systemic and topical therapy because recent literature indicates that dapsone is highly effective with an impressive complete remission rate of 81.6% (Genovese et al., 2019). Moreover, the clinical presentation and response differences between children and adults further enhance the efficacy of treatment, emphasizing the necessity of individualized therapy in the management of these multifaceted autoimmune dermatoses.

6.1.8. Prognosis and Potential Complications

The result of vesiculobullous diseases, i.e., pemphigus and bullous pemphigoid, is immensely different depending upon timeliness and suitability of diagnosis and patients' response to treatment. Early treatment is necessary because the complications of these autoimmune disorders evolve rapidly; for instance, in the absence of early treatment, patients can have extensive skin damage and secondary infection due to loss of skin barrier function (Leuci et al., 2019). In addition, the chronic nature of these diseases is capable of inducing significant morbidity, both of the skin as well as mucous membranes, that could contribute towards psychosocial challenges in patients (Taş Aygar & Gönül, 2023). Treatment over a long period typically demands immunosuppressive medications, which, though unavoidable, are accompanied by risks of related complications, such as increased susceptibility to infections and potential for organ damage. Thus, understanding of the fine balance between effective treatment and managing concomitant risk is important in optimizing patient outcomes.

Test Your Knowledge

1. What clinical sign is classically associated with pemphigus?
2. How does pemphigus foliaceus differ from pemphigus vulgaris?

6.2. Bullous Pemphigoid: An Overview

Learning Outcome

1. Understand Definition and Classification of Bullous Pemphigoid;
2. Explain Etiology and Risk Factors;
3. Focus on Pathophysiology of Bullous Pemphigoid;
4. Describe Clinical Manifestations and Symptoms;
5. Learn Diagnostic Methods and Criteria;
6. Discuss Treatment Options and Management Strategies;
7. Know Prognosis and Potential Complications.

Bullous pemphigoid is an autoimmune blistering disease that is primarily characterized by the formation of large, tense blisters that typically affect the skin and mucous membranes. This condition is due to the immune system's inappropriate reaction, in which antibodies react against structures of the basement membrane zone, most notably the bullous pemphigoid antigens 180 and 230.

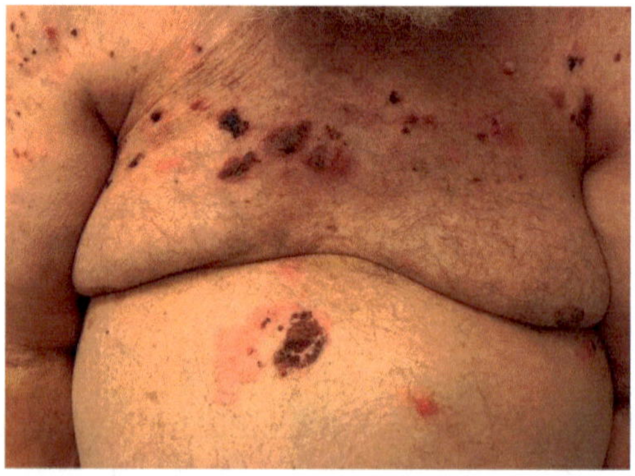

Figure 6.5. Bullous pemphigoid is a significant autoimmune blistering disorder primarily characterized by the formation of large, tense blisters that typically occur on the skin and mucous membranes.

Source: https://www.dermatologyadvisor.com/wp-content/uploads/sites/20/2025/01/bullous-skin-lesion-1.jpg.

Pruritus and the development of blisters that are prone to rupture and cause painful erosions may be components of the clinical presentation. The mechanism of bullous pemphigoid is distinct from other vesiculobullous disorders, such as pemphigus, in its subepidermal rather than intraepidermal separation, thereby underlining its classification in the pemphigoid group of diseases (Taş Aygar & Gönül, 2023). Successful treatment typically involves corticosteroids and immunosuppressive agents, underlining the importance of early diagnosis and treatment to prevent complications (Ayvaz et al., 2018) (Figure 6.5).

6.2.1. Definition and Classification of Bullous Pemphigoid

Bullous pemphigoid is an autoimmune blistering illness characterized by the presence of subepidermal blisters that primarily affect the skin of older people. This condition occurs when antibodies are targeted against specific proteins of the basement membrane zone, destroying adhesion between the epidermis and dermis. In the clinical context, it is present as tense blisters that may be pruritic, and the diagnosis largely relies on the correlation of clinical presentation, histopathology, and immunofluorescence. In vesiculobullous disease classification, bullous pemphigoid is typically grouped with other autoimmune conditions, such as pemphigus vulgaris, an intraepidermal blistering disorder with distinct immunological pathways. The differential features are noteworthy because bullous pemphigoid has a more favorable prognosis than the other blistering disorders. Proper and timely diagnosis is crucial to symptom control and prevention of complications of these diseases (Ayvaz et al., 2018; Leuci et al., 2019).

6.2.2. Etiology and Risk Factors

Etiology and risk factors of vesiculobullous diseases, particularly pemphigus and bullous pemphigoid, are multifactorial in nature and intricate. Pemphigus is typically produced due to autoimmune phenomena, through which autoantibodies bind with desmosomal proteins resulting in cell adhesion loss in the epidermis, but bullous pemphigoid presents with autoantibody production against hemidesmosomes, specifically BP230 and BP180. The autoimmune mechanism most commonly arises in older age but sometimes manifests in children as well, indicating a potential genetic susceptibility due to familial behavior (Yayla et al., 2018). Environmental stimuli such as drug exposure or UV light triggers can also augment these disorders via triggering of immune dysregulation. Systemic causes such as stress or comorbid autoimmune conditions may also be contributing factors in these disorders, and thus their etiology should be considered in an integrated manner (Raghuwanshi et al., 2023). Proper management of these risk factors is crucial for accurate diagnosis and control, which in turn leads to better patient outcomes (Figure 6.6).

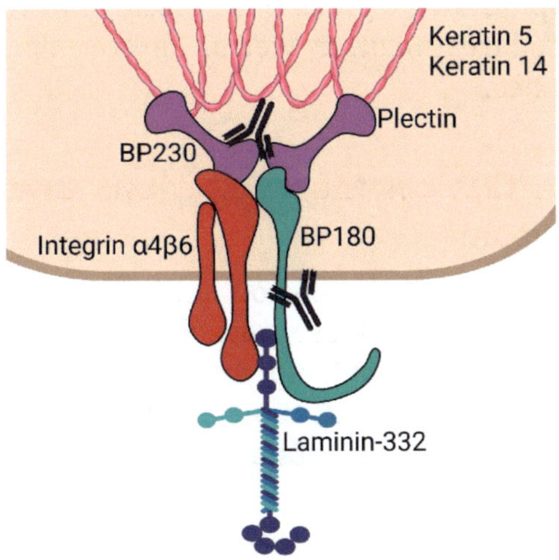

Figure 6.6. Bullous pemphigoid involves the formation of autoantibodies against hemidesmosomes, notably BP230 and BP180.

Source: https://www.mdpi.com/antibodies/antibodies-11-00044/article_deploy/html/images/antibodies-11-00044-g001.png.

6.2.3. Pathophysiology of Bullous Pemphigoid

The pathophysiology of bullous pemphigoid (BP) is basically an autoimmune phenomenon that involves the production of autoantibodies against specific hemidesmosomal proteins, specifically BP230 and BP180. These proteins play a key role in the structural integrity of the epidermal-dermal junction, and their perturbation through the targeting by autoantibodies leads to cellular adhesion followed by subepidermal blister formation. BP clinically appears as tense, large blisters on various regions of the body, usually on an erythematous base, frequently involving flexural regions, the abdomen, and mucous membranes in a subset of patients (Yayla et al., 2018). This autoimmune attack not only further highlights the pivotal role of the immune system in skin integrity but also the complexity of treatment, where systemic steroids are a first-line approach, with localized disease being possibly responsive to topical corticosteroids (Nechba et al., 2015). Understanding this pathophysiologic process is necessary to enable targeted treatments as well as improved patient outcomes.

6.2.4. Clinical Manifestations and Symptoms

The clinical presentation and the signs of vesiculobullous disease, particularly pemphigus and bullous pemphigoid, are characterized by blistering that affects both skin and mucosal surfaces extensively. Blistering in pemphigus vulgaris is preceded by painful oral mucosal lesions, with extensive buccal mucosa involvement seen in 89.7% of patients, reflecting the severity of the condition from the onset and hindering oral hygiene and nutrition (Jayasri, 2012). Conversely, bullous pemphigoid is noted for tense blisters on the skin, with mucosal symptoms in approximately 27% of the cases (Mohanapriya, 2020). The erosive characteristics of the blisters are very morbid as they are prone to secondary infection and discomfort that hinders diet consumption as well as overall quality of life. These presentations need to be understood for the early diagnosis and effective intervention in the control of these autoimmune disorders (Figure 6.7).

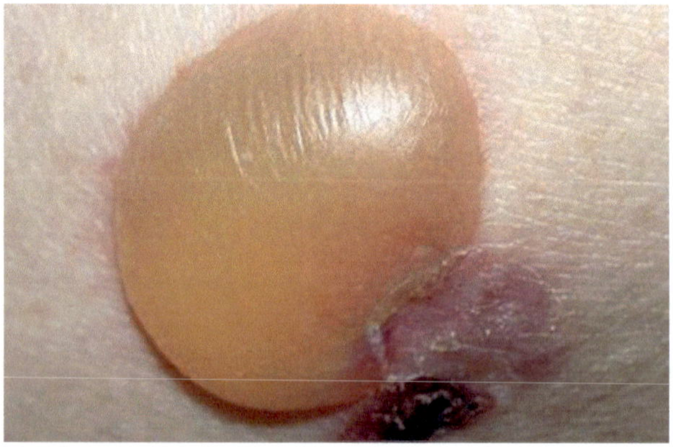

Figure 6.7. The erosive nature of these blisters poses significant morbidity, as they are prone to secondary infections and create discomfort that may hinder both dietary intake and overall quality of life.

Source: https://cached.imagescaler.hbpl.co.uk/resize/scaleWidth/815/cached.offlinehbpl.hbpl.co.uk/news/PGH/3155D832-F947-5C97-88AD22D7B4621DA4.jpg.

6.2.5. Diagnostic Methods and Criteria

Proper diagnosis of vesiculobullous illnesses such as pemphigus and bullous pemphigoid should involve a process that combines clinical evaluation and recent diagnostic techniques. These diseases tend to share similar clinical manifestations, making them hard to distinguish; histopathological examination then becomes crucial to ensure accurate diagnosis. Studies indicate that pemphigus vulgaris is the most frequent vesiculobullous condition, making careful evaluation and classification of vesiculobullous lesions crucial (Patel et al., 2023). Moreover, direct immunofluorescence

(DIF) is a major diagnostic tool in the determination of diagnoses by identifying specific autoantibodies present in such conditions. Studies indicate that 80% of the cases had positive DIF results, highlighting its utility in practice (Kumar et al., 2019). Thus, the concordance of histopathological and immunofluorescence findings not only enhances diagnostic accuracy but also guides treatment plans, ultimately maximizing patient outcomes in patients with these disabling dermatoses.

6.2.6. Treatment Options and Management Strategies

Treatment of vesiculobullous diseases such as pemphigus and bullous pemphigoid must be individualized, considering differential clinical presentations and patient profiles. The therapeutic pillar is corticosteroids, which remain the first-line drug for pemphigus due to their efficacy in immunosuppression.

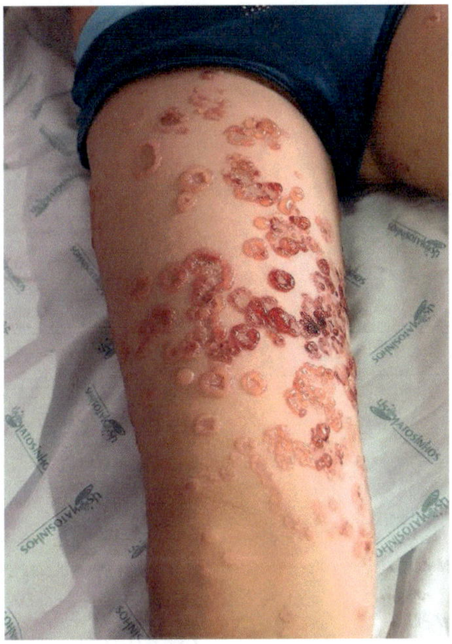

Figure 6.8. Dapsone has been shown to be effective in cases of linear IgA bullous dermatosis, achieving remission in a majority of patients.

Source: https://assets.cureus.com/uploads/figure/file/561090/article_river_72434b30ac7411edb1e41bc19ff4cd0a-Figure1.png.

However, long-term corticosteroid therapy can cause severe side effects; therefore, steroid-sparing agents like mycophenolate mofetil and azathioprine are used by clinicians, particularly in patients who require chronic therapy (Genovese et al., 2019). Similarly, dapsone also proves to be useful in the treatment of linear IgA bullous dermatosis, with remission in the majority of patients (Genovese et al., 2019). The cornerstone of effective treatment thus remains achieving a balance between effective suppression of the immune system and minimizing side effects, ultimately leading to improved outcomes in all age groups and presenting symptoms. Ongoing research on novel therapies is required to enhance treatment modalities in such challenging diseases (Figure 6.8).

6.2.7. Prognosis and Potential Complications

The prognosis of patients who are diagnosed with vesiculobullous diseases such as pemphigus and bullous pemphigoid can significantly vary based on several variables, including the specific subtype of disease, early diagnosis, and provision of adequate treatment. Early management is necessary as delay in treatment can lead to increased morbidity and development of severe complications such as secondary infection and extensive scarring that reduce quality of life. Most significantly, uncontrolled or chronic conditions exert systemic effects, emphasizing the chronic nature of the diseases (Leuci et al., 2019). Moreover, variations in intraepidermal and subepidermal separations, seen in most bullous diseases, affect expected patient outcomes; intraepidermal types tend to be at greater risk for complications due to their aggressive nature (Taş Aygar & Gönül, 2023). Therefore, knowledge of the prognosis and complications of these conditions is crucial to their optimal management and patient education.

Test Your Knowledge

1. How does the clinical presentation of bullous pemphigoid differ from pemphigus?
2. Which histopathological features are characteristic of bullous pemphigoid?

6.3. Diagnosis and Differential Diagnosis

Learning Outcome

1. Understand Importance of Accurate Diagnosis;
2. Explain Clinical Evaluation and Patient History;
3. Focus on Laboratory Tests and Skin Biopsies;
4. Describe Immunofluorescence Studies;
5. Learn Differential Diagnosis of Vesiculobullous Diseases;
6. Discuss Role of Dermatopathology;
7. Know Challenges in Diagnosis;
8. Understand Emerging Diagnostic Techniques.

Diagnosis and differential diagnosis of vesiculobullous diseases, particularly pemphigus and bullous pemphigoid, constitute an n-dimensional process that includes clinical evaluation, histopathological examination, and immunofluorescence testing. Clinically, the illness appears as characteristic vesicles and bullae, and therefore it is necessary to examine the lesions and their morphologic appearance and distribution closely to exclude several conditions. Histopathological examination is important with the anatomic plane of the cleft as the primary point of focus; the lesions are intraepidermal, e.g., pemphigus vulgaris, or subepidermal, as seen in bullous pemphigoid (Ates, 2018). Also, direct immunofluorescence can prove to be informative as it provides a definitive diagnosis through the identification of certain autoantibodies seen in such conditions (Kumar et al., 2019). Thus, a comprehensive evaluation of all these factors is required to achieve proper diagnosis and guide appropriate treatment modalities for the patients afflicted with these diseases.

6.3.1. Importance of Accurate Diagnosis

Proper diagnosis is of utmost importance in vesiculobullous diseases, such as pemphigus and bullous pemphigoid, since it has direct implications regarding the outcome of patients, treatment modalities, and overall outcome. Because of the overlap and diversity of clinical presentations of various mucocutaneous diseases, misdiagnosis will more likely lead to improper therapy that can further compromise the health of patients. For instance, while clinical presentation may initially suggest certain common autoimmune disorders, definitive diagnosis would be based on histopathological analysis and immunofluorescence tests, which distinguish them from one another according to their clinical presentations. The great significance of early and precise diagnosis is emphasized by the fact that morbidity and mortality rates are extremely variable depending on the disease, as well as on treatment speed, as emphasized in recent assessments of autoimmune mucocutaneous disorders (Leuci et al., 2019). Additionally, where oral mucosa presents the first signs, dentists and specialists are primarily accountable for early detection, with their implication in the overall diagnostic process (Silva et al., 2023).

6.3.2. Clinical Evaluation and Patient History

Clinical evaluation and patient history play a key role in the diagnosis of vesiculobullous diseases, such as pemphigus and bullous pemphigoid. A thorough assessment begins with an extensive patient history, noting the onset, duration, and provoking factors for symptoms such as age and sex, as these conditions fall in the older age range of 21–60 years (Adityan, 2007). Notably, clinical observations of blister morphology, such as intraepidermal vs. subepidermal bullae, can guide differential diagnoses. The utility of complete clinical evaluation is also emphasized by clinical presentation versus histopathological and immunofluorescence correlations, achieving a correlation rate of more than 70% in certain studies (Kumar et al., 2019). Such an assessment in multiple dimensions is required not merely to confirm diagnosis but also to value the disease's broader quality-of-life implications and potential systemic associations and direct ideal therapeutic planning and follow-up (Figure 6.9).

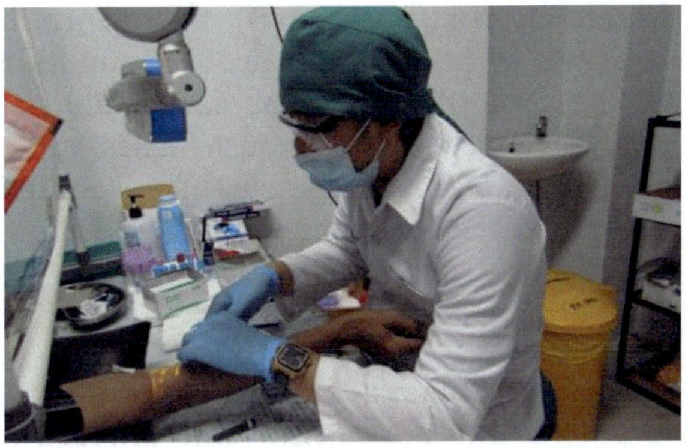

Figure 6.9. Clinical evaluation and patient history play critical roles in diagnosing vesiculobullous diseases, such as pemphigus and bullous pemphigoid.

Source: https://images.unsplash.com/photo-1601839777132-b3f4e455c369?crop=entropy&cs=tinysrgb&fit=max&fm=jpg&ixid=M3w3MDgyMDR8MHwxfHNlYXJjaHwxfHxCdWxsb3VzJTIwZGlzZWFzZXMlMkMlMjBTa2luJTIwYmlvcHN5JTJDJTIwRGlhZ25vc2lzJTJDJTIwVHJlYXRtZW50fGVufDB8MHx8fDE3NDk5MjMxOTZ8MA&ixlib=rb-4.1.0&q=80&w=500&?utm_source=numberanalytics&utm_medium=referral.

6.3.3. Laboratory Tests and Skin Biopsies

Laboratory tests and skin biopsies form a crucial basis in the diagnosis of vesiculobullous diseases such as pemphigus and bullous pemphigoid to identify the nature of the condition accurately. Skin biopsies are needed to identify the level of skin separation, either intraepidermal or subepidermal, that is crucial for differentiation between these autoimmune disorders. Furthermore, examination of the inflammatory cell component and acantholysis is significant and provides insight into the disease process and pathology (Ates, 2018). Direct immunofluorescence (DIF) is yet another essential laboratory investigation that enhances diagnostic precision, particularly if clinical presentations are heterogeneous or atypical (Mohanapriya, 2020). By integrating the results of histopathological examinations with those of DIF, clinicians can establish a definitive diagnosis, which in turn makes way for appropriate treatment regimens and eventually improved patient outcomes.

6.3.4. Immunofluorescence Studies

Immunofluorescence studies have an important role to play in diagnosing and differential diagnosis of vesiculobullous diseases, particularly pemphigus and bullous pemphigoid.

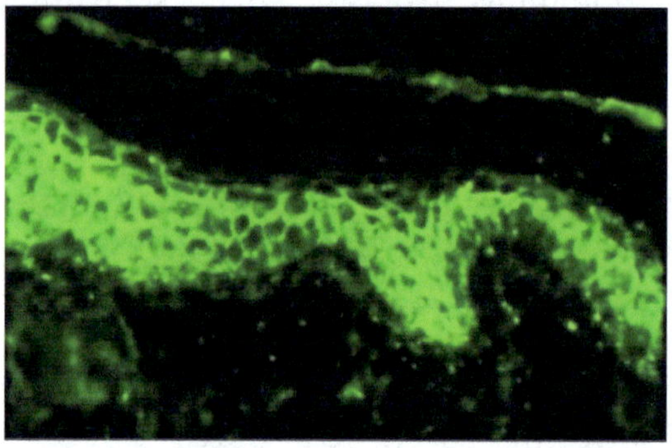

Figure 6.10. Immunofluorescence studies serve a crucial role in the diagnosis and differentiation of vesiculobullous diseases, particularly pemphigus and bullous pemphigoid.

Source: https://www.researchgate.net/publication/7801835/figure/fig4/AS:281123633549356@1444036506042/Direct-immunofluorescence-of-pemphigus-vulgaris-PV-IgG-and-complement-component.png.

These techniques allow for the determination of specific autoantibodies in the skin, thereby enhancing the clinical relevance of the observed lesions. An example would be direct immunofluorescence (DIF), which may accentuate the deposition of complement proteins and immunoglobulins, a hallmark of bullous pemphigoid and pemphigus vulgaris. DIF was positive in 80% of cases of pemphigus vulgaris in clinical practice, making it a valuable tool for diagnosis in distinguishing the condition from bullous conditions with comparable presentations (Kumar et al., 2019). DIF has also been useful in differential diagnosis between bullous pemphigoid and epidermolysis bullosa acquisita, highlighting its applicability to clinical practice (Ali et al., 2021). Therefore, inclusion of immunofluorescence tests in diagnostic protocols is indispensable for accurate diagnosis and treatment of such challenging skin conditions (Figure 6.10).

6.3.5. Differential Diagnosis of Vesiculobullous Diseases

Vesiculobullous diseases constitute a category of illnesses that might present with blistering cutaneous lesions, and a subtle differential diagnosis is needed to deliver adequate treatment. The challenge is faced by the inconsistent clinical presentation of conditions such as pemphigus and bullous pemphigoid, in which atypical presentations obscure the underlying condition. Accurate diagnosis relies on an interdisciplinary approach of integrating clinical presentation with histopathological detail and direct immunofluorescence (DIF) testing. As seen, the comprehensive assessment that brings together the aforementioned diagnostic modalities yields a more reliable result with DIF being particularly important when histopathological results are inadequate, to allow proper classification of immunobullous diseases (Mohanapriya, 2020). Pemphigus, in addition, is characterized by suprabasilar blisters owing to autoimmune activity, differentiated from other vesiculobullous disorders by careful examination (Takayama & Busch, 1991). Thus, a broad differential diagnosis is necessary to forecast the outcome and frame effective treatment strategies.

6.3.6. Role of Dermatopathology

Dermatopathology plays an important part in the clinical diagnosis and management of vesiculobullous diseases, such as pemphigus and bullous pemphigoid, through correlating clinical data with histopathological and immunofluorescence testing. The multiplicative nature of blistering illnesses that can have varying clinical presentations makes accurate diagnosis challenging. Consequently, dermatopathologists make direct immunofluorescence (DIF) an important weapon to assist in classifying these conditions, especially when clinical and histologic presentations are ambiguous. As demonstrated in the literature, an integration of clinical picture, histopathology inspection, and DIF yields more accurate diagnosis, ultimately contributing to successful treatment regimens and improving patient outcomes (Mohanapriya, 2020). Moreover, identification of the pathology of the involved diseases—i.e., the degree of blister formation—permits practitioners to classify diverse subtypes and treat accordingly (Taş Aygar & Gönül, 2023). Thus, dermatopathology plays a vital role in their treatment (Figure 6.11).

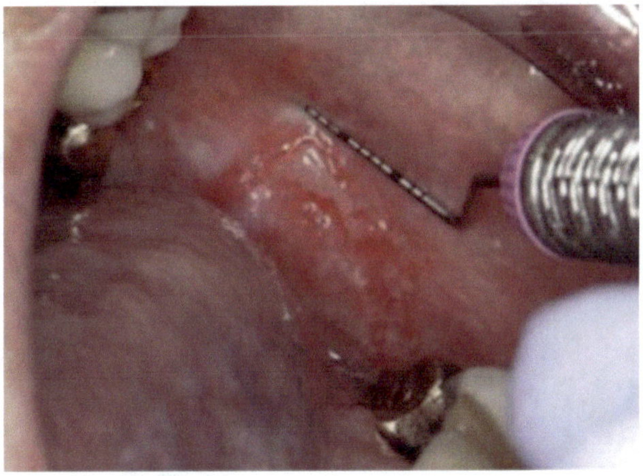

Figure 6.11. Dermatopathology plays a crucial role in the diagnosis and management of vesiculobullous diseases, such as pemphigus and bullous pemphigoid, by integrating clinical findings with histopathological and immunofluorescence studies.

Source: https://www.tandfonline.com/cms/asset/fd694e99-f8ee-4440-9119-cdde276c039c/ucda_a_2422148_f0003_oc.jpg.

6.3.7. Challenges in Diagnosis

Diagnosis of vesiculobullous disease, particularly pemphigus and bullous pemphigoid, is difficult because they have a similar clinical presentation and gradations in their presentation. Clinicians often have to grapple with distinguishing between numerous subepithelial blistering conditions, especially if oral lesions and skin diseases can mimic other diseases. This ambiguity is compounded by the requirement for precise immunological tests to obtain the diagnosis, as the onset of autoantibodies plays a major role in such conditions (Abhinaya & Arvind, 2020). Additionally, the potentially catastrophic result of an incorrect diagnosis, such as complications due to complex treatment or disease worsening, emphasizes the need for appropriate evaluation (Ojha & Yadav, 2020). Therefore, while early diagnosis is necessary for effective management, the multifactorial nature of vesiculobullous diseases necessitates thorough and sometimes multifactorial diagnostic examination.

6.3.8. Emerging Diagnostic Techniques

The development of newer diagnostic techniques has drastically changed the diagnosis of vesiculobullous disorders, particularly pemphigus and bullous pemphigoid. Complete diagnostic modalities such as direct immunofluorescence, electron microscopy, and molecular genetic analysis have optimized our understanding of these autoimmune diseases. Direct immunofluorescence helps demonstrate the presence of autoantibodies against epithelial antigens and plays a crucial role in distinguishing among various blistering diseases (Adityan, 2007). Furthermore, the application of enzyme-linked immunosorbent assays (ELISAs) has facilitated the identification of specific antibodies associated with such diseases, thus improving diagnostic efficacy (Leuci et al., 2019). Not only do such developments go toward making proper diagnoses, but they also allow for better disease progression and treatment outcomes monitoring. Thus, combining these novel diagnostic approaches is needed to maximize patient outcomes by means of early and accurate detection of the underlying autoimmune mechanisms.

Test Your Knowledge

1. What diseases must be considered in the differential diagnosis of pemphigus vulgaris?
2. How is dermatitis herpetiformis differentiated from other bullous diseases?

6.4. Treatment and Management Strategies

Learning Outcome

1. Understand Overview of Treatment Goals;
2. Explain Pharmacological Treatments;
3. Focus on Non-pharmacological Management Strategies;
4. Describe Role of Patient Education and Support;
5. Learn Monitoring and Follow-up Care;
6. Discuss Management of Complications;
7. Know Impact of Lifestyle Changes on Disease Management;
8. Understand Multidisciplinary Approach to Treatment.

Treatment and management of vesiculobullous disorders like pemphigus and bullous pemphigoid necessitate a general approach specifically tailored to the patient's clinical presentation, in addition to the prognosis of the disease.

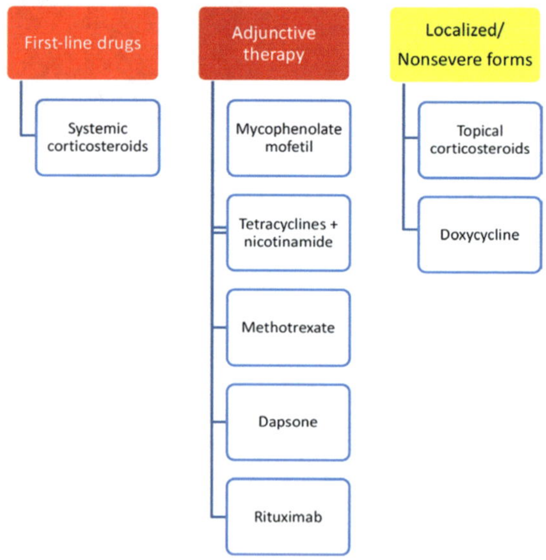

Figure 6.12. Corticosteroids for treatment and management strategies for vesiculobullous diseases.

Source: https://www.researchgate.net/publication/342846748/figure/fig7/AS:911784135389186@1594397686584/Treatment-options-for-bullous-pemphigoid.ppm.

A prompt and accurate diagnosis is paramount, given the complexities entailed in distinguishing between various autoimmune disorders manifesting on the cutaneous and mucosal surfaces (Leuci et al., 2019). Corticosteroids remain a cornerstone in the treatment of these diseases, often supported by immunosuppressants to inhibit disease activity and prevent relapses. Further, new therapies such as biologic agents are under study to disrupt targeted mechanisms in the pathogenesis of these diseases, with promise to treat refractory disease (Silva et al., 2023). Besides these, comprehensive care also entails the prevention of secondary complications such as infections and skin integrity, necessitating the need for a multidisciplinary approach to optimize patient outcomes and quality of life in those who have these disabling diseases (Figure 6.12).

6.4.1. Overview of Treatment Goals

The clinical goals of vesiculobullous disorders, i.e., pemphigus and bullous pemphigoid, are to achieve control of the disease, restore symptomatology, and maximize the quality of life in the patient. The primary goals are the suppression of autoantibody production, healing of cutaneous lesions, and prevention of complications such as infection or dysphagia due to oral disease. Effective management strategies have commonly involved the use of systemic immunosuppressive therapy, which, while capable of controlling disease activity, is most commonly supported by a risk for adverse side effects, as described in populations where rates of up to 50% of patients were noted with complications of azathioprine treatment (Al-Johani, 2010). Moreover, local agent therapy can alleviate symptoms, yet with unpredictable efficacy depending on the specific vesiculobullous disease (Diercks & Pas, 2022). Lastly, an individualized treatment plan is most crucial to optimize therapeutic outcomes and ensure greater patient well-being.

6.4.2. Pharmacological Treatments (e.g., Corticosteroids and Immunosuppressants)

Pharmacologic vesiculobullous disease treatment, particularly pemphigus and bullous pemphigoid, relies predominantly on the use of corticosteroids and immunosuppressants. Corticosteroids are considered a first-line treatment due to their potent anti-inflammatory effects, which control well the painful blistering of these conditions. However, prolonged corticosteroid use is associated with high risks, such as adrenal suppression and susceptibility to infections. To prevent these, clinicians will often use immunosuppressive agents, such as azathioprine or mycophenolate mofetil, which not only enhance the therapeutic efficacy but also allow for a lower corticosteroid dose. Specifically, treatment planning can be complicated by underlying hematologic malignancies in some patients, since the latter conditions are recognized to have a profound influence on immune function and increase the prevalence of autoimmune complications (Leuci et al., 2019; Maglie et al., 2020). Careful assessment of each patient's individual circumstances is thus of prime importance to guarantee optimal therapeutic outcome in vesiculobullous diseases (Figure 6.13).

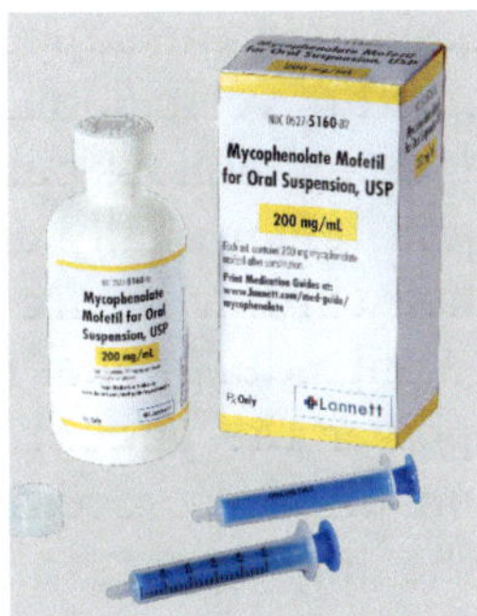

Figure 6.13. Mycophenolate mofetil.

Source: https://www.lannett.com/wp-content/uploads/2021/09/Mycophenolate-Oral-Suspension-200mg-mL-160mL-Package-Image.png.

6.4.3. Non-pharmacological Management Strategies

In the management of vesiculobullous conditions such as pemphigus and bullous pemphigoid, non-pharmacologic interventions play a crucial part in quality of life enhancement for patients and complement standard therapy. Among these interventions are patient education, topical skin hygiene procedures, and psychological counseling, all of which can moderately decrease symptoms and alleviate the psychosocial burden of chronic cutaneous diseases. Focusing on gentle skin cleansing, the application of non-irritating moisturizers, and avoiding known offenders can lower the frequency and severity of flare-ups. Additionally, the inclusion of support groups gives patients emotional strength, allowing them to deal with the distress these conditions tend to create, as they tend to occur in delicate areas such as the oral mucosa, resulting in pain and functional impairment (Al-Johani, 2010). Also, in the education of the potential side effects of pharmacologic therapy to encourage the requirement for combination of these approaches toward an all-encompassing treatment plan.

6.4.4. Role of Patient Education and Support

Adept patient education and support are critical in the management of vesiculobullous diseases such as pemphigus and bullous pemphigoid. The illnesses are quite emotionally and physically taxing due to their chronic nature and potential complications. Long educational programs can be able to empower the patient by informing them about their disease processes, treatment options, and the importance of adhering to prescribed therapies. It is also important for patients to be aware of drug side effects, such as the risk of drug-induced flares, as diseases can rapidly change according to these changes, as seen in recurrent drug-induced BP (Ambur et al., 2021). Besides, treatment of concomitant symptoms, like oral symptoms of desquamation of the gingiva, can make early intervention methods and quality of life better (Stoopler et al., 2003). Thus, the development of an educated patient base is significant to significantly enhance outcomes and improve general well-being in patients affected by such diseases (Figure 6.14).

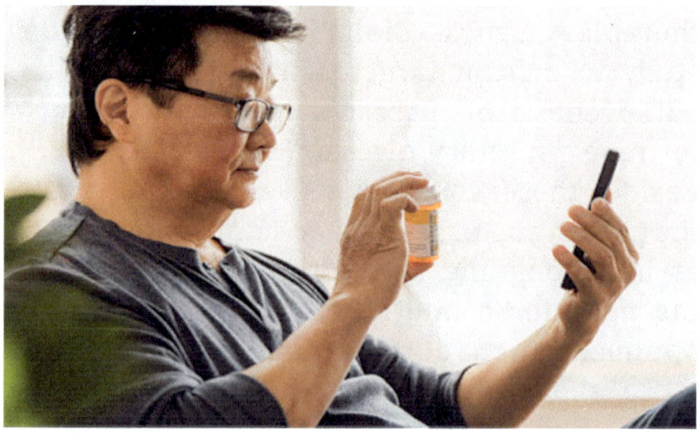

Figure 6.14. Effective patient education and support are crucial in managing vesiculobullous diseases such as pemphigus and bullous pemphigoid.

Source: https://images.ctfassets.net/1ny4yoiyrqia/3q5CzgmDszD0kaK0KZbytK/5d2998152013aba8b3225256afe902b6/bullous-pemphigoid-self-care-side-effects.png?w=450&h=450.

6.4.5. Monitoring and Follow-up Care

Monitoring and follow-up are essential in the treatment of vesiculobullous disorders such as pemphigus and bullous pemphigoid. Autoimmune in nature, these conditions need continuous evaluation to gauge the response to treatment and alter therapies based on need to minimize complications. For instance, patients must be monitored with serological tests from time to time to measure the levels of pathogenic autoantibodies, particularly desmoglein 1 and 3, which have a central role in disease expression. Employing enzyme-linked immunosorbent assays (ELISAs) enables practitioners to assess the degree of disease and hence plan management (Diercks & Pas, 2022). Moreover, indirect immunofluorescence microscopy can also assist in following circulating antibodies, thereby augmenting diagnostic accuracy during follow-up visits. Dermatological maintenance checks are also necessary to preserve skin integrity and efficient control of blistering, with a better quality of life for the patient and potential reduction in disease morbidity secondary to early clinical treatment (Diercks & Pas, 2022).

6.4.6. Management of Complications

Complications of vesiculobullous diseases, such as pemphigus and bullous pemphigoid, must be controlled through an interrelated approach to both clinical diagnosis and pathophysiologic mechanisms involved. Complications range from secondary infection and fluid loss to adverse reactions to systemic therapy, making close and individualized treatment strategies necessary. Complete management often includes the use of immunosuppressive therapy to repress disease activity while minimizing potential for complications of treatment. Histopathological study, as stated, is crucial to diagnose accurately and guide treatment, enabling timely intervention that can optimally better the patient outcome (Patel et al., 2023). Besides, awareness of the history of the disease, for instance, analogies drawn from the traditional Ayurvedic system such as Vishphot, can provide richness to existing treatment modalities, enabling an improved knowledge base of vesiculobullous disorders (Raghuwanshi et al., 2023). Adequate management of these complexities is crucial in improving patient quality of life and minimizing morbidity related to such conditions (Figure 6.15).

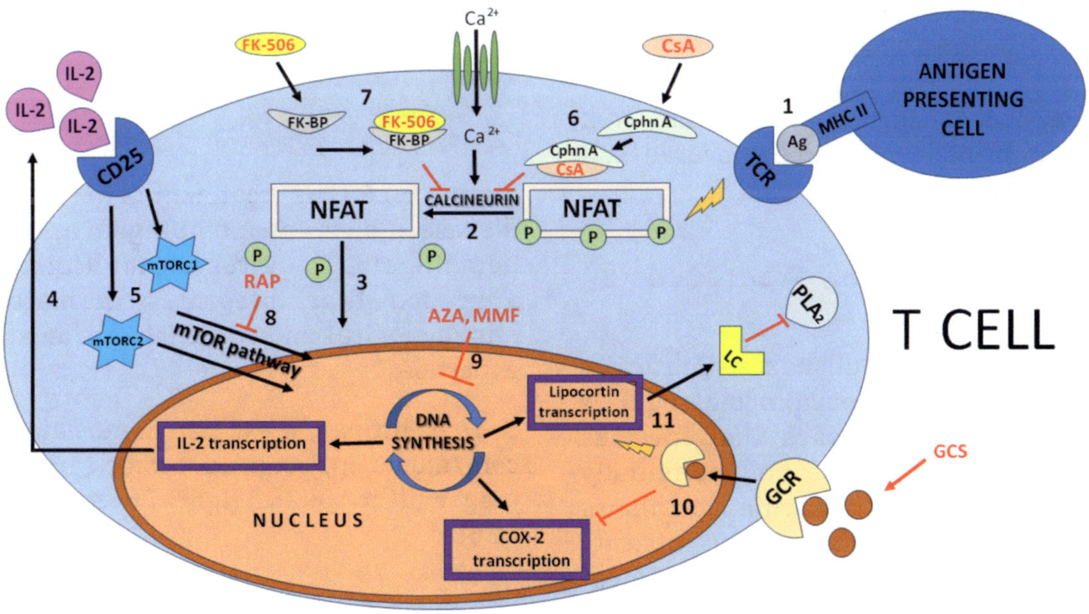

Figure 6.15. The use of immunosuppressive agents to control disease activity while minimizing the potential for treatment-related complications.

Source: https://pub.mdpi-res.com/jcm/jcm-12-06935/article_deploy/html/images/jcm-12-06935-g001.png?1699172726.

6.4.7. Impact of Lifestyle Changes on Disease Management

Lifestyle changes play an important role in managing vesiculobullous diseases like pemphigus and bullous pemphigoid. Evidence suggests that psychological well-being and stress are major contributing factors towards the deterioration of autoimmune diseases, which have been found to be linked to emotional and behavioral processes. As suggested by recent studies, the oral mucosa might present symptoms of stress-related illness, substantiating the theory that patients must be treated in a manner that includes psychological care as part of multimodal treatment (Avramova & Bonev, 2024). In addition, the premise of healthier lifestyle choices, such as good nutrition and abstinence from smoking or irritating causes, may minimize the severity and rate of disease occurrences. Of note, systemic patients are more likely to carry a higher incidence of mucosal lesions within the oral mucosa, again pointing towards the value of treating not just the skin but also the mucosal manifestations (Suliman et al., 2011). Through the encouragement of these beneficial changes, patients can gain both quality-of-life improvement overall and improved treatment results.

6.4.8. Multidisciplinary Approach to Treatment

Management of vesiculobullous disease such as pemphigus and bullous pemphigoid requires a multidisciplinary approach that involves dermatologic, immunologic, and potentially rheumatologic input. Such coordination allows for widespread management of the intricate pathologies of the illnesses, with development of blisters secondary to destructive autoimmune processes. Successful therapy protocols typically involve a therapy regimen of systemic corticosteroids and immunosuppressants. This is dependent on the individual patient requirements and severity of the illness. Further, consultation with dermatologists for skin care and rheumatologists for co-morbid autoimmune disease management enhances patient outcomes through the treatment of short- and long-term complications of the disease. As stressed, the immunological aspects, such as the antibodies to the individual antigens, must be elucidated more clearly to effectively diagnose and manage the diseases, persistently upholding the team method of treatment (Ayvaz et al., 2018; Taş Aygar & Gönül, 2023) (Figure 6.16).

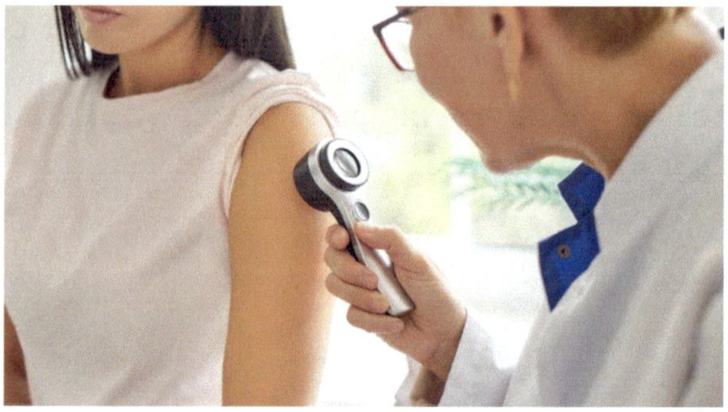

Figure 6.16. The treatment of vesiculobullous diseases, such as pemphigus and bullous pemphigoid, requires a multidisciplinary approach that integrates dermatological, immunological, and potentially rheumatological expertise.

Source: https://www.britishjournalofnursing.com/media/jpejscdh/adobestock_1339561165.jpeg?width=1002&height=564&v=1dbcfc8cf0ff560.

Test Your Knowledge

1. What supportive measures are important in managing pemphigus patients?
2. What are the potential complications of long-term corticosteroid use?

SUMMARY

Vesiculobullous diseases, and most notably pemphigus and bullous pemphigoid, present a significant challenge for dermatological and immunological medicine. These autoimmune conditions not only adversely affect patients' quality of life through their incapacitating symptoms but also attest to the complexity of immune system malfunction. Advances in diagnostic technology, such as indirect immunofluorescence microscopy, have enhanced our ability to identify individual autoantibodies, which are crucial for accurate diagnosis and treatment of these conditions (Diercks & Pas, 2022). Moreover, novel therapeutic strategies continue to emerge, with improved patient outcomes while mitigating the inherent risk of employing immunosuppressive medications. More studies are needed to decipher the pathophysiology of these diseases so that potentially more effective and tailored treatment plans can be developed that can lower morbidity and enhance the overall well-being of the patients, thus making further studies important in this context.

In the summary of the vital concerns regarding vesiculobullous diseases such as pemphigus and bullous pemphigoid, it is significant to state their classification as autoimmune disorders that result in blistering of the skin. Pemphigus vulgaris has been identified as the most common type, with significant occurrence among females between the age group of 21–60 years, revealing the age-related effect of these diseases (Adityan, 2007). The incidence of the research that was carried out was found to be low for overall incidence, yet the psychological and physical effect on the victims may be substantial. Diagnostic tests like Tzanck smears and immunofluorescence were found to be pivotal in differentiating these diseases, as were findings indicating bullous pemphigoid patients possessing increased levels of serum APRIL, which would mean its potential as a biomarker and therapeutic intervention (Watanabe et al., 2007). These advances highlight the imperative to further study the pathogenesis and the therapy of these multifactorial disorders.

KEY TERMS FROM THIS CHAPTER

- Heterogeneous group
- Blisters
- Stimuli
- Pemphigus
- Autoimmune diseases
- Subepidermal splitting
- Epidermis
- Autoantibodies
- Bullae
- Epidermal adhesion
- Vesiculobullous diseases
- Bullous pemphigoid
- Pemphigus foliaceous
- Nomenclature
- Cell adhesion
- Desmogleins

CRITICAL THINKING QUESTIONS

1. **Which of the following is an example of an autoimmune vesiculobullous disorder?**
   a. Impetigo
   b. Pemphigus vulgaris
   c. Herpes simplex
   d. Scabies
2. **The Nikolsky sign is positive in which of the following conditions?**
   a. Bullous pemphigoid
   b. Herpes zoster
   c. Pemphigus vulgaris
   d. Erythema multiforme
3. **The autoantibodies in pemphigus vulgaris are directed against:**
   a. Desmoglein 1 and 3
   b. Hemidesmosomes
   c. Collagen type VII
   d. Keratin
4. **Which of the following diseases shows subepidermal blistering?**
   a. Pemphigus vulgaris
   b. Bullous pemphigoid
   c. Impetigo
   d. Darier disease
5. **Which of the following is true about bullous pemphigoid?**
   a. Occurs mostly in young adults
   b. Involves mucosal surfaces more than the skin
   c. Blisters are tense and not easily ruptured
   d. Has antibodies against desmoglein 3

Short Answer Questions

1. What are the primary autoantibodies involved in pemphigus vulgaris?
2. Which layer of the skin is affected in pemphigus vulgaris?
3. What are the target antigens in bullous pemphigoid?
4. What is the age group most commonly affected by bullous pemphigoid?
5. What are the major clinical signs used in diagnosing vesiculobullous diseases?
6. How is a Tzanck smear helpful in diagnosis?
7. What is the first-line treatment for pemphigus vulgaris?
8. What are the roles of immunosuppressants in autoimmune blistering diseases?

Answers to Critical Thinking Questions

1. (b); 2. (c); 3. (a); 4. (b); 5. (c)

REFERENCES

1. Leuci, S., Ruoppo, E., Adamo, D., Calabria, E., & Mignogna, M. D. (2019). Oral autoimmune vesicobullous diseases: Classification, clinical presentations, molecular mechanisms, diagnostic algorithms, and management. *Periodontology 2000*, *80*(1), 77–88. https://doi.org/10.1111/prd.12263(accessed on 23rd July 2025).
2. Adityan, M. S. (2007). A clinicopathological study of autoimmune vesiculobullous diseases. https://core.ac.uk/download/235664077.pdf (accessed on 23rd July 2025).
3. Al-Johani, K. (2010). Outcomes of therapy of immunologically-mediated diseases of the oral mucosa. https://core.ac.uk/download/1849368.pdf (accessed on 23rd July 2025).
4. Ali, J., Ali, S. M., Aslam, A., et al. (2021). Morphological spectrum of vesiculobullous skin lesions: An institutional perspective. https://core.ac.uk/download/478214654.pdf (accessed on 23rd July 2025).
5. Suliman, N. M., Astrøm, A. N., Ali, R. W., Salman, H., & Johannessen, A. C. (2011). Oral mucosal lesions in skin diseased patients attending a dermatologic clinic: a cross-sectional study in Sudan. *BMC oral health*, *11*, 24. https://doi.org/10.1186/1472-6831-11-24(accessed on 23rd July 2025).
6. Ambur, A. B., Nathoo, R., & Saeed, S. (2021). A Case of Drug-Induced Bullous Pemphigoid With an Isomorphic Response and Updated Review of Koebnerization in Bullous Diseases. *Cureus*, *13*(12), e20647. https://doi.org/10.7759/cureus.20647(accessed on 23rd July 2025).
7. Budianti, Windy Keumala; Fitri, Eyleny Meisyah; Meilinda, Puti Rineska; Novianto, Endi; Anindya, Shafira; and Debinta, Arlha Aporia (2021) "Clinical characteristics and treatment regimen of pemphigus patients: A retrospective study," *Journal of General - Procedural Dermatology and Venereology Indonesia*: Vol. 5: Iss. 2, Article 2. DOI: 10.19100/jdvi.v5i2.235 (accessed on 23rd July 2025).
8. Abhinaya, L. M., & Arvind, M. (2020). mmune Mediated Sub-Epithelial Blistering Disorders: Case Series. *The Journal of Contemporary Issues in Business and Government*, *26*(2), 1766–1777. Retrieved from https://cibgp.com/index.php/1323-6903/article/view/443 (accessed on 23rd July 2025).
9. Watanabe, R., Fujimoto, M., Yazawa, N., Nakashima, H., Asashima, N., Kuwano, Y., Tada, Y., Maruyama, N., Okochi, H., & Tamaki, K. (2007). Increased serum levels of a proliferation-inducing ligand in patients with bullous pemphigoid. *Journal of dermatological science*, *46*(1), 53–60. https://doi.org/10.1016/j.jdermsci.2006.12.008 (accessed on 23rd July 2025).
10. Ayvaz, H. H., Gönül, M., & Atay, S. (2018). Bullous Systemic Lupus Erythematosus and Cicatricial Pemphigoid. InTech. doi: 10.5772/intechopen.74069(accessed on 23rd July 2025).
11. Ates, D. (2018). Histomorphology and direct immunofluorescence findings of autoimmune bullous disease. https://core.ac.uk/download/322435686.pdf (accessed on 23rd July 2025).
12. Kumar, S. S., Atla, B., Patnala, G. P., Sarat Srinivas, K. S., Samantra, S., & Priyanka, A. L. N. (2019). Clinical, histopathological and immunofluorescent study of vesicobullous lesions of skin. *International Journal of Research in Medical Sciences*, *7*(4), 1288–1295. https://doi.org/10.18203/2320-6012.ijrms20191341 (accessed on 23rd July 2025).

13. Taş Aygar, G., & Gönül, M. (2023). Skin Blister Formation and Subepidermal Bullous Disorders. IntechOpen. doi: 10.5772/intechopen.110472(accessed on 23rd July 2025).
14. Nechba, R.B., Kadiri, M.E., Bennani-Ziatni, M., Zeggwagh, A.A., & Mesfioui, A. (2015). Difficulty in managing polypharmacy in the elderly: Case report and review of the literature. *Journal of Clinical Gerontology and Geriatrics, 6*, 30-33.(accessed on 23rd July 2025).
15. Avramova, N. T., & Bonev, B. K. (2024). The Role of Psychogenic Factors in the Etiopathogenesis of Autoimmune Disorders in the Oral Cavity. *Journal of Mind and Medical Sciences, 11*(1), 10-16. https://doi.org/10.22543/2392-7674.1450(accessed on 23rd July 2025).
16. Takayama, A. K., & Busch, D. S. (1991). Pemphigus: An autoimmune complex in dogs and cats. https://core.ac.uk/download/38907930.pdf (accessed on 23rd July 2025).
17. Silva, W. R., de Lima-Souza, R. A., Silva, L. P., Filho, L. G., Montenegro, L. T., & Iglesias, D. P. (2023). Mucocutaneous diseases with manifestations in the head and neck region: 24 years of experience in a Dermatology service. *Medicina oral, patologia oral y cirugia bucal, 28*(2), e126–e130. https://doi.org/10.4317/medoral.25549(accessed on 23rd July 2025).
18. Stoopler, E. T., Sollecito, T. P., & DeRossi, S. S. (2003). Desquamative gingivitis: early presenting symptom of mucocutaneous disease. *Quintessence international (Berlin, Germany : 1985), 34*(8), 582–586.(accessed on 23rd July 2025).
19. Diercks, G. F. H., & Pas, H. H. (2022). Indirect immunofluorescence microscopy. https://core.ac.uk/download/589894592.pdf (accessed on 23rd July 2025).
20. Maglie, R., Genovese, G., Solimani, F., Guglielmo, A., Pileri, A., Portelli, F., Hertl, M., Marzano, A. V., & Antiga, E. (2020). Immune-Mediated Dermatoses in Patients with Haematological Malignancies: A Comprehensive Review. *American journal of clinical dermatology, 21*(6), 833–854. https://doi.org/10.1007/s40257-020-00553-9(accessed on 23rd July 2025).
21. Yayla, D., Hizli, P., & Yayla, Y. (2018). Bullous Pemphigoid. InTech. doi: 10.5772/intechopen.73543(accessed on 23rd July 2025).
22. Jayasri, J. (2012). A clinic-epidemiological study of oral lesions in acquired bullous dermatoses. https://core.ac.uk/download/235664032.pdf (accessed on 23rd July 2025).
23. Genovese, G., Venegoni, L., Fanoni, D., Muratori, S., Berti, E., & Marzano, A. V. (2019). Linear IgA bullous dermatosis in adults and children: a clinical and immunopathological study of 38 patients. *Orphanet journal of rare diseases, 14*(1), 115. https://doi.org/10.1186/s13023-019-1089-2(accessed on 23rd July 2025).
24. Mathew, T. (2007). A validation of ELISA test for detection of desmoglein 1 & 3 antibodies as a diagnostic test of pemphigus. https://core.ac.uk/download/235664148.pdf (accessed on 23rd July 2025).
25. Mohanapriya, L. (2020). Clinical and immunohistopathological study of dermatological lesions in a tertiary care centre. https://core.ac.uk/download/386332433.pdf (accessed on 23rd July 2025).
26. Mortazavi, H., Baharvand, M., Rahmani, S., & Safi, Y. (2016). Diagnostic features of common oral ulcerative lesions: An updated decision tree. https://core.ac.uk/download/194242479.pdf (accessed on 23rd July 2025).

27. Ojha, N., & Yadav, O. P. (2020). Benign mucous membrane pemphigoid: A case report. Int Healthc Res J. 2020;4(2):34-37 https://core.ac.uk/download/327113213.pdf (accessed on 23rd July 2025).

28. Porro, A. M., Caetano, L.deV., Maehara, L.deS., & Enokihara, M. M. (2014). Non-classical forms of pemphigus: pemphigus herpetiformis, IgA pemphigus, paraneoplastic pemphigus and IgG/IgA pemphigus. *Anais brasileiros de dermatologia*, *89*(1), 96–106. https://doi.org/10.1590/abd1806-4841.20142459(accessed on 23rd July 2025).

29. Patel, K., Vasudha Bhagat, Jahanvi Vyas, & Prashant Patel. (2023). Histomorphological study of vesiculobullous lesions of skin: a study of 66 cases at tertiary care center. *International Journal of Research in Medical Sciences*, *11*(2), 606–610. https://doi.org/10.18203/2320-6012.ijrms20230172(accessed on 23rd July 2025).

30. Vivek Raghuwanshi, Sushil Kumar Jha, Suman Prasad Sahu, Neha Yadav, Sujeet Kumar. Bullous Disorder - An Ayurvedic review study. J Ayurveda Integr Med Sci [Internet]. 2023 Jun. 28 [cited 2026 Jan. 20];8(5):129-34. Available from: https://jaims.in/jaims/article/view/2420(accessed on 23rd July 2025).

CONNECTIVE TISSUE DISEASES

7

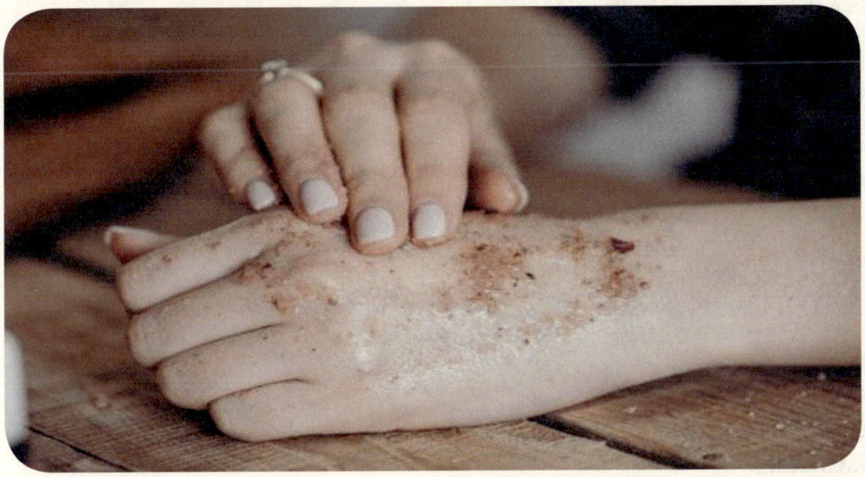

Introduction

The connective tissue diseases, including lupus, dermatomyositis, and scleroderma, are a diverse array of autoimmune diseases that affect patients' quality of life and health in a substantial manner. The diseases often have overlapping clinical features, and thus, diagnosis and treatment are complicated. For instance, Sharp and colleagues' discovery of mixed connective tissue disease (MCTD) in 1972 not only highlighted the interrelation and similarity of most autoimmune rheumatic diseases but also sparked a number of controversies regarding whether MCTD represents an independent disease (Ciang et al., 2017). Furthermore, interstitial lung disease (ILD) is one of the prevalent conditions associated with these connective tissue diseases and poses additional challenges due to its high morbidity and mortality risk (Castelino & Varga, 2010). Comprehension of the complex interactions among these diseases is vital for the formulation of effective therapeutic protocols and enhancing patient outcomes, thus emphasizing the need for further research in this area.

LEARNING OBJECTIVES

After studying this chapter, you will be able to:

1. Understand Systemic Lupus Erythematosus (SLE);
2. Explain Dermatomyositis;
3. Describe Scleroderma.

7.1. Systemic Lupus Erythematosus (SLE)

Learning Outcome

1. Understand the Definition and Classification of Lupus;
2. Explain Etiology and Risk Factors;
3. Focus on Common Symptoms and Manifestations;
4. Describe Diagnostic Criteria and Methods;
5. Learn Treatment Options and Management Strategies;
6. Discuss Complications Associated with Lupus;
7. Know Psychological Impact on Patients;
8. Understand the Role of Lifestyle Modifications.

Systemic Lupus Erythematosus (SLE) is the most complex and multifaceted autoimmune disease within the category of connective tissue diseases. With the development of autoantibodies and an extensive range of clinical manifestations, SLE can affect nearly any organ system, leading to renal dysfunction, cutaneous manifestations, and neurological impairment.

The convergence of environmental stimulus and genetic susceptibility adds to the etiologic confusion of diseases, complicating the process of diagnosis and treatment. As Febyani et al. (2011) emphasize, the presence of overlapping syndromes and features such as sclerodermatomyositis shows how complicated it is to delineate SLE from other autoimmune conditions.

Furthermore, gastrointestinal disturbances, like dysphagia, may happen as a consequence of SLE's inflammatory processes that significantly impact the patient's nutritional status and quality of life, as in Di Piazza et al. (2017). It is crucial to understand SLE's multifarious manifestations to better devise effective treatment strategies and improve patient outcomes as a whole (Figure 7.1).

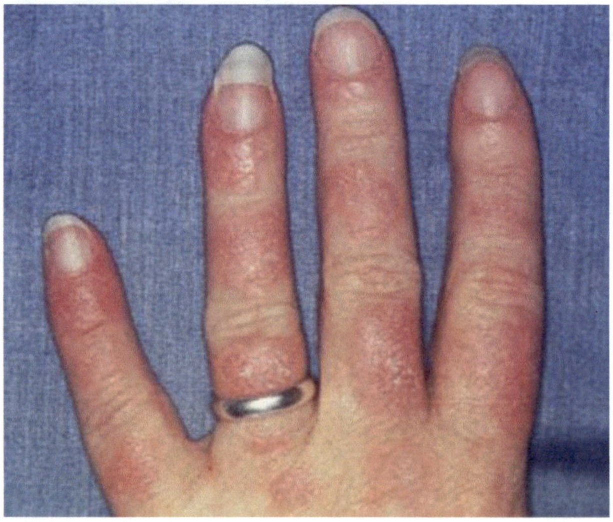

Figure 7.1. Systemic lupus erythematosus (SLE) represents one of the most complex and multifaceted autoimmune diseases within the category of connective tissue disorders.

Source: https://img.medscapestatic.com/pi/meds/ckb/24/39224tn.jpg.

7.1.1. Definition and Classification of Lupus

Lupus, an autoimmunity disease of complex nature, is best described by systemic lupus erythematosus (SLE), affecting all organ systems. The lupus classification includes a number of subforms, most frequent among them being SLE, often appearing with features such as arthralgia, rash, and fatigue, but also with severe forms like nephritis and nervous system involvement. Pain is particularly conspicuous in patients, as it may occur due to musculoskeletal involvement and plays an important role in their general distress and compromised quality of life (Di Franco et al., 2015). In addition, some biomarkers, including anti-C1q antibodies, have been associated with renal disease activity in SLE patients, suggesting their possible use as clinical markers for the observation of disease activity and organ damage (Makda, 2013). Understanding of these definitions and classifications is required to guide effective treatment plans and improve patient outcomes across the spectrum of connective tissue diseases.

7.1.2. Etiology and Risk Factors

The etiology of connective tissue diseases such as lupus, dermatomyositis, and scleroderma is multifactorial and involves intricacies of genetic predispositions, environmental triggers, and dysregulation of the immune system. Genetic processes also come into play, as certain alleles and polymorphisms have been found to be associated with an increased susceptibility, and this would suggest that inherent qualities could influence disease expression. Environmental insults like infections, chemicals, and exposure to ultraviolet light may precipitate or enhance these diseases in genetically predisposed individuals. The immune dysregulation is also the basis for the autoimmune characteristics of these diseases, whereby the body mistakenly attacks its own connective tissues. This autoimmune process may lead to profound inflammation and subsequent damage to numerous organs, the gastrointestinal tract being particularly susceptible. With these autoimmune illnesses present, such symptoms as dysphagia, secondary to ineffective swallowing, can lead to serious complications such as malnutrition and aspiration pneumonia, and so clearly point to the urgent need for early diagnosis and treatment (Elmasry, 2014; Di Piazza et al., 2017) (Figure 7.2).

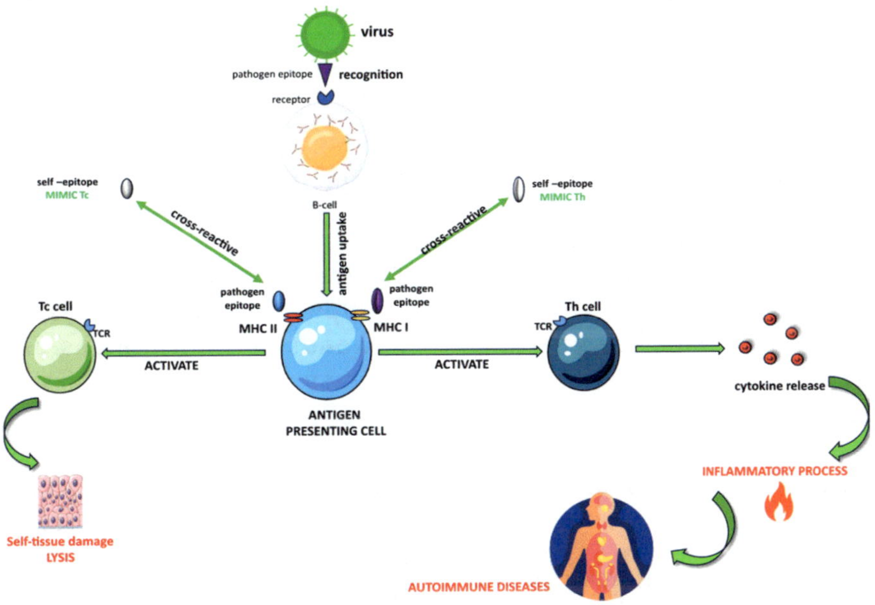

Figure 7.2. Dysregulation of the immune system contributes to the autoimmune nature of these conditions, whereby the body mistakenly attacks its own connective tissues.

Source: https://www.mdpi.com/cimb/cimb-46-00220/article_deploy/html/images/cimb-46-00220-g001.png.

7.1.3. Common Symptoms and Manifestations

Connective tissue disorders such as lupus, dermatomyositis, and scleroderma are characterized by a wide variety of common symptoms with a great impact on the patients' quality of life. Among them, fatigue, arthralgias, and skin changes frequently emerge as prominent features. Specifically, in dermatomyositis, typical skin manifestations, including periorbital erythema and Gottrons papules, are described alongside symptoms such as myalgia and dysphagia, which can lead to severe complications, including malnutrition and aspiration pneumonia (Di Piazza et al., 2017). Scleroderma is typically found with Raynaud's phenomenon and sclerodactyly, contributing to the usual disease clinical presentation. Also, overlap syndromes, where two or more connective tissue diseases overlap, may complicate the clinical presentation, augmenting the heterogeneity of symptoms and requiring particular treatment approaches (Di Piazza et al., 2017). Therefore, it is crucial to be aware of these symptoms for early diagnosis and effective management of such conditions.

7.1.4. Diagnostic Criteria and Methods

The clinical tests and procedures for diseases of connective tissue, including lupus, dermatomyositis, and scleroderma, play a critical role in accurate diagnosis and ensuing treatment of these complex diseases. Clinicians are prone to applying a combination of laboratory testing, clinical examination, and advanced imaging studies. Importantly, nailfold capillaroscopy has emerged as a useful tool, especially for revealing microvascular changes indicative of disease progression.

It has been proven by studies that dramatic capillaroscopy pattern changes, i.e., the existence of giant capillaries and avascular areas, are associated with the evolution of connective tissue diseases in patients presenting initially with Raynaud's phenomenon (Meli et al., 2018). Moreover, Piotto et al. (2012) highlight that normal capillaroscopy findings are frequent, yet particular patterns can aid diagnosis for juvenile dermatomyositis and scleroderma, indicating the usefulness of techniques in practice. Such diagnostic tools play an important role in establishing patient management based on individual needs and improving long-term results (Figure 7.3).

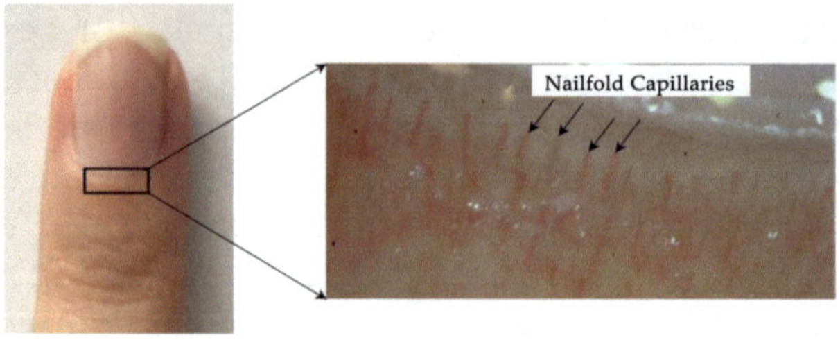

Figure 7.3. Nailfold capillaroscopy has emerged as an important tool, especially for its ability to reveal microvascular changes indicative of disease progression.

Source: https://media.springernature.com/full/springer-static/image/art%3A10.1038%2Fs41598-025-85277-8/MediaObjects/41598_2025_85277_Fig1_HTML.png.

7.1.5. Treatment Options and Management Strategies

The treatment of connective tissue diseases such as lupus, dermatomyositis, and scleroderma demands a multidimensional approach to address the diversity in presentations and complications of the illnesses. Pharmacologic therapies commonly involve the use of immunosuppressive medications, with mycophenolate mofetil (MMF) emerging as a major substitute for cyclophosphamide in treating interstitial lung disease (ILD) due to rheumatic conditions due to its promising side-effect profile and efficacy (Vacchi et al., 2021). In addition, neurologic features, such as peripheral neuropathy, may be seen in the setting of these diseases and necessitate unique interventions aimed at early diagnosis and tailored treatment to obtain optimal outcomes (Snoussi et al., 2018). Overall, utilization of patient-centered care modalities that involve pharmacologic and non-pharmacologic therapy is essential for improving quality of life in the patient and for managing the multifaceted complexities involved with connective tissue diseases.

7.1.6. Complications Associated with Lupus

Lupus, a prevalent autoimmune connective tissue disorder, is associated with several complications that are directly related to the patient's quality of life. One of the notable risks is multi-organ system involvement, particularly gastrointestinal tract involvement, which may manifest in dysphagia and severe conditions such as aspiration pneumonia and malnutrition. Dysphagia may follow both the disease process and the effects of pharmacologic management, the causes of which require close monitoring in managing the patient (Di Piazza et al., 2017). Other research that utilized nailfold capillaroscopy has proven that most patients with lupus have normal capillary morphology, but that significant variation occurs when lupus is complicated by other autoimmune diseases, such as juvenile dermatomyositis or scleroderma. This highlights the complexity of lupus and the necessity of tailored diagnostic approaches to properly monitor disease activity and its associated complications (Piotto et al., 2012) (Figure 7.4).

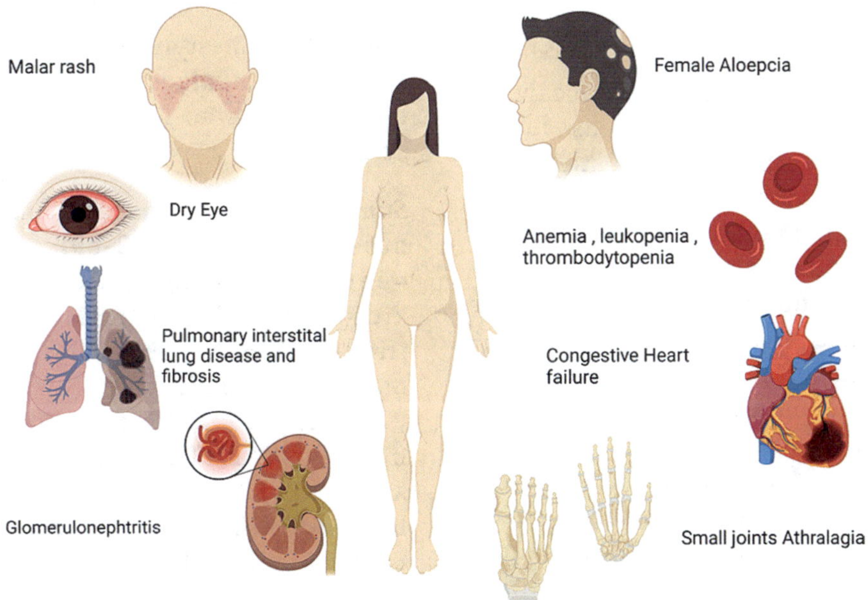

Figure 7.4. Lupus, a prevalent form of autoimmune connective tissue disease, is associated with various complications that significantly impact patients' quality of life.

Source: https://assets.cureus.com/uploads/figure/file/635428/article_river_72d8cda0f3b311edb92717f2100a0cc6-Untitled.png.

7.1.7. Psychological Impact on Patients

Psychological impacts of the connective tissue diseases, such as lupus, dermatomyositis, and scleroderma, are significant factors that influence patients' overall well-being. Chronic illnesses, by their nature, have an emotional impact, hence leading to elevated rates of depression and anxiety among those afflicted. Trieste et al. (2022) highlight that the diseases not only impact bodily health but also disrupt psychological, social, and economic lives, altering family life and relationships between families. In addition, the psychological effect can manifest in the symptoms of decreased quality of life and fatigue, making it important to evaluate these elements when calculating patient care. Orofacial manifestations of such diseases can be taken as initial signs of the disease conditions, further highlighting how multifaceted symptoms can cause intensification of feelings of frustration or isolation. Addressing the psychological dimension is crucial to improving patient outcomes and building resilience, highlighting the need for supportive interventions combined with medical treatments.

7.1.8. Role of Lifestyle Modifications

Lifestyle changes are pivotal in the care of connective tissue diseases such as lupus, dermatomyositis, and scleroderma. Patients are also encouraged to adopt a healthy, balanced diet rich in anti-inflammatory foods, exercise regularly, and adequate stress management to alleviate symptoms and improve well-being. For instance, avoidance of known precipitants—smoking and cold—can help limit attacks of Raynaud's phenomenon, a common complication of these disorders (Matucci-Cerinic et al., 2018). Moreover, patients with rheumatoid arthritis and inflammatory myopathy are typically advised to consider potential dietary adaptations and exercise regimens tailored to their condition (Cerqueira, 2016). These adaptations not only supplement usual medical treatments but also motivate patients to take an active role in their health, provoking a sense of control and potentially improving the quality of their lives. This combined approach highlights the crucial role of including lifestyle changes within the overall treatment plan for patients with these debilitating diseases (Figure 7.5).

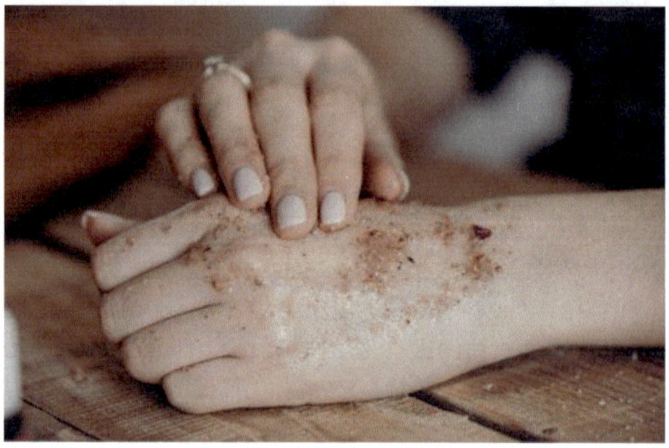

Figure 7.5. Lifestyle modifications play a crucial role in the management of connective tissue diseases such as lupus, dermatomyositis, and scleroderma.

Source: https://images.u nsplas h.com/photo-1669979963553-c9b 9e347f08a?crop=entropy&cs=tinysrgb&fit=m ax&fm=jpg&ixid=M3w3MDgyMDR8MHwxfHNlYXJjaHwxfHxkZXJtYXRvb G9naWNh bC UyMG1hbmlmZXN0YXRpb25zJTJDJTIwY29ubmVjdGl2ZSUyMHRpc3N1ZSUy MGRpc2Vhc2VzJTJDJTIwQ1REJTIwc2tpbiUyMHN5bXB0b21zJT JDJTIw ZGVybWF0b215b3NpdGlzJTJDJTI wc2NsZXJvZGVybWF8ZW58MHwwfHx8MTc0OTkyODY3NXww&ixlib= rb-4.1.0&q=80&w=500&?utm_source=numberanalytics&utm_medium=referral.

Test Your Knowledge

1. What organ systems are commonly involved in SLE?
2. What is the significance of the butterfly (malar) rash in SLE?

7.2. Dermatomyositis

Learning Outcome

1. Understand Definition and Classification of Dermatomyositis;
2. Explain Etiology and Potential Triggers;
3. Focus on Characteristic Skin Rashes and Muscle Weakness;
4. Describe Diagnostic Approaches and Criteria;
5. Learn Treatment Modalities and Rehabilitation;
6. Discuss Associated Conditions and Comorbidities;
7. Know Long-term Prognosis and Outcomes;
8. Understand the Importance of Patient Education.

Dermatomyositis, an idiopathic inflammatory myopathy, is associated with distinctive findings beyond muscle weakness, often including concurrent skin involvement in the form of heliotrope rash and Gottrons papules. This autoimmune disease affects not only skeletal muscle, leading to progressive weakness and atrophy, but also involves intricate interactions with other connective tissues, defining its systemic nature. Therapeutic drugs are still few and contentious; corticosteroids are in routine usage, but effectiveness is awaiting confirmation by formal randomized controlled trials. More recent treatments, including intravenous immunoglobulin, hold some promise, but long-term effectiveness is not known (Aggarwal & Oddis, 2012). The complexities of dermatomyositis demand continuing research to better understand its pathogenesis and optimize therapy, underscoring the value of an integrated care plan in managing this complicated disease in the context of all the connective tissue diseases (Griger et al., 2017).

7.2.1. Definition and Classification of Dermatomyositis

Dermatomyositis is a rare autoimmune connective tissue disease with muscle weakness and typical rashes on the skin, hence distinguishing it from other inflammatory myopathies. Classification of dermatomyositis is necessary to ensure proper diagnosis and treatment, and it is typically based on the availability of specific clinical, serological, and histopathological features. The patient typically presents with proximal muscle weakness and cutaneous findings in the form of heliotrope rash and Gottrons papules. Serologic tests, particularly anti-Jo-1 and other myositis-specific autoantibodies, also aid in classification. Dermatomyositis may be an idiopathic disease or a disease associated with other connective tissue diseases, like systemic lupus erythematosus, making it crucial to have an extensive differential diagnosis. Some recent studies have examined the utility of nailfold capillaroscopy for distinguishing dermatomyositis from other connective tissue disorders and for potentially enhancing diagnostic sensitivity (Wu et al., 2013; Hanly et al., 2015). This sophisticated process of discrimination is central to therapeutic and prognostic practice (Figure 7.6).

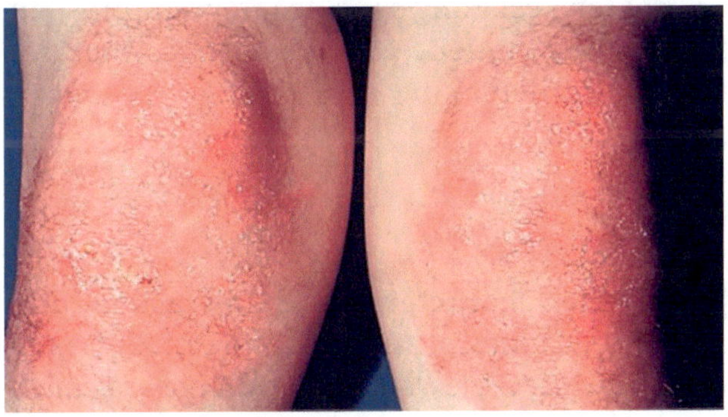

Figure 7.6. Dermatomyositis is a rare autoimmune connective tissue disease characterized by muscle weakness and distinctive skin rashes, which distinguishes it from other inflammatory myopathies.

Source: https://i0.wp.com/post.healthline.com/wp-content/uploads/2021/02/648x364_Dermatomyositis.jpg?w=1155&h=764.

7.2.2. Etiology and Potential Triggers

The etiology of connective tissue disorders such as lupus, dermatomyositis, and scleroderma also remains multifactorial and complex, with some autoimmune reactions triggered by environmental and genetic factors. This sophistication is brought to the forefront by the role of serum autoantibodies, which are central to the diagnosis and classification of the diseases. Recent studies have focused on the emergence of new biomarkers that are pertinent in explaining the pathogenesis and progression of connective tissue diseases (Ceribelli, 2016). These also include viral infections, drug contact with certain drugs, and UV light, which have been identified as probable inducers resulting in the onset of abnormal immune responses and tissue destruction (Lupu et al., 2024). Moreover, the convergence of genetic predisposition with environmental exposure makes the clinical presentation of these conditions more complicated, thereby making it difficult to treat. Identification of these etiologic precipitants is crucial for designing specific interventions and maximizing patient outcomes in connective tissue disorders.

7.2.3. Characteristic Skin Rashes and Muscle Weakness

When the characteristic skin rashes and muscle weakness, as in connective tissue disorders, are viewed, some disorders, such as dermatomyositis and scleroderma, have very typical manifestations. Dermatomyositis, for instance, is often marked by cutaneous alteration in the pattern of periorbital erythema and Gottrons papules, distinctive features of diagnosis combined with the grave muscle weakness which can ensue (Navaratnam et al., 2011). The muscle weakness is not merely a symptom but a multifaceted element of the disease, which generally leads to increasing disability. In addition, overlap syndromes, like sclerodermatomyositis, can have muscle weakness and skin changes consistent with scleroderma, significantly complicating clinical presentation (Febyani et al., 2011). Overlapping symptoms require careful assessment since they complicate the clinician's ability to distinguish among separate connective tissue diseases, eventually influencing treatment modalities and patient outcomes. Accurate diagnosis and treatment of these complex conditions depend on an understanding of these skin and muscle manifestations (Figure 7.7).

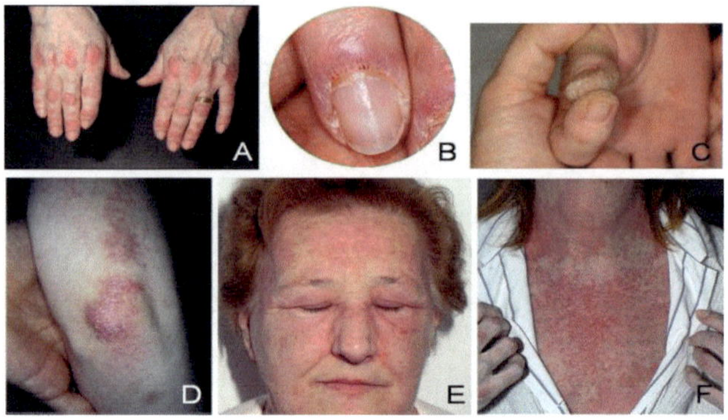

Figure 7.7. Dermatomyositis, for instance, is often marked by skin changes such as periorbital erythema and Gottrons papules, which are significant diagnostic features alongside the profound muscle weakness that can ensue.

Source: https://ars.els-cdn.com/content/image/1-s2.0-S0896841114000341-gr1.jpg.

7.2.4. Diagnostic Approaches and Criteria

After the diagnosis of connective tissue diseases such as lupus, dermatomyositis, and scleroderma, the assigned diagnostic approaches and criteria tend to largely rely on ever-evolving diagnostic techniques in a bid to enhance precision. In lupus, to take an example, the American College of Rheumatology has established definite criteria, clinical manifestations and serological abnormalities, to guide towards accurate diagnosis. Similarly, the criteria for the classification of systemic sclerosis are being revised to facilitate better discrimination between scleroderma and its imitators, such as systemic lupus erythematosus and myositis, on clinical grounds by skin thickening and the presence of some autoantibodies, which the latter was proven through good discriminant validity of these findings (Johnson et al., 2012). Furthermore, a decision rule study in rheumatoid arthritis demonstrated heterogeneity of diagnostic accuracy with administrative data, emphasizing the importance of valid diagnostic frameworks to distinguish such complex conditions (Hanly et al., 2015). Hence, having a persistent interest in refining diagnostic criteria is needed to improve patient outcomes.

7.2.5. Treatment Modalities and Rehabilitation

Effective management of autoimmune connective tissue diseases such as lupus, dermatomyositis, and scleroderma requires an integrated treatment modality approach and rehabilitation.

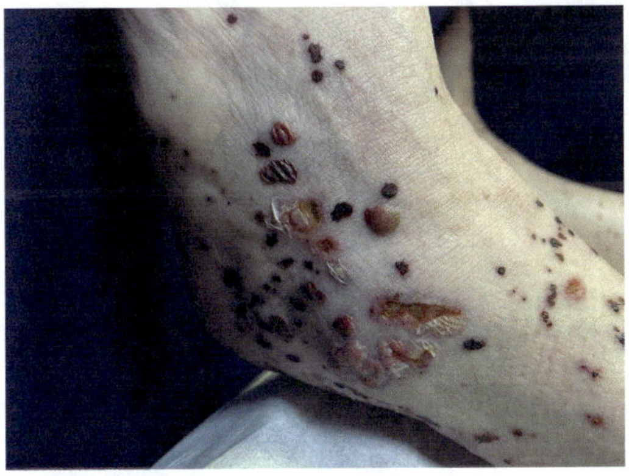

Figure 7.8. Effective management of connective tissue diseases such as lupus, dermatomyositis, and scleroderma requires a comprehensive approach to treatment modalities and rehabilitation.

Source: https://www.medical.theclinics.com/cms/10.1016/j.mcna.2021.04.011/asset/c32244ed-559c-4ba1-8023-ba573711e4f8/main.assets/gr8_lrg.jpg.

Management can involve the administration of immunosuppressive medication and corticosteroids to reduce systemic inflammation and stop the development of the disease. Particularly, treatment of interstitial lung disease, one of the severe complications of these conditions, is extremely difficult; recent studies, the most recent of which come from the INBUILD trial, show that antifibrotic drugs are promising for patients with CTD-related ILD (Vacchi et al., 2020). In addition, the complexity of systemic sclerosis (SSc) illustrates the need for specially tailored rehabilitation interventions; oral symptoms can contribute profoundly to compromised quality of life, affecting both function and psychological health (Abdouh, 2020). A multidisciplinary intervention featuring pharmacological treatment, physical therapy, and psychosocial rehabilitation is thus mandatory in an attempt to improve patient outcomes and general quality of life (Figure 7.8).

7.2.6. Associated Conditions and Comorbidities

Connective tissue diseases such as lupus, scleroderma, and dermatomyositis are frequently associated with a very broad spectrum of associated conditions and comorbidities that account for patient morbidity. For instance, interstitial lung disease (ILD) is one of the significant problems in these disorders, being a common reason for respiratory compromise and reduced quality of life.

Mycophenolate mofetil (MMF) has become a significant treatment option for the treatment of RD-related ILD due to its efficacy and favorable side effect profile compared to others; its use is, however, grounded on poor scientific evidence (Vacchi et al., 2021). In addition, intravenous CYC has also been found to be more efficient in improving lung function in ILD associated with idiopathic inflammatory myopathy, and making the correct choice of immunosuppressive drugs based on patient needs (Moreno-Torres et al.,

2023). Understanding these conditions is vital in formulating integrated strategies for managing the underlying condition and its complications.

7.2.7. Long-term Prognosis and Outcomes

The long-term outcome and prognosis of patients with connective tissue disease, such as lupus, dermatomyositis, and scleroderma, depend on many factors, including the presence of specific autoantibodies. Each of these conditions has high morbidity and mortality, the latter typically being due to internal organ involvement, which needs long-term evaluation. For instance, the presence of anti-Scl70 autoantibodies in scleroderma correlates with a higher risk for pulmonary involvement, including interstitial lung disease, with a poor prognosis (Kuwana et al., 2021). Similarly, some autoantibodies of dermatomyositis, such as anti-MDA5, have been correlated with rapidly progressive interstitial lung disease and have a poor prognosis (Mulhearn et al., 2020). Therefore, identification of these autoantibodies not only helps in diagnosis but also in predicting clinical outcome and management on a long-term basis in the affected. With these correlations, clinicians can tailor interventions to maximize quality of life as well as management of disease as a whole (Figure 7.9).

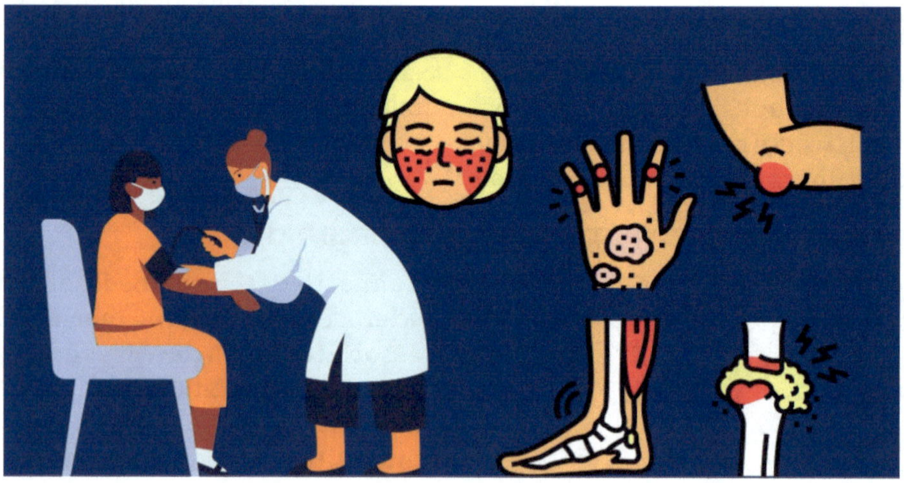

Figure 7.9. The long-term prognosis and outcomes of patients with connective tissue diseases, such as lupus, dermatomyositis, and scleroderma, are influenced by various factors, including the presence of specific autoantibodies.

Source: https://careclinic.io/wp-content/uploads/2023/12/living-with-scleroderma-jpg.webp.

7.2.8. Importance of Patient Education

Patient education is important in the management of connective tissue diseases such as lupus, dermatomyositis, and scleroderma because it educates patients with the knowledge to manage their complex conditions. Successful learning leads to better self-care and adherence to treatment schedules, ultimately leading to better health outcomes. Symptomatic awareness, like Raynaud's phenomenon (usually found in patients with systemic sclerosis), can lead to serious complications like digital ischemic lesions and highlights the need for education of the patient regarding their drug regimen (Tolosa Vilella et al., 2009). Similarly, knowledge about the risks of interstitial lung disease, a serious manifestation of autoimmune rheumatic diseases, enables patients to recognize warning signals at an early stage, enabling timely intervention (Good et al., 2024). Through specific education programs, health workers can enhance awareness and enable individuals to take an active role in their health, leading to a better quality of life and morbidity reduction associated with these disabling diseases.

Test Your Knowledge

1. What is the significance of muscle enzyme levels in diagnosis?
2. How is dermatomyositis diagnosed (clinical, lab, biopsy)??

7.3. Scleroderma

Learning Outcome

1. Understand Definition and Types of Scleroderma;
2. Explain Pathophysiology and Immune Response;
3. Focus on Common Symptoms and Organ Involvement;
4. Describe Diagnostic Techniques and Challenges;
5. Learn Treatment Options and Management Approaches;
6. Discuss Impact on Daily Living and Functionality;
7. Know Psychological and Emotional Considerations;
8. Understand Support Systems and Resources for Patients;
9. Explain Emerging Research and Therapeutic Strategies.

Scleroderma is a complex and multifaceted autoimmune connective tissue disease affecting the skin and visceral organs mainly by hyperplastic collagen deposition and fibrosis. The condition, which presents with manifestations such as Raynaud's phenomenon and sclerodactyly, is very variable in presentation and thus presents challenges in diagnosis, particularly when it overlaps with another rheumatic disorder such as dermatomyositis, as in the case of the entity of sclerodermatomyositis, where both conditions' features are seen (Navarathnam et al., 2011). The digestive system is most commonly involved, and dysphagia is the frequent complaint secondary to esophageal dysfunction, which can result in severe complications such as malnutrition or aspiration pneumonia (Di Piazza et al., 2017). Besides this, the heterogeneity in clinical manifestations warrants a cautious attitude towards diagnosis and therapy and emphasizes the importance of watchfulness among clinicians for the onset of appropriate intervention and smooth management of affected individuals.

7.3.1. Definition and Types of Scleroderma

Scleroderma, or systemic sclerosis, is a connective tissue disease characterized by overproduction of collagen, leading to thickened skin and organ fibrosis. It exists predominantly in two types: localized and systemic scleroderma. Localized scleroderma affects only the skin, typically in the form of patches or bands of induration, while systemic scleroderma can affect one or more organs such as the lungs, kidneys, and gastrointestinal tract, having a significant impact on overall health. This systemic variant can further be classified into limited and diffuse scleroderma, the former being slower in evolution with extremity and facial skin disease and the latter having a sudden onset of skin and organ disease. These distinctions are significant to know, as one may observe from research on connective tissue disorders, which indicates varying prognoses and treatment responses based on the specific scleroderma diagnosed (Martin et al., 2011; Navaratnam et al., 2011). Successful management and improved patient outcomes rely on this knowledge (Figure 7.10).

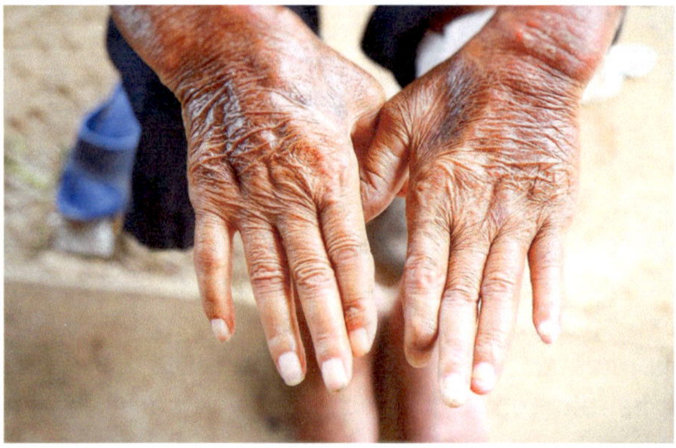

Figure 7.10. Scleroderma, or systemic sclerosis, is a complex connective tissue disease characterized by the excessive accumulation of collagen, leading to skin thickening and organ fibrosis.

Source: https://post.medicalnewstoday.com/wp-content/uploads/sites/3/2022/07/scleroderma-skin-slide1.jpg.

7.3.2. Pathophysiology and Immune Response

Pathophysiology of the connective tissue diseases, such as lupus, dermatomyositis, and scleroderma, is essentially founded on dysregulated immune responses against the body's own tissues. It is in these autoimmune diseases that a dysfunctional self-reactivity is the cause of autoantibody production, which can significantly influence connective tissues and other organ systems. This process can particularly be exemplified in systemic lupus erythematosus (SLE), in which heterogeneous autoantibodies correlate with specific clinical manifestations and complications, including renal involvement and hematological disorders (Mulhearn et al., 2020). Parallel with this, dermatomyositis is characterized by skin and muscle pathology involving immune-mediated damage, whereas scleroderma is characterized by fibroblast activation and increased collagen deposition that ends in fibrosis (Ciang et al., 2017). The recognition of such mechanisms not only explains disease progression but also points towards probable therapeutic targets, paving the way for more effective management strategies in patients with these multifactorial conditions.

7.3.3. Common Symptoms and Organ Involvement

In connective tissue diseases, classical presentations and organ involvement in confounding and overlapping combinations are common, which complicate diagnosis as well as therapy. For instance, the patient presents with arthralgia, myalgia, and skin changes indicative of scleroderma, pointing to a combination syndrome like sclerodermatomyositis, where the features of dermatomyositis and scleroderma merge (Navaratnam et al., 2011). Gastrointestinal issues are also frequent, with dysphagia, secondary to the muscular dysfunction of the mechanism of swallowing, being particularly frequent. This symptom can cause severe complications like aspiration pneumonia and malnutrition (Di Piazza et al., 2017). The extreme concurrence of symptoms justifies the use of an extensive evaluation method because organ involvement could extensively differ and is responsible for significant implications on the management of the patient. In general, it is very important for medical professionals to be aware of these symptoms so that they can develop appropriate treatment plans for patients of such complicated diseases (Figure 7.11).

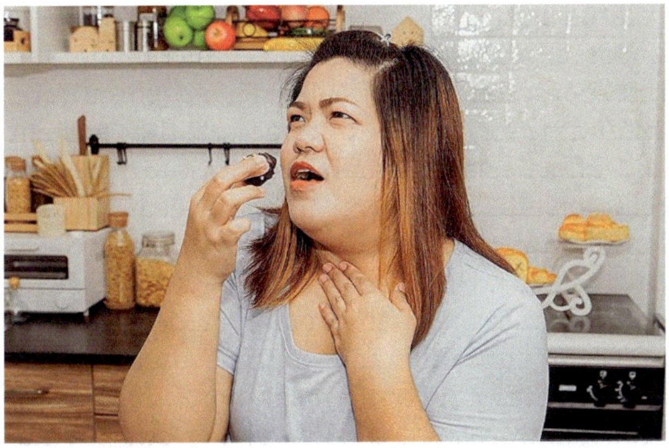

Figure 7.11. Gastrointestinal complications are also prevalent, particularly dysphagia, which arises from the muscular dysfunction affecting the swallowing mechanism.

Source: https://scx2.b-cdn.net/gfx/news/2025/swallowing-disorder-no.jpg.

7.3.4. Diagnostic Techniques and Challenges

The arena of diagnostic means for connective tissue diseases, such as lupus, dermatomyositis, and scleroderma, has advanced methodology and unparalleled challenges. One of the biggest problems is the heterogeneity of the diseases, often complicating the clinical diagnosis. Autoantibodies are typical of the diseases and are very informative because they not only diagnose the diseases but also provide prognostic details about potential complications of the diseases, like the implication of internal organs (Mulhearn et al., 2020). Nailfold videocapillaroscopy has also turned out to be a significant tool in assessing scleroderma-related microangiopathy, facilitating physicians to analyze capillary morphology and provide forecasts for disease progression (Pizzorni et al., 2016). However, the practice of conducting tests for autoantibodies is filled with pitfalls like false positives and negatives, thus potentially leading to misdiagnosis. Hence, it is crucial to have an apparent understanding of both the modes of diagnosis and limits to facilitate effective disease control in the patient with connective tissue diseases.

7.3.5. Treatment Options and Management Approaches

Effective management of connective tissue diseases (CTDs) such as lupus, dermatomyositis, and scleroderma demands an integrated approach, particularly when dealing with complications like interstitial lung disease (ILD). Treatment strategies are primarily centered around immunosuppressive medications, with mycophenolate mofetil (MMF) now being a viable replacement for cyclophosphamide in the management of RD-associated ILD, due to its better side effect profile (Vacchi et al., 2021).

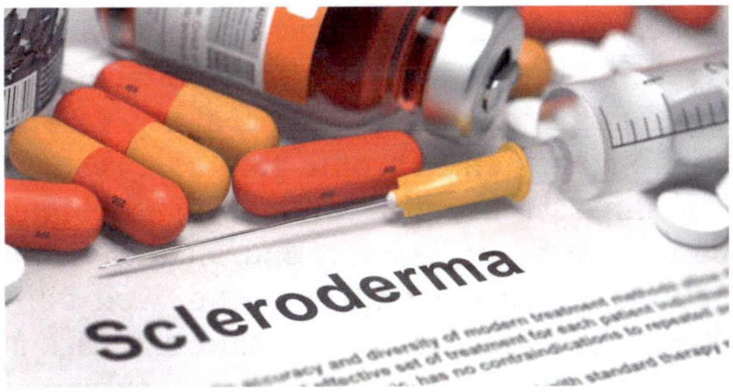

Figure 7.12. Treatment strategies primarily involve immunosuppressive agents, with mycophenolate mofetil (MMF) emerging as a viable alternative to cyclophosphamide for patients with RD-related ILD, thanks to its lower side effect profile.

Source: https://m3.healio.com/~/media/images/news/print/healio-rheumatology/2022/03_march/adobestock_83601828_og.jpg.

Nonetheless, the preferred treatment in CTD-ILD remains confounded by a lack of prospective data and variability of responses to treatment among different individuals (Vacchi et al., 2020). Recent advances, such as outcomes from the INBUILD trial, have also established the basis for antifibrotic therapy consideration, providing new therapeutic options for managing this disabling aspect of CTDs. Ultimately, a personalized approach from an interdisciplinary team, depending upon the individual patient's unique needs and disease presentation, is required in optimizing treatment outcomes and overall quality of life (Figure 7.12).

7.3.6. Impact on Daily Living and Functionality

The impact of connective tissue diseases such as lupus, dermatomyositis, and scleroderma on everyday life and functionality is enormous, and more often than not, it has a two-way impact both on physical functions and the psychological state of an individual. These conditions may lead to a great level of mobility limitation due to fatigue, joint pain, and muscle weakness, further decreasing the capacity to perform activities of daily living such as dressing, cooking, or even social engagement. Chronic pain as a result of these illnesses usually results in psychological issues such as depression and anxiety, which tend to increase symptoms and well-being difficulties. According to clinical observations, musculoskeletal examinations are extremely crucial for comprehending the functional impairment of patients to help healthcare practitioners offer tailored interventions and treatment strategies. Lastly, the complexity of these disorders emphasizes the critical need for holistic patient management strategies to address both physical and emotional health (Cerqueira, 2016).

7.3.7. Psychological and Emotional Considerations

The psychological and emotional consequences of connective tissue diseases, such as lupus, dermatomyositis, and scleroderma, cannot be overstated, as these chronic conditions critically affect patients' quality of life. Patients become increasingly anxious and depressed due to the volatile nature of their symptoms, leading to a loss of ability for everyday functioning and interpersonal interaction. These conditions extend their reach outside of the patient and affect family dynamics and interpersonal relationships as patients learn to accommodate new limitations and treatment regimens (Trieste et al., 2022). Of these, systemic sclerosis (SSc) demonstrates the interconnected nature of bodily symptoms and mental disturbance, with studies observing meaningful impacts on oral health-related quality of life and mental wellbeing (Abdouh, 2020). A clear understanding of these emotional problems is necessary in the development of efficient holistic treatment approaches addressing physical and mental health concerns in treating these conditions (Figure 7.13).

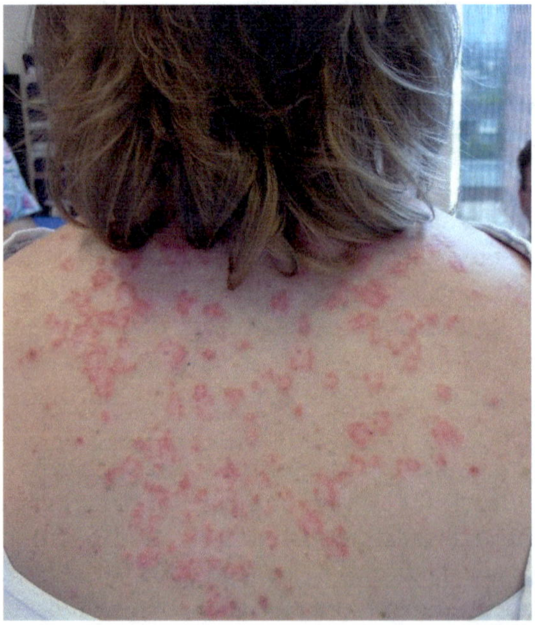

Figure 7.13. The psychological and emotional ramifications of connective tissue diseases, such as lupus, dermatomyositis, and scleroderma, cannot be overstated, as these chronic conditions profoundly affect patients' quality of life.

Source: https://www.sanovadermatology.com/wp-content/uploads/2016/07/DSCN0397-e1469763494904.jpg.

7.3.8. Support Systems and Resources for Patients

Dealing with the intricacies of connective tissue diseases such as lupus, dermatomyositis, and scleroderma demands good support systems and interventions for patients.

Treatment is highly dependent on education and awareness levels among patients and doctors to recognize and treat the varied presentations of such diseases. For instance, orofacial manifestations may be the first signs of systemic involvement, underscoring the need for specialized management by multi-disciplinary teams of rheumatologists and dental professionals. Facilities such as patient advocacy groups also play a vital role in providing emotional support and facilitating access to necessary health care services, both of which are essential for effective disease control. These networks not only facilitate greater patient understanding of their condition but also stimulate active involvement in the decision-making process, leading to lower morbidity and increased quality of life.

7.3.9. Emerging Research and Therapeutic Strategies

Therapeutic strategies for connective tissue diseases (CTDs) like lupus, dermatomyositis, and scleroderma have increasingly more encouraging progress, particularly for addressing associated complications like interstitial lung disease (ILD). There is new evidence supporting the utility of mycophenolate mofetil (MMF) as a first-line replacement for cyclophosphamide in treating RD-associated ILD, with an excellent side effect profile and adequate immunosuppression (Vacchi et al., 2021). Full multidisciplinary clinics for CTD-ILD care are being established more and more, enabling early diagnosis and tailored therapies (Castelino & Varga, 2010). Furthermore, additional research on the pathogenic mechanisms of CTD-ILD is revealing critical information on the effector cells and inflammatory mediators implicated, paving the way for selective therapies. All these efforts constitute an important step towards personalized therapies, which ultimately hold the promise to enhance patient outcome in this complex setting of connective tissue disorders.

Test Your Knowledge

1. What are the gastrointestinal manifestations of systemic sclerosis?
2. How is pulmonary arterial hypertension assessed in systemic sclerosis?

SUMMARY

The assessment of connective tissue disease, including lupus, dermatomyositis, and scleroderma, portrays the complexity and clinical significance of these disorders. The diverse pathophysiologic mechanisms and genetic underpinnings account for the heterogeneous presentations that are encountered by clinicians. Research has revealed that environmental etiology and geographic variation influence disease occurrence, as expressed in the higher incidence of scleroderma in certain locations, suggesting the need for more geographically specific studies to identify etiologic factors (Borman, 1975). Furthermore, new technologies in the diagnosis of the conditions, such as nailfold capillaroscopy, have contributed important information regarding monitoring and control of such conditions, particularly in children, where evidence has been found to be variable in clinical presentation and disease activity (Piotto et al., 2012). In general, a multidisciplinary treatment strategy with augmented research activity, patient education, and tailor-made therapeutic interventions is warranted to improve patient outcomes and quality of life in patients with these disabling conditions. The research into connective tissue diseases, especially lupus, dermatomyositis, and scleroderma, illustrates a large degree of similarity between autoimmune pathology and diverse clinical presentations. At the root of these diseases is the presence of autoantibodies, whose role is not just in diagnosis but also in guiding prognosis and clinical care is considerable (Mulhearn et al., 2020). The autoantibodies are typically disease-specific and correlate with various complications, particularly pertaining to involvement of internal organs. As mentioned, identification of the exact autoantibodies may enlighten the course of the disease and its severity, and thus the targeted therapies (Mulhearn et al., 2019). Discussion of the subject also points to the complexity of diagnosis of such diseases, e.g., the logistics and shortcomings of autoantibody analysis. Overall, a thorough understanding of these points is required in order to advance the treatment protocols of patients with connective tissue disorders, ultimately improving their quality of life and clinical course.

KEY TERMS FROM THIS CHAPTER

- Connective tissue diseases
- Dermatomyositis
- Mixed connective tissue disease (MCTD)
- Interstitial lung disease (ILD)
- Systemic Lupus Erythematosus (SLE)
- Organ system
- Neurological impairment
- Dysphagia
- Lupus
- Scleroderma
- Autoimmune rheumatic diseases
- Therapeutic protocols
- Autoantibodies
- Renal dysfunction
- Sclerodermatomyositis
- Nutritional status

CRITICAL THINKING QUESTIONS

1. Which of the following is a characteristic autoantibody in systemic lupus erythematosus (SLE)?

a. Anti-centromere antibody

b. Rheumatoid factor

c. Anti-dsDNA antibody

d. Anti-CCP antibody

2. The "butterfly rash" in SLE typically involves which areas?

a. Forearms and chest

b. Nose and cheeks

c. Chin and forehead

d. Neck and scalp

3. Which of the following is most specific for systemic sclerosis (scleroderma)?

a. Anti-dsDNA antibody

b. Anti-Scl-70 (anti-topoisomerase I) antibody

c. Anti-Ro antibody

d. Anti-mitochondrial antibody

4. CREST syndrome is a limited form of systemic sclerosis. What does the "C" stand for?

a. Cyanosis

b. Calcinosis

c. Conjunctivitis

d. Cirrhosis

5. Which autoantibody is most specific for Rheumatoid Arthritis?

a. ANA

b. Anti-dsDNA

c. Anti-CCP antibody

d. Anti-Sm antibody

Short Answer Questions

1. What are the hallmark clinical features of SLE?
2. What is the role of anti-dsDNA and anti-Sm antibodies in SLE?
3. What are the classical cutaneous manifestations of dermatomyositis?
4. What is the difference between dermatomyositis and polymyositis?
5. What is the difference between limited and diffuse systemic sclerosis?
6. What are the features of CREST syndrome?

Answers to Critical Thinking Questions

1. (c); 2. (b); 3. (b); 4. (b); 5. (c)

REFERENCES

1. Abdouh, I. (2020). *The Nature and Impact of Oral Disease of Systemic Sclerosis.* https://core.ac.uk/download/336583022.pdf (accessed on 23rd July 2025).
2. Aggarwal, R., & Oddis, C. V. (2012). Inclusion body myositis: therapeutic approaches. *Degenerative neurological and neuromuscular disease, 2,* 43–52. https://doi.org/10.2147/DNND.S19899(accessed on 23rd July 2025).
3. Johnson, S. R., Fransen, J., Khanna, D., Baron, M., van den Hoogen, F., Medsger, T. A., Jr, Peschken, C. A., Carreira, P. E., Riemekasten, G., Tyndall, A., Matucci-Cerinic, M., & Pope, J. E. (2012). Validation of potential classification criteria for systemic sclerosis. *Arthritis care & research, 64*(3), 358–367. https://doi.org/10.1002/acr.20684(accessed on 23rd July 2025).
4. Navaratnam, V., Ali, N., Smith, C. J., McKeever, T., Fogarty, A., & Hubbard, R. B. (2011). Does the presence of connective tissue disease modify survival in patients with pulmonary fibrosis?. *Respiratory medicine, 105*(12), 1925–1930. https://doi.org/10.1016/j.rmed.2011.08.015(accessed on 23rd July 2025).
5. Meli, M., Gitzelmann, G., Koppensteiner, R., & Amann-Vesti, B. R. (2006). Predictive value of nailfold capillaroscopy in patients with Raynaud's phenomenon. *Clinical rheumatology, 25*(2), 153–158. https://doi.org/10.1007/s10067-005-1146-1(accessed on 23rd July 2025).
6. Tolosa Vilella, C., Simeón Aznar, C. P., & Gabarró Julià, L. (2009). El fenómeno de Raynaud [Raynaud's phenomenon]. *Medicina clinica, 132*(18), 712–718. https://doi.org/10.1016/j.medcli.2008.11.017(accessed on 23rd July 2025).
7. Di Franco, M., Bazzichi, L., Casale, R., Sarzi-Puttini, P., & Atzeni, F. (2015). Pain in systemic connective tissue diseases. *Best practice & research. Clinical rheumatology, 29*(1), 53–62. https://doi.org/10.1016/j.berh.2015.05.006(accessed on 23rd July 2025).
8. Snoussi, M., Frikha, F., & Bahloul, Z. (2019). Peripheral Neuropathy in Connective Tissue Diseases. IntechOpen. doi: 10.5772/intechopen.82271(accessed on 23rd July 2025).
9. Matucci-Cerinic, C., Nagaraja, V., Prignano, F., Kahaleh, B., & Bellando-Randone, S. (2018). The role of the dermatologist in Raynaud's phenomenon: a clinical challenge. *Journal of the European Academy of Dermatology and Venereology : JEADV, 32*(7), 1120–1127. https://doi.org/10.1111/jdv.14914(accessed on 23rd July 2025).
10. Martin, N., Krol, P., Smith, S., Murray, K., Pilkington, C. A., Davidson, J. E., Wedderburn, L. R., & Juvenile Dermatomyositis Research Group (2011). A national registry for juvenile dermatomyositis and other paediatric idiopathic inflammatory myopathies: 10 years' experience; the Juvenile Dermatomyositis National (UK and Ireland) Cohort Biomarker Study and Repository for Idiopathic Inflammatory Myopathies. *Rheumatology (Oxford, England), 50*(1), 137–145. https://doi.org/10.1093/rheumatology/keq261(accessed on 23rd July 2025).
11. Borman, G. B. (1975). *Medical Geography and Its Contribution to The Etiology of Rare Systemic Connective Tissue Diseases* (Master's thesis, Massey University). https://core.ac.uk/download/157568842.pdf (accessed on 23rd July 2025).
12. Trieste, L., Cannizzo, S., Palla, I., Triulzi, I., & Turchetti, G. (2022). State of the art and future directions in assessing the quality of life in rare and complex connective tissue and musculoskeletal diseases. *Frontiers in medicine, 9,* 986218. https://doi.org/10.3389/fmed.2022.986218(accessed on 23rd July 2025).

13. Vacchi, C., Sebastiani, M., Cassone, G., Cerri, S., Della Casa, G., Salvarani, C., & Manfredi, A. (2020). Therapeutic Options for the Treatment of Interstitial Lung Disease Related to Connective Tissue Diseases. A Narrative Review. *Journal of clinical medicine*, *9*(2), 407. https://doi.org/10.3390/jcm9020407(accessed on 23rd July 2025).

14. Castelino, F. V., & Varga, J. (2010). Interstitial lung disease in connective tissue diseases: evolving concepts of pathogenesis and management. *Arthritis research & therapy*, *12*(4), 213. https://doi.org/10.1186/ar3097(accessed on 23rd July 2025).

15. Ceribelli, A. (2016). *Protein and RNA Immunoprecipitation for The Identification of Specific Serum Autoantibodies in Systemic Autoimmune Rheumatic Diseases.* https://core.ac.uk/download/187945494.pdf (accessed on 23rd July 2025).

16. Cerqueira, C. (2016). *Studies on the Role of Autoantibodies and Autoantigens in Rheumatoid Arthritis and Myositis.* https://core.ac.uk/download/70343823.pdf (accessed on 23rd July 2025).

17. Ciang, N. C., Pereira, N., & Isenberg, D. A. (2017). Mixed connective tissue disease-enigma variations?. *Rheumatology (Oxford, England)*, *56*(3), 326–333. https://doi.org/10.1093/rheumatology/kew265(accessed on 23rd July 2025).

18. Di Piazza A, Vernuccio F, Costanzo M, et al. The Videofluorographic Swallowing Study in Rheumatologic Diseases: A Comprehensive Review. *Gastroenterol Res Pract.* 2017;2017:7659273. doi:10.1155/2017/7659273(accessed on 23rd July 2025).

19. Pizzorni, C., Sulli, A., Smith, V., Lladó, A., Paolino, S., Cutolo, M., & Ruaro, B. (2016). Capillaroscopy 2016: new perspectives in systemic sclerosis. Capillaroscopy 2016: new perspectives in systemic sclerosis. *Acta reumatologica portuguesa*, *41*(1), 8–14. (accessed on 23rd July 2025).

20. Griger, Z., Nagy-Vincze, M., & Dankó, K. (2017). Pharmacological management of dermatomyositis. *Expert review of clinical pharmacology*, *10*(10), 1109–1118. https://doi.org/10.1080/17512433.2017.1353910 (accessed on 23rd July 2025).

21. Elmasry, O. A. (2014). *The Heart in Systemic Autoimmune Disorders.* https://core.ac.uk/download/478454505.pdf (accessed on 23rd July 2025).

22. Moreno-Torres, V., Martín-Iglesias, D., Vivero, F., González-Echavarri, C., García-Moyano, M., Enghelmayer, J. I., Malfante, P., Gaser, A., Ruiz-Irastorza, G., & EPIMAR cohort Investigators (2023). Intravenous cyclophosphamide improves functional outcomes in interstitial lung disease related to idiopathic inflammatory myopathies. *Seminars in arthritis and rheumatism*, *59*, 152164. https://doi.org/10.1016/j.semarthrit.2023.152164(accessed on 23rd July 2025).

23. Kuwana M, Gil-Vila A, Selva-O'Callaghan A. Role of autoantibodies in the diagnosis and prognosis of interstitial lung disease in autoimmune rheumatic disorders. *Ther Adv Musculoskelet Dis.* 2021;13:1759720X211032457. Published 2021 Jul 27. doi:10.1177/1759720X211032457(accessed on 23rd July 2025).

24. Good, S., Sparks, J., & Volkmann, E. (2024). Screening, diagnosis, and monitoring of interstitial lung disease in autoimmune rheumatic diseases: A narrative review. https://core.ac.uk/download/618291919.pdf (accessed on 23rd July 2025).

25. Hanly, J. G., Skedgel, C., & Thompson, K. (2015). The use of administrative health care databases to identify patients with rheumatoid arthritis. https://core.ac.uk/download/41991036.pdf (accessed on 23rd July 2025).

26. Piotto, D. G., Len, C. A., Hilário, M. O., & Terreri, M. T. (2012). Nailfold capillaroscopy in children and adolescents with rheumatic diseases. *Revista brasileira de reumatologia, 52*(5), 722–732.(accessed on 23rd July 2025).

27. Wu, P. C., Huang, M. N., Kuo, Y. M., Hsieh, S. C., & Yu, C. L. (2013). Clinical applicability of quantitative nailfold capillaroscopy in differential diagnosis of connective tissue diseases with Raynaud's phenomenon. *Journal of the Formosan Medical Association = Taiwan yi zhi, 112*(8), 482–488. https://doi.org/10.1016/j.jfma.2012.02.029(accessed on 23rd July 2025).

28. Makda, M. A. (2013). The prevalence of anti-C1q antibodies in black South Africans with systemic lupus erythematosus and their clinical significance. https://core.ac.uk/download/39671407.pdf (accessed on 23rd July 2025).

29. Mulhearn, B., Tansley, S. L., & McHugh, N. J. (2020). Autoantibodies in connective tissue disease. *Best practice & research. Clinical rheumatology, 34*(1), 101462. https://doi.org/10.1016/j.berh.2019.101462(accessed on 23rd July 2025).

30. Lupu, A., Sasaran, M. O., Jechel, E., Azoicai, A., Alexoae, M. M., Starcea, I. M., Mocanu, A., Nedelcu, A. H., Knieling, A., Salaru, D. L., Burlea, S. L., Lupu, V. V., & Ioniuc, I. (2024). Undercover lung damage in pediatrics - a hot spot in morbidity caused by collagenoses. *Frontiers in immunology, 15*, 1394690. https://doi.org/10.3389/fimmu.2024.1394690(accessed on 23rd July 2025).

31. Febyani M, Purbo DH, Hamijoyo L, Sutedja. E, Suwarsa O, Sclerodermatomyositis,. Indonesian Journal of Rheumatology;. 2011. 13.https://core.ac.uk/download/228794365.pdf (accessed on 23rd July 2025).

VASCULITIS AND PURPURA

8

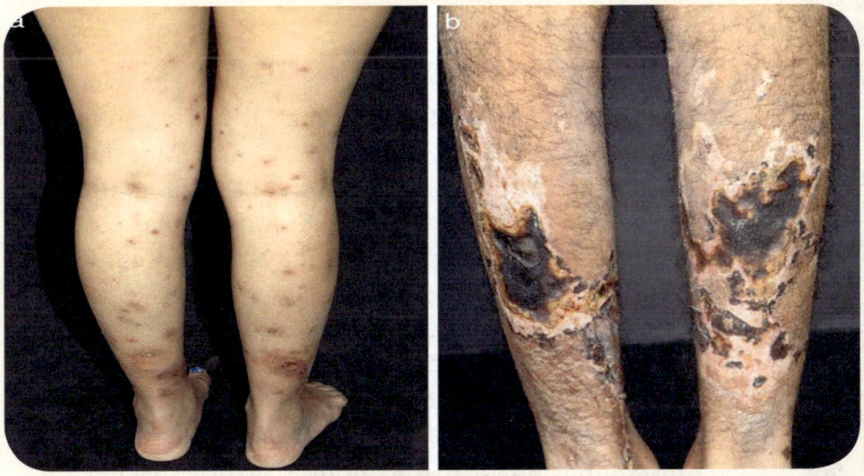

LEARNING OBJECTIVES

After studying this chapter, you will be able to:

1. Understand Types of Vasculitis;
2. Explain Pathophysiology of Vasculitis;
3. Describe Causes and Types of Purpura;
4. Focus on Diagnosis and Treatment.

Introduction

Purpura and vasculitis are significant clinical presentations that are related to the inflammation of blood vessels and produce a wide range of symptoms and complications that affect various organ systems. These conditions should be well known because they may be secondary to drug reactions or underlying systemic illness. For example, patients on immune checkpoint inhibitors (ICPi) can experience immune-related adverse events that need careful management maneuvers to minimize toxicity, thus necessitating an expert consensus on treatment guidance (Schneider et al., 2021). Additionally, current-day challenges such as the COVID-19 pandemic have highlighted emergent presentations of vasculitis associated with viral infections, for example, the purpuric vasculitic pattern experienced by patients (Genovese et al., 2020). This chapter tries to explore the complexities of vasculitis and purpura, examining their pathophysiology, clinical relevance, and the management of such complicated conditions.

8.1. Types of Vasculitis

Learning Outcome

1. Understand Large Vessel Vasculitis;
2. Explain Medium Vessel Vasculitis;
3. Focus on Small Vessel Vasculitis;
4. Describe Primary vs. Secondary Vasculitis;
5. Learn Systemic vs. Localized Vasculitis;
6. Discuss Common Types: Giant Cell Arteritis;
7. Know Common Types: Takayasu arteritis;
8. Understand Common Types: ANCA-associated Vasculitis;
9. Explain Rare Forms of Vasculitis.

Vasculitis is a heterogeneous group of disorders characterized by inflammation of the blood vessels that involve multiple organ systems.

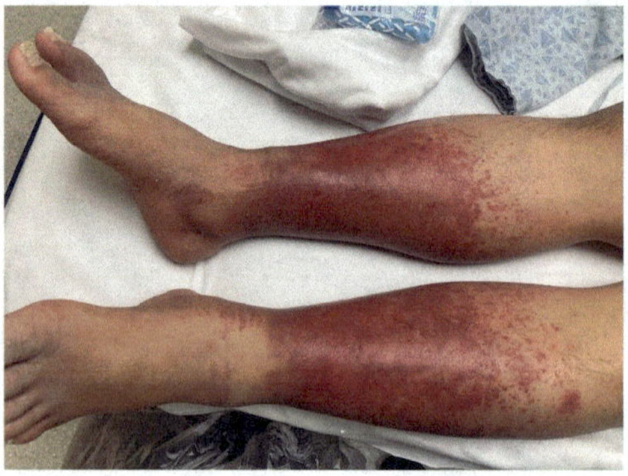

Figure 8.1. Cryoglobulinaemic vasculitis.

Source: https://www.jem-journal.com/cms/10.1016/j.jemermed.2022.09.004/asset/2676334c-112f-4e88-a54a-3ef896995ccc/main.assets/gr1_lrg.jpg.

Among these, cryoglobulinaemic vasculitis is particularly noted as it is most often secondary to infections like hepatitis C and leads to serious complications like glomerulonephritis and potential renal failure. Identification of the etiologic cause is most crucial as antiviral therapy depicts a pathway for effective treatment of this disease (Braun et al., 2007). The other extreme is RPGN, which also threatens the kidney with irreparable damage by acute inflammatory processes in glomeruli. With treatment, albeit conventional with glucocorticoids and cyclophosphamide, the lack of widespread clinical trials in severe cases is a testament to the challenges in managing RPGN effectively (Greenhall & Salama, 2015). Knowledge of these types of vasculitides is paramount to developing targeted treatments and improving patient outcomes in the context of vasculitis and purpura (Figure 8.1).

8.1.1. Large Vessel Vasculitis

Large vessel vasculitis (LVV) is a serious category of vasculitides whereby there is inflammation of the great vessels, i.e., the aorta and its major branches. This condition predominantly affects older persons and could have nonspecific symptoms and signs such as fever, malaise, and weight loss, rendering it hard to diagnose at an early stage. LVV pathogenesis is complex and could involve immunological mechanisms such as cell-mediated and immune complex-mediated inflammation, which produces severe vascular damage and tissue ischemia in infected tissue (Guillevin & Dörner, 2007). Due to the potential for serious complications like stroke and organ ischemia, early diagnosis and prompt treatment are required. Histopathological analysis is critical in making a final diagnosis, clearing the way for targeted therapies that can minimize vascular injury and improve patient outcomes (Gupta et al., 2020). The heterogeneity of LVV emphasizes the importance of an integrated management approach in the setting of the overall context of purpura and vasculitis.

8.1.2. Medium Vessel Vasculitis

Medium vessel vasculitis is a severe form of vascular inflammation of medium-sized arteries that causes severe organ damage as a result of decreased blood supply. These conditions, like polyarteritis nodosa (PAN), are covered in this category and have a very diverse range of clinical manifestations, with the kidneys, skin, and nervous system most commonly affected. The interaction between medium vessel vasculitis and secondary initiators is particularly significant; for instance, infections like hepatitis C can induce cryoglobulinaemia, which may induce vaso-occlusive processes and organ damage (Braun et al., 2007). In addition, new evidence suggests that certain drugs of abuse, such as levamisole-adulterated cocaine, can induce unique forms of vasculitis with severe dermatologic and renal manifestations like leukocytoclastic vasculitis and necrotizing glomerulonephritis, making the clinical presentation complex (Nolan & Jen, 2015). Understanding these nuances is central to the successful diagnosis and treatment of medium vessel vasculitis (Figure 8.2).

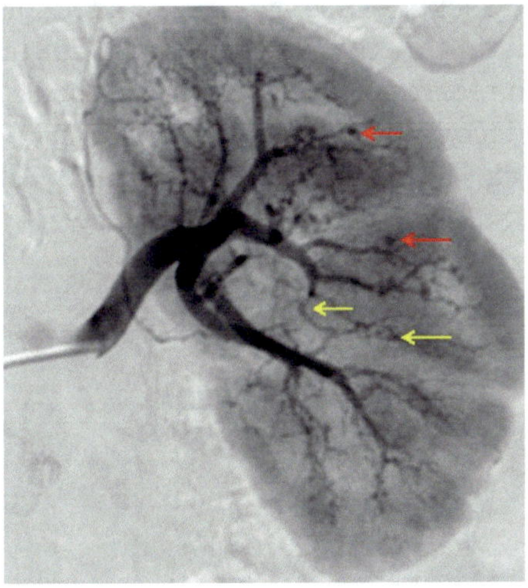

Figure 8.2. Polyarteritis nodosa (PAN).

Source: https://www.techvir.com/cms/10.1053/j.tvir.2014.11.005/asset/d725aa20-338f-4835-ab0d-6d5d7598857e/main.assets/gr1_lrg.jpg.

8.1.3. Small Vessel Vasculitis

Small vessel vasculitis is a cluster of disorders characterized by small vessel inflammation and create noteworthy clinical presentation. The most significant among them is Henoch-Schönlein purpura (HSP), which favors children but may also affect adults. HSP is predominantly immunmediated by IgA-containing immune complex deposition in target tissues, with presentation of abdominal pain, purpura, and glomerulonephritis. Small vessel vasculitis is characterized by its heterogeneity and can be exemplified in a condition like cryoglobulinaemia that is secondary to infections such as hepatitis C and could lead to serious renal complications such as end-stage renal failure (Braun et al., 2007). Moreover, viral causes, like in a rotavirus-induced case of HSP, represent the multifaceted interaction between inciting agents and the induction of small vessel vasculitis and therefore should be treated with careful regulation to avoid concomitant morbidities (Adderley, 2017).

8.1.4. Primary vs. Secondary Vasculitis

The primary/secondary distinction in vasculitis is critical to the management as well as the etiology of such inflammatory processes. Primary vasculitis, such as Granulomatosis with polyangiitis or Polyarteritis nodosa, are idiopathic without an associated underlying disease, typically with systemic presentation and potential organ damage. Secondary vasculitis, on the other hand, arises as a complication of other diseases, such as infections or autoimmune disorders, that can lead to presentations that are similar to the primary counterparts. For instance, Henoch-Schönlein purpura (HSP), a form of secondary vasculitis, typically occurs in the aftermath of infection and is typified by a symptom syndrome including purpura and kidney disease (Adderley, 2017). Additionally, RPGN can occur in the context of secondary vasculitis and must be treated promptly to prevent irreversible kidney injury (Greenhall & Salama, 2015). Such variations highlight the significance of an intensive approach in diagnosis and treatment, thus the complexity of the vasculitis categories (Figure 8.3).

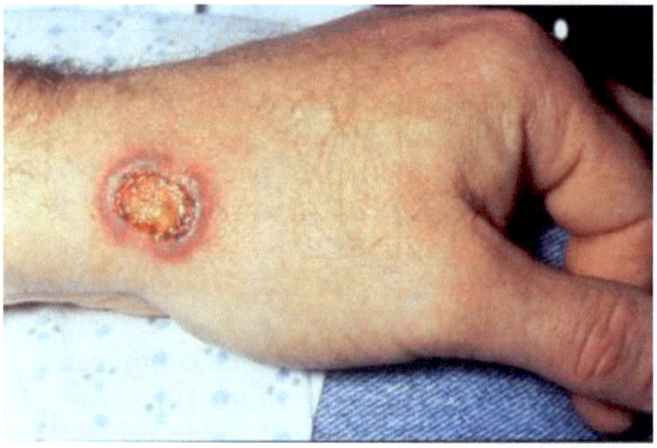

Figure 8.3. Granulomatosis with polyangiitis.

Source: https://img.medscapestatic.com/pi/meds/ckb/49/39249tn.jpg.

8.1.5. Systemic vs. Localized Vasculitis

Understanding the variation between systemic and localized vasculitis is necessary to guarantee correct diagnosis and treatment procedures in patients afflicted by these conditions. Systemic vasculitis targets more than one organ system, usually leading to highly disabling complications that may greatly reduce quality of life; for example, cryoglobulinemic vasculitis, commonly seen with hepatitis C, may cause severe systemic manifestations such as skin ulcers, which necessitate complex management strategies that include both systemic and local therapies (Giuggioli et al., 2015). In contrast, localized vasculitis is more likely to be confined to specific areas of the vessels and can have less severe manifestations, involving only subcutaneous or cutaneous tissue. Difficulty in management of localized forms is quite frequently the potential for secondary complications if left untreated, and prioritization of certain therapies may be essential (Walter et al., 2016). Therefore, the management of vasculitis in a clinical environment must be specific to the condition and severity to obtain optimal patient outcomes.

8.1.6. Common Types: Giant Cell Arteritis

Giant cell arteritis (GCA), also referred to as temporal arteritis, is a prevalent form of large vessel vasculitis that predominantly affects older adults, typically over the age of 50. Involving inflammation of the arterial wall, and more so the cranial arteries, GCA can lead to serious complications, including blindness and aneurysm of the aorta if left untreated. They present typically without headache, scalp tenderness, jaw claudication, or systemic signs like fever and fatigue. The co-occurrence of GCA with polymyalgia rheumatica highlights the interrelated nature of the vasculitides and further complicates the clinical challenge of diagnosis. Recent gene research has revealed potential correlations of HLA alleles and susceptibility to various vasculitides, suggesting a need for future research on genetic susceptibility to diseases like GCA (Ana Márquez et al., 2015; Eleftheriou et al., 2015). Recognition of such typical presentations is critical for early detection and effective management of the disease (Figure 8.4).

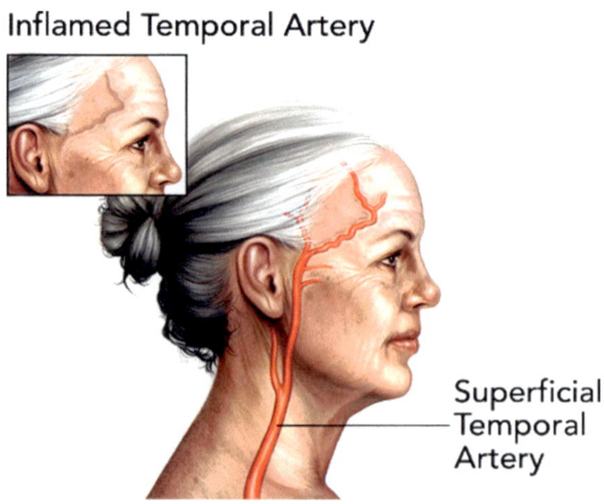

Figure 8.4. Giant cell arteritis (GCA).

Source: https://www.actemra.com/content/dam/gene/actemra/gca/images/what-is-gca/mobile/actemra-artery-head-mobile.genecoreimg.480.png.

8.1.7. Common Types: Takayasu arteritis

Takayasu arteritis, a rare large-vessel vasculitis, occurs predominantly in young women and is characterized by aorta and its major branches' inflammation. Takayasu arteritis results in very severe vascular complications, i.e., stenosis and aneurysm, leading to impaired blood supply to organs, and therefore, it is associated with the classically nonspecific presentations such as fatigue, loss of weight, and claudication of limbs, which render early diagnosis challenging. Despite its extreme rarity, Takayasu arteritis mirrors the larger category of systemic vasculitides occurring in pediatric age groups, as underscored by recent publications with vasculitis classification into types based on vessel size and location, recognizing idiopathic causes even in children (Pereira & Amaro, 2012; Eleftheriou et al., 2015). Early diagnosis and treatment are critical to disease containment and organ protection, highlighting ongoing research and awareness in clinical practice.

8.1.8. Common Types: ANCA-associated Vasculitis

ANCA-associated vasculitis (AAV) is a significant subgroup of the broader vasculitis group, characterized by ANCA-positivity and by the consequent inflammation of small to medium-sized blood vessels. The more generalized varieties of AAV are Granulomatosis with Polyangiitis (GPA) and Microscopic Polyangiitis (MPA), which have varying clinical manifestations but share common pathological processes. AAV predominantly affects organs such as the kidneys, lungs, and skin, thereby giving rise to dangerous complications unless detected early and treated. Inflammation response in AAV can be due to immune-mediated mechanisms, potentially leading to endothelial cell activation and subsequent vascular dysregulation, a pathway classically observed in systemic conditions like rheumatoid arthritis and systemic lupus erythematosus, linking AAV with increased cardiovascular risks (Dörner et al., 2007; Gupta et al., 2020). Effective management relies on a thorough knowledge of such conditions to minimize morbidity and improve patient outcomes (Figure 8.5).

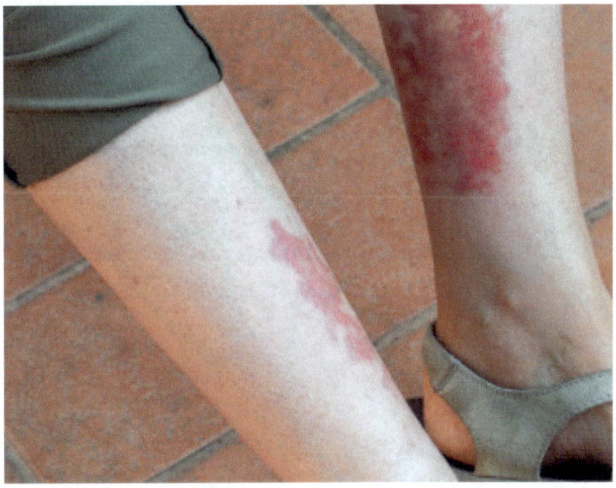

Figure 8.5. ANCA-associated vasculitis (AAV).

Source: https://www.the-rheumatologist.org/wp-content/uploads/2019/03/THR_0319_pg58a.png.

8.1.9. Rare Forms of Vasculitis

Uncommon forms of vasculitides may considerably complicate clinical presentations, usually resulting in severe health consequences. A prime example is cryoglobulinemic vasculitis, commonly linked to hepatitis C virus infection, which has the potential to trigger debilitating manifestations such as cutaneous vasculitis and glomerulonephritis, eventually at risk of end-stage renal failure (Braun et al., 2007). This highlights the need for appropriate therapeutic intervention, especially with the emergence of antiviral therapeutic drugs to treat the underlying viral pathology. Levamisole-induced vasculitis is another concern due to levamisole-contaminated cocaine abuse. The syndrome manifests in the form of retiform purpura and may have profound renal consequences, including pauci-immune glomerulonephritis, wherein there is a wide spectrum of drug-induced organ toxicity (Carlson et al., 2014). These rare variants need greater caution and specialist management to avoid the severe effects on patient health.

Test Your Knowledge

1. What is ANCA-associated vasculitis, and which conditions fall under it?
2. How do primary vasculitis syndromes differ from secondary vasculitis?

8.2. Pathophysiology of Vasculitis

Learning Outcome

1. Understand Immune System Involvement;
2. Explain Genetic Predispositions;
3. Focus on Environmental Triggers;
4. Describe Inflammatory Processes;
5. Learn Vascular Damage Mechanisms;
6. Discuss Role of Cytokines and Chemokines;
7. Know Consequences of Vascular Inflammation;
8. Understand Interaction with Other Diseases;
9. Explain Diagnostic Challenges in Understanding Pathophysiology.

The pathophysiology of vasculitis entails a complex interplay among immune dysregulation, inflammation, and endothelial damage, which profoundly affects the vascular system. The disease in its systemic form occurs by leukocyte and immune complex infiltration into vessel walls with various degrees of necrosis and thrombosis. Eosinophilic granulomatosis with polyangiitis (EGPA) is particularly significant in highlighting the complex interplay between vasculitis and neurological manifestations. For instance, the association of this condition with posterior reversible encephalopathy syndrome (PRES) indicates the potential implications of vasculitis-induced endothelial damage on treatment with immunosuppressive drugs (Marra et al., 2015). Furthermore, purpura is a clinical feature of vasculitis and reflects underlying vascular damage. As purpura is caused by diverse etiologies, its characteristics and classification are important so that it may be controlled effectively (Lamadrid-Zertuche et al., 2018). Its intricate pathophysiology needs to be explored more through more research studies so that the fine mechanisms are unraveled.

8.2.1. Immune System Involvement

The immune system plays a pivotal role in the pathogenesis of vasculitis and purpura with inflammatory involvement of blood vessels followed by cutaneous involvement. In particular, various forms of vasculitis are associated with dysregulation of anti-neutrophil cytoplasmic antibodies (ANCA). These antibodies can target rare antigens within neutrophil granules to cause leukocytoclastic vasculitis in targeted areas, such as in levamisole-contaminated cocaine, with patients showing typical skin lesions and renal dysfunction with elevated p-ANCA (Nolan & Jen, 2015). Moreover, vasculitis can even manifest its influence in the central and peripheral nervous system, like in patients with Henoch-Schönlein purpura, where it may appear as confusion and neurological dysfunction (Garzoni et al., 2017). This intricate relationship between the immune processes and vascular inflammation testifies to the multifactorial etiology of vasculitis and emphasizes the necessity for specific therapeutic interventions in the management of such diseases (Figure 8.6).

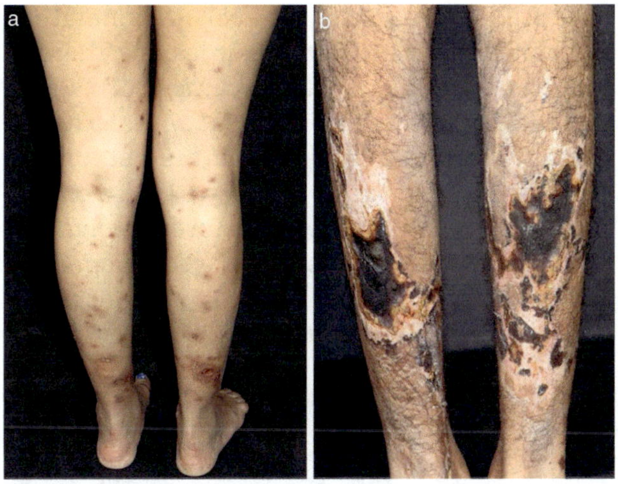

Figure 8.6. The immune system plays a pivotal role in the pathogenesis of vasculitis and purpura, characterized by inflammation of blood vessels and subsequent skin manifestations.

Source: https://static.elsevier.es/multimedia/03650596/0000009500000003/v4_202007210853/S0365059620300969/v4_202007210853/en/main.assets/gr3.jpeg.

8.2.2. Genetic Predispositions

It is crucial to consider genetic predispositions to describe the multifaceted pathogenesis of vasculitis and purpura. According to several studies, some genetic markers have the ability to make someone more susceptible to these conditions, impacting the severity as well as the presentation of symptoms. Particularly, research on cryoglobulin-associated vasculitis has pointed to significant associations with single-nucleotide polymorphisms (SNPs) located near the NOTCH4 and MHC class II genes that indicate the role of inherited traits in disease susceptibility (Zignego et al., 2014). Moreover, skin lesions are also common presenting symptoms in rheumatic diseases in children, such as IgA vasculitis and Kawasaki disease, and this shows that genetic factors may influence not just the etiology of vasculitis but also its presentations (Di Ludovico et al., 2024). Thus, increased understanding of these genetic predispositions can be used to direct targeted therapies and increase diagnostic accuracy in the management of vasculitides and purpura and ultimately improve patient outcomes.

8.2.3. Environmental Triggers

Environmental precipitants also play an important role in the pathogenesis of purpura and vasculitis, particularly in conditions such as Henoch-Schönlein purpura (HSP) and leukocytoclastic vasculitis (LCV).

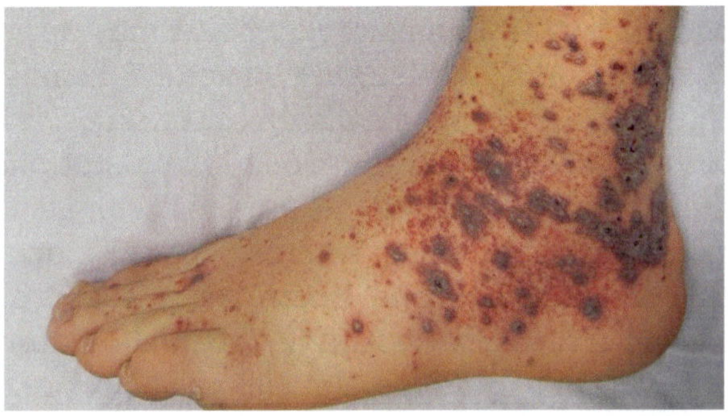

Figure 8.7. Leukocytoclastic vasculitis (LCV).

Source: https://post.healthline.com/wp-content/uploads/2019/12/Cutaneous-small-vessel-vasculitis-1296x728-gallery_slide2.jpg.

A retrospective analysis of HSP patients revealed that common environmental precipitants include upper respiratory tract infections, heavy exercise, and seasonality, which demonstrated peak incidence in autumn and winter months (Wang et al., 2016). These stimuli can trigger concomitant inflammatory pathways, leading to the characteristic cutaneous and joint manifestations of the disease. Similarly, LCV, characteristically drug- or infection-related, is a model for the manner in which environmental agents precipitate vasculitis. In one example, trimethoprim/sulfamethoxazole was given to an elderly woman, with the development of a purpuric rash, demonstrating the role of environmental agents in precipitating vascular inflammation (Shivarajpur et al., 2025). Understanding these environmental triggers holds the key to management and prevention of vasculitis and purpura (Figure 8.7).

8.2.4. Inflammatory Processes

Inflammatory processes form the core of the pathogenesis of vasculitis and purpura since they underscore the body's immune reaction to infection or trauma. Inflammatory processes are characterized by vascular inflammation, which can result in an assortment of clinical features ranging from cutaneous lesions to systemic presentation and organ impairment. In vasculitis, the inflammatory process may target blood vessels with resultant structural damage and secondary ischemia of adjacent tissues. It is most apparent with cutaneous manifestations, where characteristic lesions are the harbinger of underlying vascular compromise, the solution to a proper diagnosis and treatment (Kang et al., 2023). Further, understanding the inflammatory processes at play allows clinicians to better read clinical presentations and laboratory findings, thus ultimately leading to treatment decisions. A nuanced comprehension of inflammatory processes is thus essential to unpack the complexity of vasculitis and purpura, as well as negotiate proximal healthcare inequalities (Konorev, 2008).

8.2.5. Vascular Damage Mechanisms

Insight into the mechanisms of vascular injury in vasculitis and purpura will allow us to develop appropriate therapies. Vascular inflammation has different etiologies, leading to dysfunction of the normal endothelium and varied clinical presentations. For instance, levamisole-contaminated cocaine exposure has been linked with severe vascular injury, characterized by retiform purpura and autoimmunity to different body organ systems, most significantly the kidney, where it can cause pauci-immune glomerulonephritis (Carlson et al., 2014). Furthermore, recent advances in neuroimaging techniques have helped us to more accurately distinguish between inflammatory and non-inflammatory vascular lesions, thereby improving the diagnostic accuracy for PCNSV and other such diseases (Mansueto et al., 2022). The advances not only explain the pathogenic processes behind vascular injury but also enable us to intervene on time, therefore highlighting the close inter-relationship between diagnostic precision and treatment outcome in vasculitis and purpura (Figure 8.8).

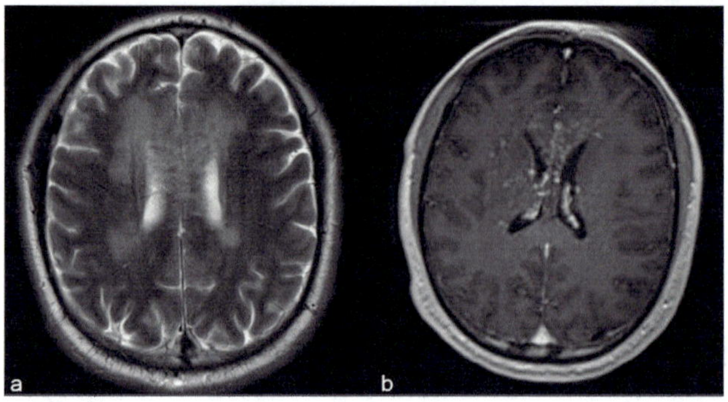

Figure 8.8. Recent advances in neuroimaging techniques have improved our ability to distinguish inflammatory from non-inflammatory vascular lesions, enhancing diagnostic accuracy for conditions like primary central nervous system vasculitis (PCNSV)

Source: https://www.jns-journal.com/cms/10.1016/j.jns.2021.117422/asset/b6344355-0b0b-4e46-89ba-b5e4600abddf/main.assets/gr2_lrg.jpg.

8.2.6. Role of Cytokines and Chemokines

Cytokines and chemokines play an imperative role in the pathophysiology of vasculitis and purpura, as these signaling molecules mediate the inflammation of these conditions. Higher concentrations of some chemokines, such as interferon-γ-inducible protein-10 (IP-10) and monocyte chemoattractant protein-1 (MCP-1), have been linked with increased monocyte function in acute stages of diseases such as Kawasaki and Henoch-Schönlein purpura (Chung et al., 2004). This suggests that monocytes are significant in the inflammatory process in vasculitis. In addition, the interaction of cytokines, chemokines, and endothelial cells underscores the sophistication of inflammatory processes, wherein glucocorticoids can modulate such effects through the regulation of endothelial cell function and cytokine production (Zielińska et al., 2016). The understanding of the particular functions of these molecules can direct therapeutic approaches, which in turn can eventually enable improved control of vasculitis and purpura.

8.2.7. Consequences of Vascular Inflammation

Inflammation of the vasculature, as in vasculitis, produces serious and complex effects on an individual's health.

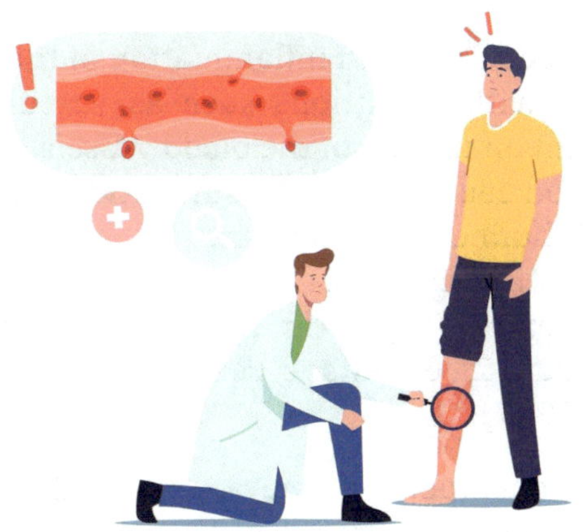

Figure 8.9. Vascular inflammation, as seen in conditions such as vasculitis, leads to significant and multifaceted consequences that can severely impact an individual's health.

Source: https://health.veininstitutenj.com/hubfs/iStock-1300907023.jpg.

Among the most notable are the eruption of skin lesions and renal impairment, which can be a response to any number of extrinsic stimuli, including agents like levamisole-contaminated cocaine. Under these circumstances, patients have a significant presence of anti-neutrophil cytoplasmic antibodies (p-ANCA), with other atypical patterns against non-conventional antigens also present, so the clinical presentation becomes even more complicated (Nolan & Jen, 2015). Furthermore, histological examinations reveal leukocytoclastic vasculitis, which is proof of both superficial and deep dermal vessel infiltration, thus characterizing the cutaneous presentation of this disease. Renal injury typically presents as necrotizing and crescentic pauci-immune glomerulonephritis, highlighting the systemic implications of vascular inflammation and highlighting the importance of early diagnosis and treatment in avoiding its devastating effects (Konorev, 2008) (Figure 8.9).

8.2.8. Interaction with Other Diseases

The interaction between purpura and vasculitis with other diseases portends a complicated situation in which these diseases can affect and be affected by comorbid conditions. For instance, the presence of primary immunodeficiencies (PIDs) makes management of autoimmune disease challenging since the treatment must accomplish immune support and immune suppression to arrest inflammation. This double demand is ubiquitous since autoimmune cytopenias and rheumatologic conditions often occur concomitantly with vasculitis (Walter et al., 2016). Chronic inflammation brought about by infections may also worsen vascular diseases such as atherosclerosis, implying that inflammatory and serological markers may be important in forecasting vascular events among patients with vasculitis (Abbas et al., 2008). Such interactions highlight the importance of an integrated vision for handling patient history and treatment protocols when working with such complex diseases.

8.2.9. Diagnostic Challenges in Understanding Pathophysiology

The primary reason for the difficulty of diagnosing vasculitis and purpura is that the complexities of their pathophysiology have a tendency to make multifaceted symptoms that are not difficult at all be misconceived as manifestations of more common diseases. This diagnostic challenge is also exacerbated by the fact that such conditions have a relatively low prevalence, as shown by reports that illustrate stroke in children, an extraneous complication of vasculitis, as it affects only two to eight out of every 100,000 children, thereby putting clinicians at greater risk of missing it (Mekitarian Filho & Carvalho, 2009). Furthermore, developments in diagnostic methods such as modern neuroimaging modalities have played a crucial role in differentiating inflammatory disorders from other vascular lesions, but doctors are usually still left with misdiagnosis due to the unpredictable histopathological features of these conditions (Mansueto et al., 2022). Therefore, an acute recognition of the diverse clinical manifestations and use of new diagnostic methods are needed in a bid to improve outcomes in vasculitis-related disorders.

Test Your Knowledge

1. What is fibrinoid necrosis and where is it seen?
2. How does endothelial injury lead to purpura and tissue ischemia?

8.3. Purpura: Causes and Types

Learning Outcome

1. Understand Definition and Characteristics of Purpura;
2. Explain Thrombocytopenic purpura;
3. Focus on Non-thrombocytopenic Purpura;
4. Describe Causes Related to Vasculitis;
5. Learn Causes Related to Infections;
6. Discuss Causes Related to Medications;
7. Know Causes Related to Systemic Diseases;
8. Understand Idiopathic Purpura;
9. Explain Diagnostic Criteria for Purpura.

Purpura, or the development of purple spots on the skin due to bleeding underneath the skin surface, can be caused by many underlying conditions, primarily divided into non-thrombocytopenic and thrombocytopenic purpura. Non-thrombocytopenic purpura is more often associated with inflammation of the blood vessels, with conditions such as vasculitis in which inflammation of the blood vessels leads to red blood cell loss into the surrounding tissues. Cryoglobulinemic vasculitis, for instance, can cause both skin lesions and renal complications like glomerulonephritis, which, if not treated, can result in end-stage renal disease (Braun et al., 2007).

Thrombocytopenic purpura, on the other hand, is caused by a decrease in platelets, generally due to immune diseases or certain medications. Further, rapidly progressive glomerulonephritis (RPGN) can also complicate this picture since it is caused by extensive damage to the kidneys that usually occurs with purpura as part of its other major renal consequences (Greenhall & Salama, 2015). Understanding, therefore purpuras complex etiology is important for proper diagnosis and treatment (Figure 8.10).

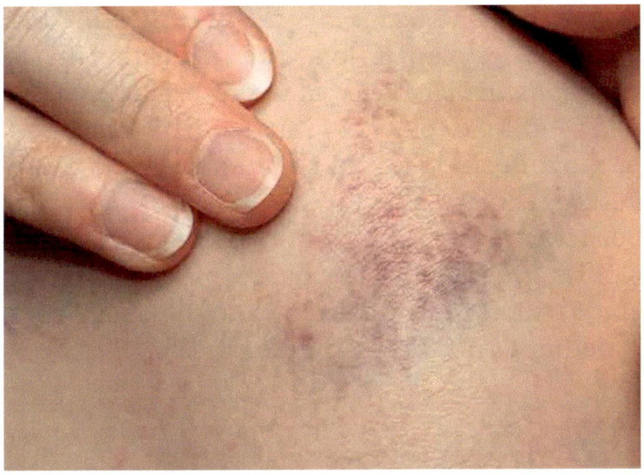

Figure 8.10. Purpura, characterized by the appearance of purple spots on the skin due to bleeding underneath, can arise from various underlying conditions, primarily classified into non-thrombocytopenic and thrombocytopenic types.

Source: https://media.post.rvohealth.io/wp-content/uploads/2020/09/bleeding-into-the-skin_thumb-1-732x549.jpg.

8.3.1. Definition and Characteristics of Purpura

Purpura is characterized by the formation of purple or red coloration on the skin or mucous membranes due to bleeding below the skin. This condition is produced by various underlying pathologies, most often in the context of vascular inflammation or dysfunction. In the context of vasculitis, purpura is a significant clinical observation, implying damage to small vessels with extravasation of blood into adjacent tissues. Inflammatory pathways of vasculitis, such as in systemic lupus erythematosus and rheumatoid arthritis, result in endothelial cell activation and, therefore, sustain vascular dysregulation, posing risk for purpura development (Guillevin & Dörner, 2007). Of particular interest is the relationship of purpura with renal disease in conditions like small vessel vasculitis, which indicates its severity since it can lead to severe morbidity, including end-stage renal disease (El-Husseini et al., 2018). Understanding these characteristics is paramount for effective diagnosis and treatment of purpura in a clinical environment.

8.3.2. Thrombocytopenic purpura

Thrombocytopenic purpura, where platelet count is reduced, causing bleeding spontaneously and purple spots on the skin, is a significant clinical issue with a connection to vasculitis and other autoimmune disorders. In systemic lupus erythematosus (SLE) disease, thrombocytopenic purpura can be a heterogeneous hematologic deviation, necessitating tailored therapeutic interventions from simple observation to drastic immunosuppression, depending on the severity of the disease (Velo-García et al., 2016).

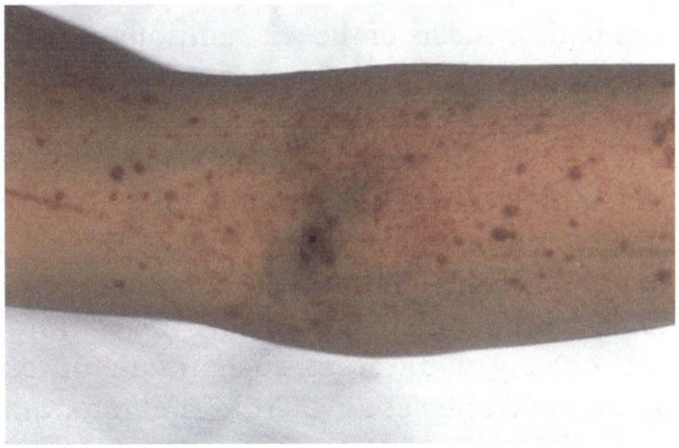

Figure 8.11. Thrombocytopenic purpura.

Source: https://www.nhlbi.nih.gov/sites/default/files/inline-images/pupura-petechiae_1.png.

In response to progress in therapeutic approaches, rituximab has been an effective second-line treatment option, with up to 60% success rates in immune thrombocytopenia, essentially before chronic evolution (Lucchini et al., 2019). However, the long-term viability of such actions remains doubtful, since a small subgroup of patients can sustain remission in the long term, and therefore, the need for ongoing studies and customized treatment protocols in treating this multi-causative disease in the context of vasculitis and purpura at large (Figure 8.11).

8.3.3. Non-thrombocytopenic Purpura

Non-thrombocytopenic purpura is a potentially life-threatening group of cutaneous manifestations of small vessel vasculitis, with post-capillary venular bleeding but without extreme platelet loss. This is typically secondary to the intrinsic inflammatory processes that target the vascular walls, leading to extravasation of red cells and purpuric lesions. Non-thrombocytopenic purpura pathogenesis can be caused by numerous autoimmune conditions leading to an abnormally formed immune response, with a central role of B-lymphocytes in the pathogenesis of these conditions, as seen through ongoing research studies that attempt to unravel their precise mechanisms (Tuscano & Sands, 2009). The challenge with managing such cases is how to balance immune enhancement and necessary immune suppression, especially in primary immunodeficiencies, whose therapeutic interventions must specifically be tailored to effectively counteract such inflammatory responses (Walter et al., 2016). Understanding this interaction is critical in developing an intervention specifically for affected individuals.

8.3.4. Causes Related to Vasculitis

Vasculitis has a multifactorial etiology involving both autoimmune and environmental aetiologies. Among the major causes are drug reactions, the most frequent of which is to drugs such as levamisole-adulterated cocaine, which has been linked to distinct pathologic findings. Patients with this exposure to the cocaine adulterant typically present with skin lesions and renal insufficiency, with an unusually frequent presence of perinuclear anti-neutrophil cytoplasmic antibodies (p-ANCA). Notably, the specific p-ANCA reacts with atypical antigens rather than the usual targets, complicating the diagnosis (Nolan & Jen, 2015). Furthermore, infections, malignancies, and certain autoimmune diseases also play a vital role in vasculitis pathogenesis. The understanding of these heterogeneous causes is critical to clinicians because management and treatment plans can be greatly variable based on the etiology, emphasizing individualized patient management (Cheung et al., 1999) (Figure 8.12).

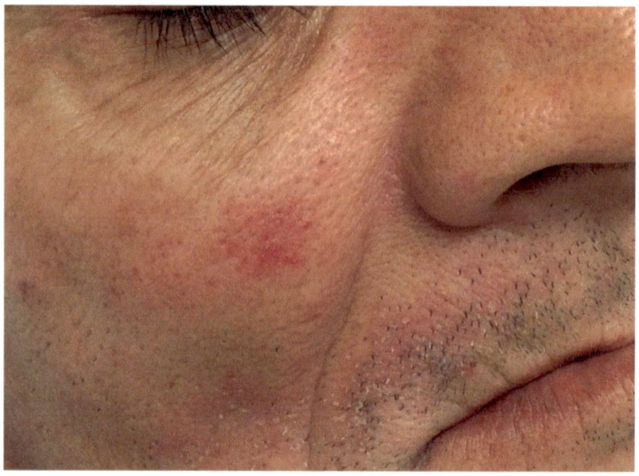

Figure 8.12. Levamisole-adulterated cocaine.

Source: https://casereports.bmj.com/content/casereports/2015/bcr-2015-211768/F2.large.jpg?download=true.

8.3.5. Causes Related to Infections

In vasculitides and purpura, infections were identified as significant precipitating factors with the potential to cause such inflammatory disorders. Surprisingly, Henoch-Schönlein purpura (HSP), primarily a small vessel vasculitis, has a tendency to follow infections such as rotavirus and Giardia. A case presentation shows an older man whose HSP was associated with these pathogens and establishes that gastrointestinal infection may cause localized immune responses leading to vasculitis manifestations like purpuric rashes and renal damage (Adderley, 2017). Similarly, cryoglobulinaemia, another aetiology of cutaneous vasculitis, has also been linked to infections, and more notably, those secondary to the hepatitis C virus. It is particularly relevant in the context of identifying underlying infective causes in patients presenting with features of vasculitis since treatment of the infection might potentially slow down the progression of vasculitis and lead to improved patient outcomes (Braun et al., 2007). Detection of such associations is key to the best management and treatment regimens.

8.3.6. Causes Related to Medications

Drugs can also play an immense role in the etiology of vasculitis and purpura, leading to a tremendous inflammatory response in the body. Some drugs, particularly antibiotics, non-steroidal anti-inflammatory drugs (NSAIDs), and antiepileptics, have been known to be precipitants of various forms of vasculitis, such as allergic vasculitis, which can cause cutaneous manifestations like purpura.

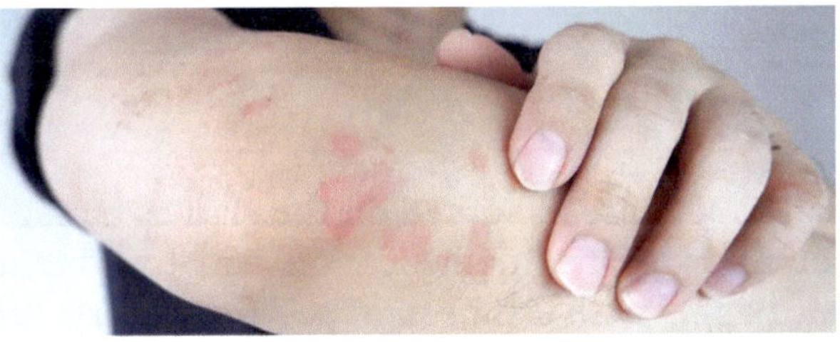

Figure 8.13. Medications can play a significant role in the onset of vasculitis and purpura, leading to notable inflammatory responses within the body.

Source: https://drmaggieyu.com/wp-content/uploads/2024/05/leukocytoclastic-vasculitis-treatment-options-and-monitoring.webp.

The mechanisms of pathogenicity are typically immune-mediated, in which the organism reacts negatively to such material, causing deposition of immune complexes that can result in small vessel injury. It has been recently suggested in the literature that infections, even drug-induced or drug-exacerbated, can potentially be linked with conditions like Henoch-Schönlein purpura (HSP), suggesting the intricacy of such interactions. As HSP predominantly concerns children, even though it is potentially worse in adults (Adderley, 2017), their identification as a drug cause is of key importance in timely management and diagnosis, especially when the treatment regimen of glucocorticoids for RPGN comes into play (Greenhall & Salama, 2015) (Figure 8.13).

8.3.7. Causes Related to Systemic Diseases

Purpura and vasculitis pathogenesis is often rooted in multifactorial systemic diseases, which provoke an inflammatory reaction targeted at the vascular system. Cryoglobulinaemia is one such classic example of such an association, where the presence of immune complexes in circulation leads to vasculitis, most typically presented in terms of skin rashes or renal impairment. Much of the cryoglobulinaemias are secondary to hepatitis C virus infection, which highlights the infectious etiologies relevant to systemic disease (Braun et al., 2007). Additionally, eosinophilic granulomatosis with polyangiitis (EGPA), being one of the ANCA-associated vasculitides, highlights involvement of systemic disease in vasculitis pathology. EGPA patients may have complex symptoms, including central nervous system involvement in the form of posterior reversible encephalopathy syndrome (PRES), which makes treatment with immunosuppressive drugs more complex (Marra et al., 2015). Overall, awareness of the systemic etiology of these conditions is essential for effective management and therapeutic interventions in such patients.

8.3.8. Idiopathic Purpura

Idiopathic purpura, a disease which is spontaneous bruising and petechiae with no apparent underlying cause, occupies a unique place in the broader picture of vasculitis and purpura. The disease is an autoimmune dysregulation whereby the immune system is inadvertently activated against blood vessel walls and consequently restricts itself to responding with inflammation to propagate hematologic diseases. Notably, its classification may interdigitate with some of the other vasculitides in which similar symptoms complicate diagnosis and treatment planning. Although idiopathic purpura is predominantly linked to children, it can persist and recur in adult populations, paralleling presentations described in comparable conditions such as Takayasu arteritis and membranoproliferative glomerulonephritis among different age groups, which have different incidences and clinical features among groups (Eleftheriou et al., 2015). Identification of idiopathic purpura in this spectrum is crucial for the development of comprehensive management protocols aimed at minimizing morbidity and maximizing patient outcomes (Figure 8.14).

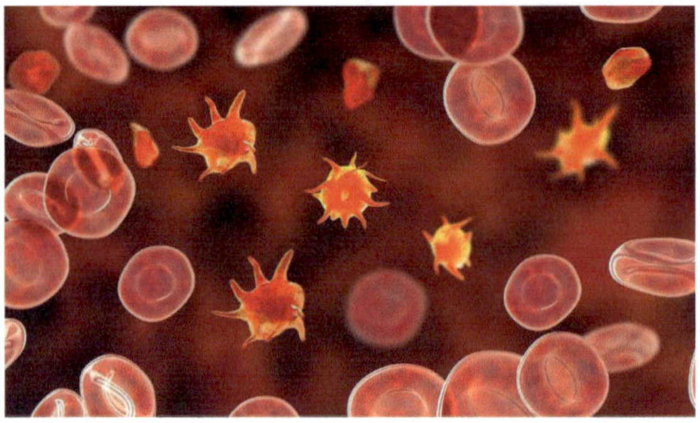

Figure 8.14. Idiopathic purpura.

Source: https://ameripharmaspecialty.com/wp-content/uploads/2021/11/blood-clotting-idiopathic-thrombocytopenic-purpura.jpg.

8.3.9. Diagnostic Criteria for Purpura

Diagnostic criteria for purpura, a condition where purple spots are observed on the skin as a result of bleeding underneath, are extremely significant for appropriate identification and treatment, especially with regard to vasculitis. Clinical assessment begins with a thorough patient history and physical examination, where the distribution, size, and character of the purpura are examined in detail. Etiologic causes can include potential precipitants like infections, medications, or allergy leading to specific forms of vasculitis. For instance, IgA vasculitis has been associated with diet, with its examples reported in cases when patients during adulthood experienced purpura upon ingestion of particular foods (Díaz et al., 2017). Additionally, recognition of the systemic signs is important, particularly in the situation where Takayasu arteritis can present with purpura accompanied by other complications of vascular disease (Eleftheriou et al., 2015). An integrated strategy enhances diagnostic efficiency, which results in timely and proper therapeutic measures.

Test Your Knowledge

1. What is senile purpura, and what is its pathophysiology?
2. How does thrombocytopenia cause purpura?

8.4. Diagnosis and Treatment

Learning Outcome

1. Understand Clinical Evaluation and History Taking;
2. Explain Laboratory Tests for Vasculitis;
3. Focus on Imaging Studies for Vascular Assessment;
4. Describe Biopsy Procedures and Their Significance;
5. Learn Treatment Options for Vasculitis;
6. Discuss Treatment Options for Purpura;
7. Know Role of Corticosteroids;
8. Understand Immunosuppressive Therapies;
9. Explain Monitoring and Follow-up Care.

In vasculitis and purpura, treatment and diagnosis become mandatory in managing potentially catastrophic complications. One notable variant is cryoglobulinemic vasculitis, most frequently linked with hepatitis C virus (HCV) infections. Cryoglobulinemic vasculitis ensues upon the precipitation of cryoglobulins at temperatures below body temperature, leading to dermal and renal manifestations such as purpura and glomerulonephritis. The link between HCV with cryoglobulinemic vasculitis reiterates the need for certain therapeutic approaches. New antiviral drugs hold promise for causal treatment, targeting the underlying infection and, consequently, the associated vasculitis (Braun et al., 2007). Secondly, the complexity in the management of cryoglobulinemic vasculitis is suggested through cases where patients exhibit severe renal impairment as the disease advances, which will then need close monitoring and management interventions to prevent end-stage renal failure (Caragea et al., 2018). Thus, the interplay between diagnosis and individualized treatment remains central to optimizing patient outcomes in such complicated cases.

8.4.1. Clinical Evaluation and History Taking

Effective clinical assessment and taking an active history are essential to diagnosing and managing diseases such as vasculitis and purpura. By detailed history-taking from a patient, including the onset and duration of symptoms, clinicians can identify clinical patterns consistent with systemic disease.

That, for instance, the presence of atypical symptoms, as in hepatitis C-associated cryoglobulinemic vasculitis, underscores the need for detailed assessment; these symptoms may only appear in the context of hepatic illness, as is underscored by the critique of patient cases (Caragea et al., 2018).

Likewise, in conditions like granulomatosis with polyangiitis, a keen watch on respiratory presentations, for instance, hemoptysis, can prove to be critical in making an early diagnosis and intervention and impacting the patients' outcome directly (Sattar et al., 2019). Therefore, meticulous history taking not only leads to appropriate diagnosis but also influences subsequent follow-up treatment protocols for the management of complicated vasculitic disease (Figure 8.15).

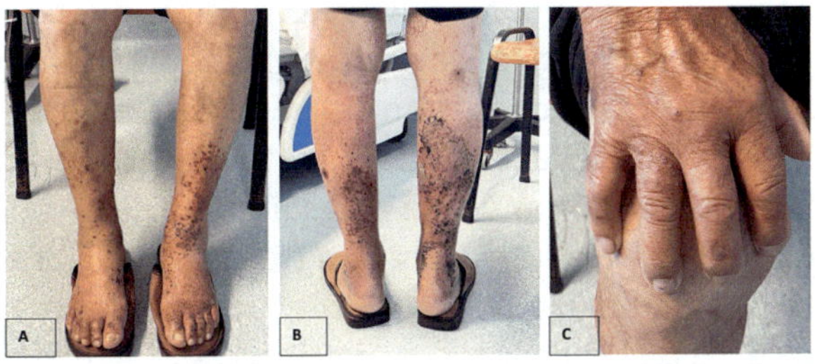

Figure 8.15. Effective clinical evaluation and thorough history taking are paramount in the diagnosis and management of conditions such as vasculitis and purpura.

Source: https://assets.cureus.com/uploads/figure/file/1113636/article_river_d0636a10448511efa697fb62f4d4e838-_figure1_Case-Report_Vasculite-IgA.png.

8.4.2. Laboratory Tests for Vasculitis

Efficient diagnosis of vasculitis is highly reliant on a combination of clinical evaluation and particular laboratory tests. Laboratory tests are able to reveal significant information on the underlying pathophysiology of the various forms of vasculitis. For instance, elevated markers of inflammation, such as erythrocyte sedimentation rate (ESR) and C-reactive protein (CRP), will usually mean active inflammation, while some autoantibodies, such as antineutrophil cytoplasmic antibodies (ANCA), will mean certain types of vasculitis. Henoch-Schönlein purpura (HSP) is a good example of how useful this type of testing can be; the condition, which presents as small vessel vasculitis, may be seen with serum creatinine elevation and abnormal urinalysis (Adderley, 2017). Furthermore, in acute hemorrhagic edema of infancy, laboratory tests usually are not informative and may indicate that the diagnosis is more clinical than lab-based (Garcia et al., 2016). Thus, an understanding of the lab picture is essential for the best possible management of vasculitis.

8.4.3. Imaging Studies for Vascular Assessment

Imaging studies have a pivotal role in the vascular assessment of vasculitis and purpura patients, serving to clarify the pathophysiology underlying the condition as well as the scope of vascular disease. Imaging techniques like magnetic resonance angiography (MRA) and computed tomography angiography (CTA) are particularly useful in the demarcation of large vessel disease, e.g., in Takayasu arteritis involving the aorta and large branches (Al-Obaidi et al., 2015). In addition, in Henoch-Schönlein purpura, neuroimaging is able to identify big structural changes, like vascular lesions and intracerebral hemorrhage, which are significant for the clinical management (Garzoni et al., 2017). Besides helping clinicians evaluate the vasculature's immediate status, these imaging techniques also aid in following disease response and evolution. Lastly, the synergy of advanced imaging techniques is responsible for a greater overall understanding of vasculitis complications, which leads to improved patient outcomes (Figure 8.16).

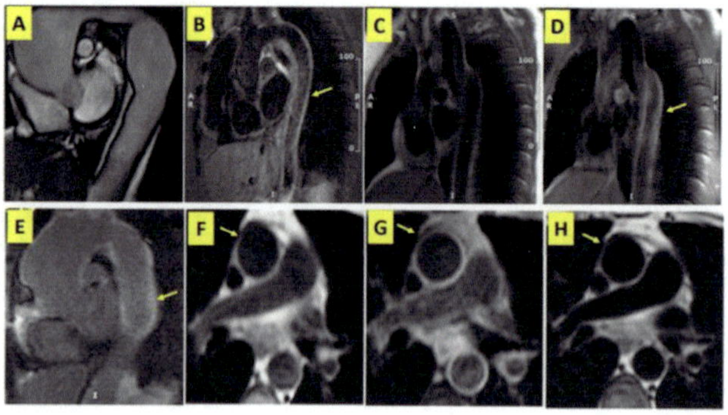

Figure 8.16. Techniques such as magnetic resonance angiography (MRA) and computed tomography angiography (CTA) are particularly useful in visualizing large vessel involvement, as seen in conditions like Takayasu arteritis.

Source: https://www.mdpi.com/diagnostics/diagnostics-13-03575/article_deploy/html/images/diagnostics-13-03575-g001-550.jpg.

8.4.4. Biopsy Procedures and Their Significance

The role of biopsy tests in the diagnosis and management of vasculitis and purpura cannot be overstated since they yield crucial evidence of the causative pathological processes. Biopsies of the affected organs or skin lesions allow for direct examination of the tissue, via which diagnostic evidence of vascular inflammation and damage specific to various forms of vasculitis can be detected. They are particularly crucial given the non-specific presentation of vasculitis, where a certain diagnosis to ascertain appropriate treatment modalities is necessitated. For instance, the differentiation between primary and secondary vasculitis is based on biopsy findings, which illustrate definitive histological observations (Hankollari et al., 2019). Further, in glomerulonephritis associated with systemic vasculitis, biopsy findings can influence management techniques, such as plasma exchange in dialysis patients, underlining the procedure's utility in augmenting renal function and the patient general prognosis (Pusey et al., 1991). Thus, biopsy remains part of optimal purpura and vasculitis management.

8.4.5. Treatment Options for Vasculitis

Effective vasculitis treatments largely rely on the etiology, clinical behavior, and severity of the disease.

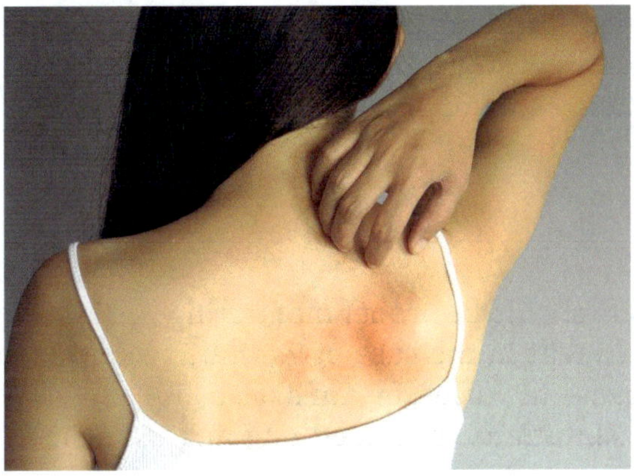

Figure 8.17. In cases of leukocytoclastic vasculitis, which presents with palpable purpura and may involve internal organs, treatment typically includes corticosteroids to reduce inflammation and suppress the immune response.

Source: https://media.post.rvohealth.io/wp-content/uploads/2020/08/allergic-vasculitis_thumb-1-732x549.jpg.

For instance, cryoglobulinaemic vasculitis, which is classically associated with infection by the hepatitis C virus, is treated using antiviral medication targeting the root viral infection, which relieves secondary manifestations as well as prevents complications in the form of renal failure (Braun et al., 2007). Treatment of leukocytoclastic vasculitis, where palpable purpura occurs and internal organs may be involved, includes corticosteroids to reduce inflammation and dampen immune function (Quack et al., 2013). Immunohistochemical drugs such as cyclophosphamide or rituximab may also be employed in cases of severe vasculitis for remission. Thus, an individualized treatment plan considering the patient-specific factors is essential in designing effective vasculitis treatment plans, illustrating the complexity of treating this multi-factorial disease (Figure 8.17).

8.4.6. Treatment Options for Purpura

The treatment of purpura, particularly that secondary to vasculitis, to a great extent depends on the aetiology and severity of the disease. In cases secondary to cryoglobulinaemia, often as a consequence of hepatitis C virus infection, antiviral therapy is very promising for its management. These novel antiviral drugs can be used to treat the viral infection as well as the resultant cryoglobulinaemic vasculitis, leading to relief of symptoms and good general health of the patient (Braun et al., 2007). Treatment of complications such as renal impairment is also critical; immunosuppressive therapy may be required to downregulate inflammation and prevent irreversible damage to the organs. As mentioned in clinical observations, patients with hepatitis C-related cryoglobulinaemic vasculitis can be characterized by alternating states of the disease, requiring proper monitoring and an individualized treatment strategy responsive to the changing condition of the patients (Caragea et al., 2018). Generally speaking, a multidisciplinary management is crucial in ensuring maximum treatment benefits for purpura.

8.4.7. Role of Corticosteroids

Corticosteroids are pivotal in the management of various forms of vasculitis and purpura by affecting the immune system and conferring immediate anti-inflammatory effects. Corticosteroids are included in treatment protocols with agents like cyclophosphamide and plasmapheresis for RPGN and significantly reduce the chance of kidney damage when administered early (Greenhall & Salama, 2015). Similarly, in Takayasu arteritis, corticosteroids are also pivotal in treating disease activity and large-vessel vasculitis symptoms (Al-Obaidi et al., 2015). Although useful, corticosteroid use with the treatment plan should be closely monitored due to potential side effects and steroid-sparing regimens for the management of chronic disease. Finally, although corticosteroids remain a staple in the management of vasculitis and purpura, ongoing research is needed to extend their use and improve patient outcomes with these complex diseases (Figure 8.18).

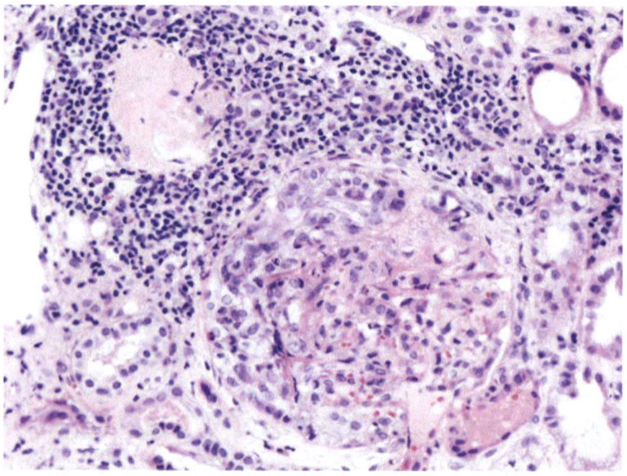

Figure 8.18. Rapidly progressive glomerulonephritis (RPGN).

Source: https://upload.wikimedia.org/wikipedia/commons/2/2e/Crescentic_glomerulonephritis_%282%29.jpg.

8.4.8. Immunosuppressive Therapies

The role of immunosuppressive therapies in the management of vasculitis and purpura remains viewed as fundamental to the complex autoimmune illnesses. These treatments are aimed at suppressing inflammatory pathways that cause vascular damage, improving patient response with a decrease in long-term complications. Specifically, studies have shown that treatments targeting B-lymphocytes, such as rituximab, have been effective in their capacity to treat a variety of autoimmune disorders, such as rheumatoid arthritis, with therapeutic implications for use in associated disorders like vasculitis and purpura (Tuscano & Sands, 2009). Furthermore, within the IgA vasculitis context, a recent observational study determined that patients were more often treated with immunosuppressive therapy compared to those with IgA nephropathy, which reflected different treatment protocols according to disease classification (Selewski et al., 2018). Hence, immunosuppressive treatments remain the cornerstone of our evolving management of these challenging conditions.

8.4.9. Monitoring and Follow-up Care

There should be proper monitoring and follow-up treatment in the case of vasculitis and purpura because the diseases can have complex, evolving presentations that need ongoing assessment.

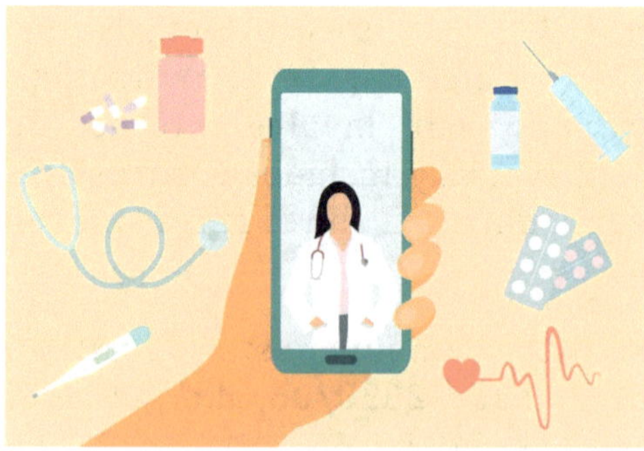

Figure 8.19. Regular follow-up visits not only enable clinicians to evaluate the progression of the disease but also allow for timely adjustments in treatment protocols.

Source: https://cdn.solutionreach.com/uploads/2023/02/04212649/resized-image-Promo-28-1.jpeg.

Follow-up visits regularly not only enable clinicians to evaluate disease progression but also afford timing for the modification of treatment. Particularly, conditions like Takayasu arteritis need to be watched carefully due to their potential for inducing serious complications in the large vasculature, particularly pertaining to pediatric settings where early intervention impacts outcomes greatly (Eleftheriou et al., 2015). Further, understanding the pathophysiology of diseases like Henoch-Schönlein purpura provides clinicians with an opportunity to identify complications and institute prophylaxis during follow-up (Thakur, 2008). By ensuring an extensive follow-up protocol, medical professionals can enhance patient outcomes and raise the standard of care provided to patients with these vascular diseases (Figure 8.19).

Test Your Knowledge

1. What imaging studies are useful in large-vessel vasculitis?
2. How is renal involvement evaluated in systemic vasculitis?

SUMMARY

The complex interplay of etiologic causes of vasculitis and purpura emphasizes the need for close observation and individualized therapy, particularly in such high-risk groups as children and adults presenting with atypical manifestations. The typical presentation of Henoch-Schönlein purpura in children emphasizes long-term impact, especially in cases of adult onset that can cause great morbidity involving renal failure and neurological involvement. Notably, a case report highlights the role of rotavirus infection as an etiologic agent in causing vasculitis with the hypothesis that infections have the potential to initiate a cascade of immune reactions leading to severe clinical manifestations (Adderley, 2017). Besides, the uncommon but serious manifestations of central and peripheral nervous system compromise in patients with Henoch-Schönlein syndrome underscore the significance of intensive neurological examination and follow-up as highlighted by recent literature (Garzoni et al., 2017). Thus, early diagnosis and personalized treatment are still critical towards preventing the undesirable outcomes of such conditions.

The study of purpura and vasculitis presents valuable observations on the pathophysiologic processes and clinical presentations of these disorders. It is noteworthy that, as rare as nervous system impairment is in Henoch-Schönlein syndrome, when it does occur, its frequency is of clinical significance, with a range of presentations from alterations in consciousness to convulsions. Imaging procedures typically identify vascular lesions and intracerebral hemorrhages that indicate the intricate interrelationship between neurological dysfunction and systemic vasculitis (Garzoni et al., 2017). In addition, cryoglobulinemic vasculitis also leads to severe implications such as non-healing cutaneous ulcers that significantly impair patients' quality of life. These ulcers correlate with more purpuric presentation and multiorgan involvement, for which the approach is multifaceted and can include immunosuppression and surgery (Giuggioli et al., 2015). These findings, in conjunction, emphasize the complexity of vasculitis and purpura management and the need for individualized therapy.

KEY TERMS FROM THIS CHAPTER

- Vasculitis
- Complications
- Immune checkpoint inhibitors (ICPi)
- COVID-19 pandemic
- Purpuric vasculitic pattern
- Glomerulonephritis
- Kidney
- Glucocorticoids
- Blood vessels
- Drug reactions
- Toxicity
- Viral infections
- Cryoglobulinaemic vasculitis
- Potential renal failure
- Glomeruli
- Cyclophosphamide

CRITICAL THINKING QUESTIONS

1. **Which of the following is a small-vessel vasculitis associated with IgA deposition?**
   a. Polyarteritis nodosa
   b. Granulomatosis with polyangiitis
   c. Henoch-Schönlein purpura (IgA vasculitis)
   d. Takayasu arteritis
2. **The characteristic skin finding in small-vessel vasculitis is:**
   a. Erythema nodosum
   b. Urticaria
   c. Palpable purpura
   d. Livedo reticularis
3. **Which of the following is commonly associated with anti-neutrophil cytoplasmic antibodies (ANCA)?**
   a. Giant cell arteritis
   b. Granulomatosis with polyangiitis
   c. Kawasaki disease
   d. Erythema multiforme
4. **Which large-vessel vasculitis is most common in elderly individuals and can cause vision loss?**
   a. Takayasu arteritis
   b. Kawasaki disease
   c. Giant cell arteritis
   d. Polyarteritis nodosa
5. **A child presents with abdominal pain, arthritis, and palpable purpura. The most likely diagnosis is:**
   a. Hemophilia A
   b. Idiopathic thrombocytopenic purpura
   c. Henoch-Schönlein purpura
   d. Thrombotic thrombocytopenic purpura

Short Answer Questions

1. What are the different types of vasculitis based on vessel size?
2. What are the key features of large-vessel vasculitis (e.g., giant cell arteritis, Takayasu arteritis)?
3. What is the role of immune complex deposition in vasculitis?
4. How does ANCA contribute to the pathogenesis of vasculitis?
5. What is purpura, and how is it classified (petechiae, ecchymoses, palpable purpura)?
6. What are the causes of non-palpable purpura?
7. What are the key investigations in suspected systemic vasculitis?
8. What is the role of ANCA testing in diagnosis?

Answers to Critical Thinking Questions

1. (c); 2. (c); 3. (b); 4. (c); 5. (c)

REFERENCES

1. Abbas, M. A., Comi, G., Corea, F., et al. (2008). Microbial risk factors of cardiovascular and cerebrovascular diseases: Potential therapeutic options. https://core.ac.uk/download/75713.pdf (accessed on 23rd July 2025).
2. Díaz JM, González AM, Alonso REB, Bruñén JMG, Repiso GA. Food-induced IgA Vasculitis (Henoch-Schönlein Purpura). *Eur J Case Rep Intern Med.* 2018;5(2):000774. Published 2018 Feb 22. doi:10.12890/2017_000774 (accessed on 23rd July 2025).
3. Adderley, A., et al. (2017). A case of *Henoch-Schönlein purpura* associated with rotavirus infection in an elderly Asian male and review of the literature. https://core.ac.uk/download/323078862.pdf (accessed on 23rd July 2025).
4. Eleftheriou, D., Varnier, G., Dolezalova, P., McMahon, A. M., Al-Obaidi, M., & Brogan, P. A. (2015). Takayasu arteritis in childhood: retrospective experience from a tertiary referral centre in the United Kingdom. *Arthritis research & therapy*, *17*(1), 36. https://doi.org/10.1186/s13075-015-0545-1 (accessed on 23rd July 2025).
5. Mansueto, G., Lanza, G., Fisicaro, F., Alaouieh, D., Hong, E., Girolami, S., Montella, M., Feola, A., & Di Napoli, M. (2022). Central and Peripheral Nervous System Complications of Vasculitis Syndromes From Pathology to Bedside: Part 1-Central Nervous System. *Current neurology and neuroscience reports*, *22*(1), 47–69. https://doi.org/10.1007/s11910-022-01172-z(accessed on 23rd July 2025).
6. Chung, H. S., Kim, H. Y., Kim, H. S., Lee, H. J., Yuh, J. H., Lee, E. S., Choi, K. H., & Lee, Y. H. (2004). Production of chemokines in Kawasaki disease, Henoch-Schönlein purpura and acute febrile illness. *Journal of Korean medical science*, *19*(6), 800–804. https://doi.org/10.3346/jkms.2004.19.6.800(accessed on 23rd July 2025).
7. Zignego, A. L., Wojcik, G. L., Cacoub, P., Visentini, M., Casato, M., Mangia, A., Latanich, R., Charles, E. D., Gragnani, L., Terrier, B., Piazzola, V., Dustin, L. B., Khakoo, S. I., Busch, M. P., Lauer, G. M., Kim, A. Y., Alric, L., Thomas, D. L., & Duggal, P. (2014). Genome-wide association study of hepatitis C virus- and cryoglobulin-related vasculitis. *Genes and immunity*, *15*(7), 500–505. https://doi.org/10.1038/gene.2014.41(accessed on 23rd July 2025).
8. Pereira, N., & Amaro, C. (2012). Primary systemic vasculitis in childhood. https://core.ac.uk/download/71737992.pdf (accessed on 23rd July 2025).
9. Serra E Moura Garcia, C., Sokolova, A., Torre, M. L., & Amaro, C. (2016). Acute Hemorrhagic Edema of Infancy. *European annals of allergy and clinical immunology*, *48*(1), 22–26. (accessed on 23rd July 2025).
10. Selewski, D. T., Ambruzs, J. M., Appel, G. B., Bomback, A. S., Matar, R. B., Cai, Y., Cattran, D. C., Chishti, A. S., D'Agati, V. D., D'Alessandri-Silva, C. J., Gbadegesin, R. A., Hogan, J. J., Iragorri, S., Jennette, J. C., Julian, B. A., Khalid, M., Lafayette, R. A., Liapis, H., Lugani, F., Mansfield, S. A., ... CureGN Consortium (2018). Clinical Characteristics and Treatment Patterns of Children and Adults With IgA Nephropathy or IgA Vasculitis: Findings From the CureGN Study. *Kidney international reports*, *3*(6), 1373–1384. https://doi.org/10.1016/j.ekir.2018.07.021(accessed on 23rd July 2025).
11. Cheung RT, Mak W, Tsang KL. MRI in vertebral artery dissection. *J Neurol Neurosurg Psychiatry.* 1999;66(5):693-694. doi:10.1136/jnnp.66.5.693a(accessed on 23rd July 2025).

12. Di Ludovico, A., Rinaldi, M., Lauriola, F., Ciarelli, F., La Bella, S., Gualdi, G., Chiarelli, F., Bailey, K., & Breda, L. (2024). The Diagnostic Role of Skin Manifestations in Rheumatic Diseases in Children: A Critical Review of Paediatric Vasculitis. *International journal of molecular sciences*, *25*(13), 7323. https://doi.org/10.3390/ijms25137323(accessed on 23rd July 2025).

13. Marra, A. M., Barilaro, G., Villella, V., & Granata, M. (2015). Eosinophilic granulomatosis with polyangiitis (EGPA) and PRES: a case-based review of literature in ANCA-associated vasculitides. *Rheumatology international*, *35*(9), 1591–1595. https://doi.org/10.1007/s00296-015-3261-x(accessed on 23rd July 2025).

14. Gupta, P., Ganorkar, S., Bhalekar, S., & Rao, R. (2020). Varied presentations of cutaneous vasculitis: a case series. *International Journal of Research in Medical Sciences*, *8*(8), 3066–3073. https://doi.org/10.18203/2320-6012.ijrms20203465(accessed on 23rd July 2025).

15. Garzoni, L., Vanoni, F., Rizzi, M., Simonetti, G. D., Goeggel Simonetti, B., Ramelli, G. P., & Bianchetti, M. G. (2009). Nervous system dysfunction in Henoch-Schonlein syndrome: systematic review of the literature. *Rheumatology (Oxford, England)*, *48*(12), 1524–1529. https://doi.org/10.1093/rheumatology/kep282(accessed on 23rd July 2025).

16. Hankollari, Joana; Duli, Marsida; Dika, Qamil; Duli, Xhenila; Bimi, Indrit; and Dervishi, Daniela, "Differential Diagnosis between the Variety of Vasculitis Forms" (2017). UBT International Conference. 288. https://knowledgecenter.ubt-uni.net/conference/2017/all-events/288(accessed on 23rd July 2025).

17. Shivarajpur, A., Londono, S., Shaw, J., Boccio, C., Melnitsky, L., McKay, J., Kohen, B., & Boccio, E. (2025). Drug-induced Leukocytoclastic Vasculitis Secondary to Trimethoprim/Sulfamethoxazole: A Case Report. *Clinical practice and cases in emergency medicine*, *9*(1), 61–64. https://doi.org/10.5811/cpcem.31056(accessed on 23rd July 2025).

18. Caragea, D. C., Săndulescu, L., Pădureanu, V., Forțofoiu, M. C., Streba, C., Boldeanu, L., Boldeanu, M. V., Popescu-Drigă, M., Ciurea, M. E., Forțofoiu, M., Rogoveanu, I., Ciurea, T., & Vere, C. C. (2018). Clinical-Evolutional Particularities of the Cryoglobulinemic Vasculitis in the Case of a Patient Diagnosed with Hepatitis C Virus in the Predialitic Phase. *Journal of Mind and Medical Sciences*, *5*(1), 135-140. https://doi.org/10.22543/7674.51.P135140(accessed on 23rd July 2025).

19. Braun, G. S., Horster, S., Wagner, K. S., Ihrler, S., & Schmid, H. (2007). Cryoglobulinaemic vasculitis: classification and clinical and therapeutic aspects. *Postgraduate medical journal*, *83*(976), 87–94. https://doi.org/10.1136/pgmj.2006.046078(accessed on 23rd July 2025).

20. Lucchini, E., Zaja, F., & Bussel, J. (2019). Rituximab in the treatment of immune thrombocytopenia: what is the role of this agent in 2019?. *Haematologica*, *104*(6), 1124–1135. https://doi.org/10.3324/haematol.2019.218883(accessed on 23rd July 2025).

21. Carlson, A. Q., Tuot, D. S., Jen, K. Y., Butcher, B., Graf, J., Sam, R., & Imboden, J. B. (2014). Pauci-immune glomerulonephritis in individuals with disease associated with levamisole-adulterated cocaine: a series of 4 cases. *Medicine*, *93*(17), 290–297. https://doi.org/10.1097/MD.0000000000000090(accessed on 23rd July 2025).

22. Mekitarian Filho, E., & Carvalho, W. B. (2009). Stroke in children. *Jornal de pediatria*, *85*(6), 469–479. https://doi.org/10.2223/JPED.1944 (accessed on 23rd July 2025).

23. El-Husseini, A., Saleh, S., Hamad, O., Mei, X., Castellanos, A. L., Davenport, D. L., Gedaly, R., & Sawaya, B. P. (2018). Outcome of Patients With Small Vessel Vasculitis After Renal

Transplantation: National Database Analysis. *Transplantation direct*, *4*(3), e350. https://doi.org/10.1097/TXD.0000000000000769(accessed on 23rd July 2025).

24. Velo-García, A., Castro, S. G., & Isenberg, D. A. (2016). The diagnosis and management of the haematologic manifestations of lupus. *Journal of autoimmunity*, *74*, 139–160. https://doi.org/10.1016/j.jaut.2016.07.001(accessed on 23rd July 2025).
25. Quack, H., Erpenbeck, L., Wolff, H. A., Sprenger, T., Seitz, C. S., Schön, M. P., Neumann, S., Stanek, K., Ghadimi, B. M., Michels, B., Middel, P., Schaefer, I. M., Liersch, T., & Conradi, L. C. (2013). Oxaliplatin-Induced Leukocytoclastic Vasculitis under Adjuvant Chemotherapy for Colorectal Cancer: Two Cases of a Rare Adverse Event. *Case reports in oncology*, *6*(3), 609–615. https://doi.org/10.1159/000357166(accessed on 23rd July 2025).
26. Walter, J. E., Farmer, J. R., Foldvari, Z., Torgerson, T. R., & Cooper, M. A. (2016). Mechanism-Based Strategies for the Management of Autoimmunity and Immune Dysregulation in Primary Immunodeficiencies. *The journal of allergy and clinical immunology. In practice*, *4*(6), 1089–1100. https://doi.org/10.1016/j.jaip.2016.08.004(accessed on 23rd July 2025).
27. Zielińska, K. A., Van Moortel, L., Opdenakker, G., De Bosscher, K., & Van den Steen, P. E. (2016). Endothelial Response to Glucocorticoids in Inflammatory Diseases. *Frontiers in immunology*, *7*, 592. https://doi.org/10.3389/fimmu.2016.00592f (accessed on 23rd July 2025).
28. Guillevin L, Dörner T. Vasculitis: mechanisms involved and clinical manifestations. *Arthritis Res Ther*. 2007;9 Suppl 2(Suppl 2):S9. doi:10.1186/ar2193(accessed on 23rd July 2025).
29. Pusey, C. D., Rees, A. J., Evans, D. J., Peters, D. K., & Lockwood, C. M. (1991). Plasma exchange in focal necrotizing glomerulonephritis without anti-GBM antibodies. *Kidney international*, *40*(4), 757–763. https://doi.org/10.1038/ki.1991.272 (accessed on 23rd July 2025).
30. Giuggioli, D., Manfredi, A., Lumetti, F., Sebastiani, M., & Ferri, C. (2015). Cryoglobulinemic vasculitis and skin ulcers. Our therapeutic strategy and review of the literature. *Seminars in arthritis and rheumatism*, *44*(5), 518–526. https://doi.org/10.1016/j.semarthrit.2014.10.004(accessed on 23rd July 2025).
31. Wang, X., Zhu, Y., Gao, L., Wei, S., Zhen, Y., & Ma, Q. (2016). Henoch-Schönlein purpura with joint involvement: Analysis of 71 cases. *Pediatric rheumatology online journal*, *14*(1), 20. https://doi.org/10.1186/s12969-016-0080-x(accessed on 23rd July 2025).
32. Lamadrid-Zertuche, A. C., Garza-Rodríguez, V., & Ocampo-Candiani, J. J. (2018). Pigmented purpura and cutaneous vascular occlusion syndromes. *Anais brasileiros de dermatologia*, *93*(3), 397–404. https://doi.org/10.1590/abd1806-4841.20187459(accessed on 23rd July 2025).
33. Genovese, G., Moltrasio, C., Berti, E., & Marzano, A. V. (2020). Skin manifestations associated with COVID-19: Current knowledge and future perspectives. *Dermatology, 237*, 1–12. https://doi.org/10.1159/000512932 (accessed on 23rd July 2025).
34. Greenhall, G. H., & Salama, A. D. (2015). What is new in the management of rapidly progressive glomerulonephritis?. *Clinical kidney journal*, *8*(2), 143–150. https://doi.org/10.1093/ckj/sfv008(accessed on 23rd July 2025).
35. Nakagawa, N., Hasebe, N., Hattori, M., Nagata, M., Yokoyama, H., Sato, H., Sugiyama, H., Shimizu, A., Isaka, Y., Maruyama, S., & Narita, I. (2018). Clinical features and pathogenesis of membranoproliferative glomerulonephritis: a nationwide analysis of the Japan renal biopsy registry from 2007 to 2015. *Clinical and experimental nephrology*, *22*(4), 797–807. https://

doi.org/10.1007/s10157-017-1513-7 (accessed on 23rd July 2025).

36. Julianna S. Kang, Julia R. Nunley, Tiffany Ho, Mavra Masood, Fnu Nutan, and Dr. Beth Rubinstein (2023). Dermatologic manifestations of rheumatic disease: Cutaneous manifestations of vasculitis's. https://core.ac.uk/download/561013875.pdf (accessed on 23rd July 2025).

37. Nolan AL, Jen KY. Pathologic manifestations of levamisole-adulterated cocaine exposure. *Diagn Pathol.* 2015;10:48. Published 2015 May 6. doi:10.1186/s13000-015-0279-z (accessed on 23rd July 2025).

38. Konorev, M. R. (2008). *Lecture Notes by Internal Diseases.* https://core.ac.uk/download/80150474.pdf (accessed on 23rd July 2025).

39. Márquez, A., Navas Parejo, A., Ubilla, B., Sevilla Pérez, B., Argila, D., Rubio, E., Galíndez-Aguirregoikoa, E., et al. (2015). Association of HLA-B*41:02 with *Henoch-Schönlein purpura* (IgA vasculitis) in Spanish individuals irrespective of the HLA-DRB1 status. https://core.ac.uk/download/pdf/81712742.pdf (accessed on 23rd July 2025).

40. Tuscano, J. M., & Sands, J. (2009). B cell reductive therapy with rituximab in the treatment of rheumatoid arthritis. *Biologics : targets & therapy*, *3*, 225–232. https://doi.org/10.2147/btt.2009.3126(accessed on 23rd July 2025).

41. Sattar, Y., Susheela, A. T., Ullah, W., Usman, N., & Zafrullah, F. (2019). Use of Plasmapheresis and Immunosuppressants to Treat Diffuse Alveolar Hemorrhage in a Patient with Granulomatosis with Polyangiitis. *Medicina (Kaunas, Lithuania)*, *55*(7), 378. https://doi.org/10.3390/medicina55070378 (accessed on 23rd July 2025).

42. Schneider, B. J., Naidoo, J., Santomasso, B., Lacchetti, C., Adkins, S., Anadkat, M. J., Atkins, M. B., et al. (2021). Management of immune-related adverse events in patients treated with immune checkpoint inhibitor therapy: ASCO guideline update. *Journal of Clinical Oncology, 39*, 4073–4126. https://doi.org/10.1200/jco.21.01440 (accessed on 23rd July 2025).

43. Thakur, S. (2008). *Henoch-Schönlein purpura (HSP).* https://core.ac.uk/download/62771964.pdf (accessed on 23rd July 2025).

SARCOIDOSIS AND GRANULOMATOUS SKIN CONDITIONS

9

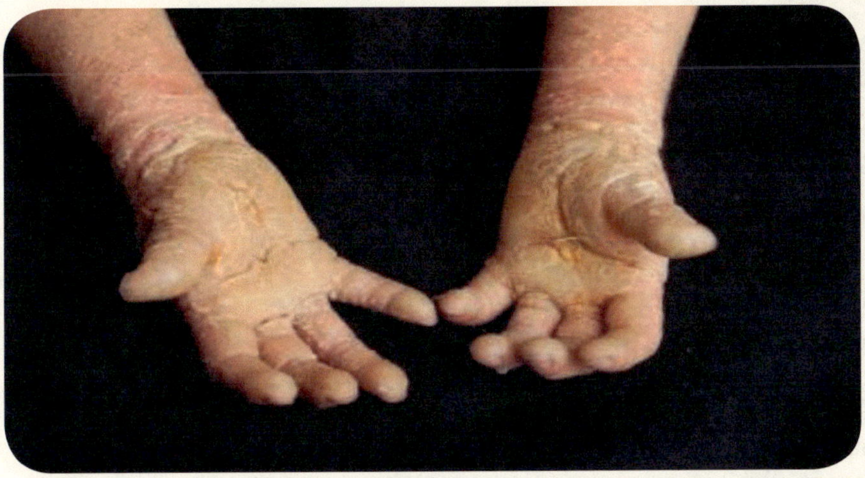

LEARNING OBJECTIVES

After studying this chapter, you will be able to:

1. Understand Pathophysiology of Sarcoidosis;
2. Explain Clinical Manifestations of Sarcoidosis;
3. Describe Granulomatous Skin Conditions;
4. Focus on Diagnosis and Management of Sarcoidosis.

Introduction

The study of sarcoidosis and its associated granulomatous skin illnesses reveals a complex ballet of systemic disease problems that affect a significant segment of the population. Sarcoidosis, as a multi-system disease, can manifest in thousands of cutaneous presentations, involving approximately 25%–30% of the affected populations. The presence of granulomas, the hallmark of this condition, reveals the immune response of the body against perceived attacks, which can be grounded in genetic and environmental factors. Furthermore, analysis of concomitant disorders, such as Crohn's disease, demonstrates concordant mechanisms in inflammatory processes, uncovering the potential for concomitant etiology and symptomatology (Woo, 2015). This primer is a good starting point for a comprehensive discussion of sarcoidosis and granulomatous skin disease pathophysiology, clinical presentation, and treatment modalities, highlighting the significance of comprehensive understanding and treatment in affected populations.

9.1. Pathophysiology of Sarcoidosis

Learning Outcome

1. Understand Immune Response in Sarcoidosis;
2. Explain Formation of Granulomas;
3. Focus on Genetic Predisposition;
4. Describe Environmental Triggers;
5. Learn Role of Cytokines;
6. Discuss Systemic Effects of Sarcoidosis;
7. Know Differences between Localized and Systemic Sarcoidosis;
8. Understand Diagnostic Criteria for Sarcoidosis;
9. Explain Challenges in Understanding the Pathophysiology.

Pathophysiology of sarcoidosis is closely related to an abnormal immune response in which granulomas—clusters of immune cells—are formed in various tissues, often in the lungs and lymphatic system. These caseating-negative granulomas have been postulated to be caused by presentation with cryptic antigens, potentially infectious or environmental, triggering an inappropriate response in genetically predisposed hosts.

The clinical manifestation of this is a chronic cough, fatigue, and skin lesions, the cutaneous manifestation typically reflecting the systemic nature of the disease, as it does in diseases like erythema nodosum. Besides, long-standing vitamin D metabolism abnormalities resulting in hypercalcemia add complexity to the disease and are responsible for its varied clinical presentations. Widespread pulmonary involvement can result in severe complications, including pulmonary hypertension, suggesting the need for targeted therapy that can avoid such effects as research is ongoing in the pathophysiology of sarcoidosis (Baughman, 2007; Nunes et al., 2007) (Figure 9.1).

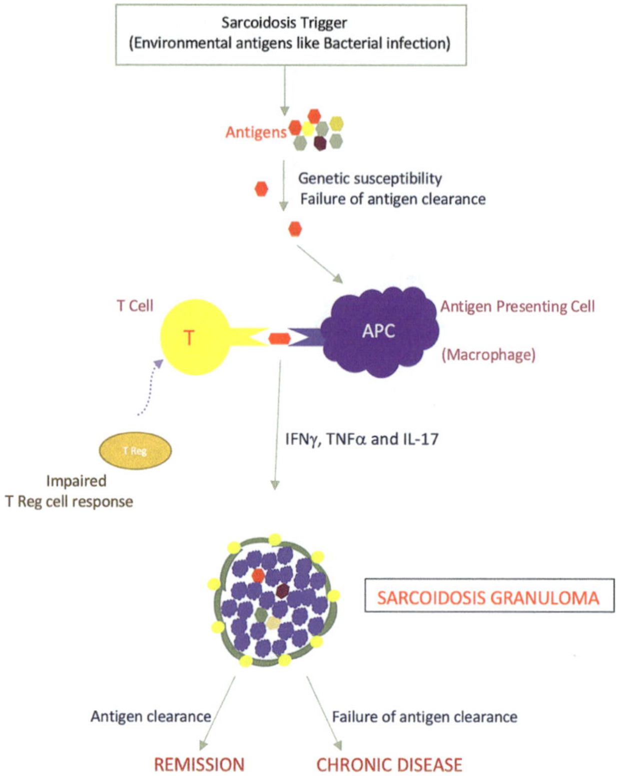

Figure 9.1. The pathophysiology of sarcoidosis.

Source: https://assets.cureus.com/uploads/figure/file/231463/article_river_bd585dd0d3d211ebb56fa5c89b5e5816-Screen-Shot-2021-06-22-at-11.24.18-PM.png.

9.1.1. Immune Response in Sarcoidosis

The immune response in sarcoidosis is characterized by a complex interplay of cellular pathways, leading to the formation of granulomas in affected tissues. Central to this process is the activation of $CD4^+$ T lymphocytes, whose function is instrumental in coordinating immune responses against suspected antigens. Some bacteria, including *Propionibacterium acnes*, have been shown to cause sarcoidosis by stimulating granulomatous reaction according to studies that have shown that *P. acnes*-sensitized mice developed large pulmonary granulomas and T-cell proliferation, specifically an elevated

CD4/CD8 ratio in bronchoalveolar lavage fluids (Iio et al., 2010). Furthermore, in the immunocompromised hosts, i.e., HIV-positive patients, the diagnosis of sarcoidosis is also confounded by overlapping manifestations and by the immunological paradox in T-cell function and in the identification of latent tuberculosis infection (Mencarini et al., 2016). This further highlights the imperative necessity of having an enhanced understanding of the immune dynamics taking place in sarcoidosis.

9.1.2. Formation of Granulomas

Granuloma formation is a feature of sarcoidosis and is of significant relevance in understanding the pathophysiology of the disease.

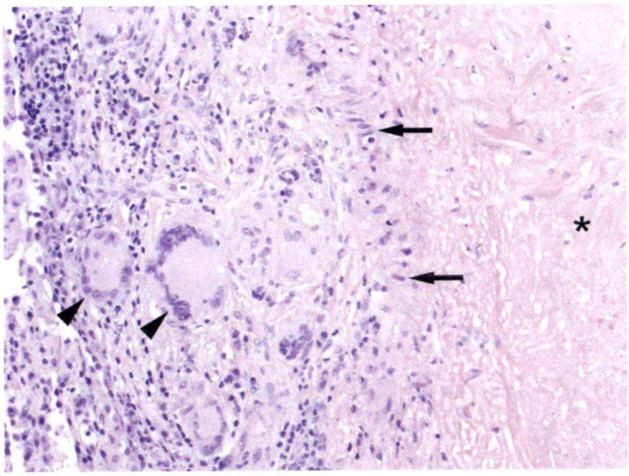

Figure 9.2. Granulomas are organized aggregates of immune cells, primarily macrophages, that arise in response to persistent antigens or irritants, a process often linked to chronic inflammation.

Source: https://ars.els-cdn.com/content/image/1-s2.0-S2405579416300328-gr1.jpg.

Granulomas are organized accumulations of immune cells, in this instance, macrophages, which form in response to the presence of enduring antigens or irritants, typically in association with chronic inflammation. The case of Propionibacterium acnes illustrates this process since it has been implicated in sarcoidosis pathogenesis; mice sensitized to such a bacterium developed epitheloid cell granulomas, illustrating the hyperresponse of immune systems to widespread environmental stimuli (Iio et al., 2010). In overlap syndromes, e.g., HIV, diagnosis is complicated, considering that overlapping features will mask sarcoidosis. The divergent clinical presentations of such patients necessitate a guarded diagnostic process in order to exclude other diseases, including reactivated tuberculosis (Mencarini et al., 2016). Therefore, the process of granuloma formation is important in diagnosing and treating sarcoidosis and skin disorders (Figure 9.2).

9.1.3. Genetic Predisposition

There is a need to recognize genetic predisposition in sarcoidosis and other granulomatous skin diseases because it reveals information on the hereditary component of these diseases. Studies show that family background is one of the causative factors in the development of sarcoidosis, with first-degree relatives diagnosed being over three times greater risk in individuals. Notably, almost 39% of susceptibility to the disease can be attributed to genes, showing the significance of genetic factors in its etiology (Rossides, 2021). In addition, genetic variation studies in granulomatous inflammatory conditions also allow us to understand the common immune mechanisms that may cause these conditions. Such a genetic model not only allows us to define susceptible populations but also sets the stage for continued study of the complex interaction between genetic susceptibility and environmental exposures in sarcoidosis and granulomatous skin disease etiology.

9.1.4. Environmental Triggers

The interaction of environmental stimuli and the induction of sarcoidosis and granulomatous cutaneous diseases has been the subject of considerable recent investigation. Involvement with certain pathogens, organic dust, and industrial toxins has been suggested as a primary cause for these conditions. As an example, the chronic inflammatory reaction to environmental antigens may result in the inappropriate activation of the immune response observed in sarcoidosis. This is consistent with findings in comparable conditions, including Crohn's disease, where pathologic mucosal responses to environmental stimuli are the rule, suggesting a shared etiology of environmental insults (Woo, 2015). Further, in inflammatory skin conditions like rosacea, environmental etiology causes triggering, in keeping with the concept of genetic susceptibility being influenced by external stimuli (Chang et al., 2015). Identification of these intersections is crucial to setting directed therapies and treatment plans, emphasizing the importance of considering the environment in the clinic (Figure 9.3).

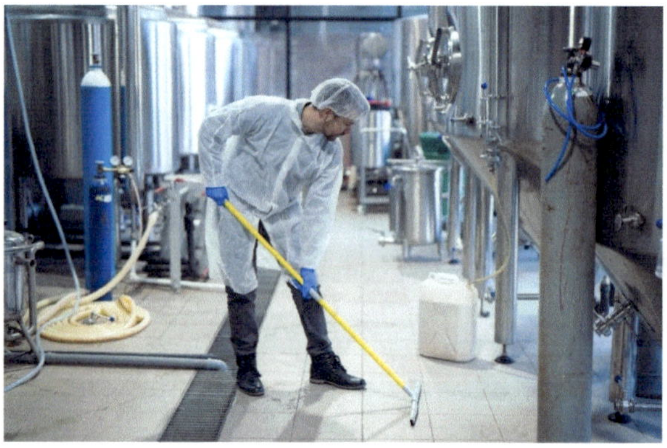

Figure 9.3. Factors such as exposure to certain pathogens, organic dust, and industrial chemicals are thought to play pivotal roles in these conditions.

Source: https://oizom.com/wp-content/uploads/2023/11/What-is-Industrial-Hygiene.webp.

9.1.5. Role of Cytokines

The function of cytokines in the pathogenesis of sarcoidosis and other granulomatous diseases of the skin is central, since these signaling molecules direct the immune response that forms granulomas. Cytokines like tumor necrosis factor-alpha (TNF-α) and interleukin-6 (IL-6) are especially noteworthy, as they are responsible for the activation and proliferation of immune cells in granulomas. Increased TNF-α concentrations, which are usually found in the affected tissues, stimulate macrophage activity and further increase the inflammatory process characteristic of sarcoidosis. This inflammatory environment explains how epithelioid cell granuloma formation occurs in the skin and other organs with manifestation as cutaneous sarcoidosis. Examples have illustrated that cytokines play a role not only in characteristic presentations but also in unusual manifestations, like psoriasiform lesions complicating management during pregnancy, to underline the complex interaction between immune signaling and clinical responses in such patients (Iio et al., 2010; Albornoz et al., 2018).

9.1.6. Systemic Effects of Sarcoidosis

The systemic effect of sarcoidosis extends far beyond its original presentation, inflicting profound effects on various organ systems and complicating the clinical scenario. The granulomatous condition very often gives rise to pulmonary involvement in the form of interstitial lung disease, which, if not well managed, may cause respiratory insufficiency. Sarcoidosis may also affect the musculoskeletal system, with arthralgia or arthritis being a possible consequence, which contributes to the poor quality of life of patients. Additionally, the disease is also said to induce systemic inflammation, exemplified by increased serum levels of angiotensin-converting enzyme (ACE), which could not only serve as indicators of disease progression but also influence treatment methods. Evidence has shown that systemic imaging modalities, such as FDG PET/CT, improve the yield of head and neck sarcoidosis detection and assess therapy responses adequately, consequently enhancing patient management (Grozdic Milojevic et al., 2019). As knowledge evolves, it is crucial to meet these systemic effects for whole-patient care in sarcoidosis patients (Piccinini et al., 2015) (Figure 9.4).

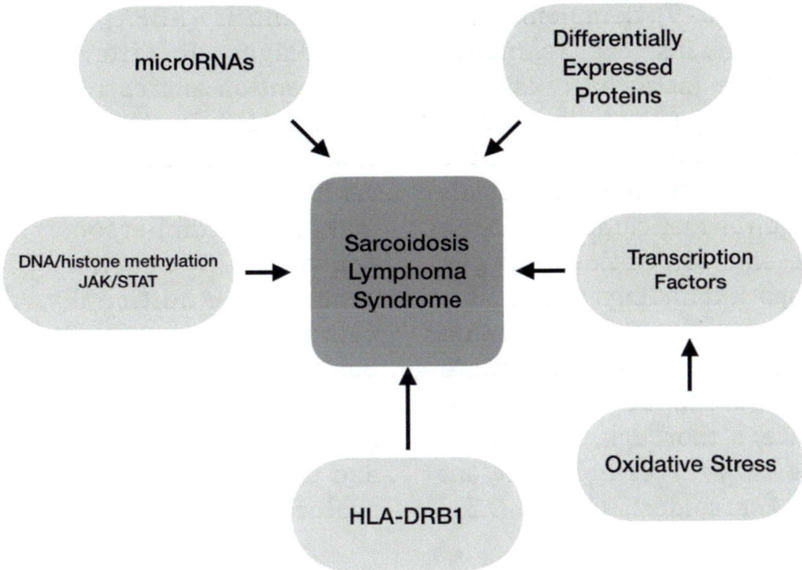

Figure 9.4. The systemic effects of sarcoidosis extend well beyond its initial presentation, significantly impacting various organ systems and complicating the clinical landscape.

Source: https://www.mdpi.com/ijms/ijms-26-00594/article_deploy/html/images/ijms-26-00594-g002.png.

9.1.7. Differences between Localized and Systemic Sarcoidosis

It is essential to comprehend the localized and systemic sarcoidosis differences for effective diagnosis and management. Localized sarcoidosis is localized to the skin, with a number of granulomatous lesions, such as erythema nodosum, which can be self-limiting and less disruptive to general health. Systemic sarcoidosis is linked to two or more organs, such as the lungs, lymph nodes, and even the heart and eyes, with a more complicated clinical presentation. Scientific literature indicates that while local forms are sensitive to local treatment, systemic sarcoidosis is aggressive in treatment, including the use of corticosteroids, in order to suppress systemic inflammation and prevent harmful complications (Darlington, 2013). Genetically controlled predisposition of individual HLA alleles, such as HLA-DRB1*04, may influence the risk of systemic disease, with every patient needing personal management (Piccinini et al., 2015). These differences emphasize the need for individualized treatment methods in the treatment of sarcoidosis.

9.1.8. Diagnostic Criteria for Sarcoidosis

Diagnostic criteria for sarcoidosis embrace multi-dimension since clinical presentation may be diverse and often mimic other diseases. Essential to diagnosis is the finding of non-caseating granulomas, as often observed on biopsy, which may occur in the skin with accompanying systemic symptoms.

Cutaneous involvement is unexpectedly prevalent, occurring in up to one-third of patients with the systemic type, and represents an important indicator of disease progression (Grozdic Milojevic et al., 2019). Complementing histopathologic diagnosis, imaging techniques such as FDG PET/CT are increasingly applied to assess disease activity, particularly in cases with complex symptomatology, e.g., that of the head and neck area (Grozdic Milojevic et al., 2019). Diagnosis requires meticulous exclusion of infectious cause and correlation between clinical manifestations and findings on imaging, reiterating the necessity of serial observation since cutaneous lesions can be followed by more extensive systemic disease in the future (Bindu & Joshi, 2014). Hence, a thorough, methodical evaluation is necessary in establishing an absolute diagnosis of sarcoidosis (Figure 9.5).

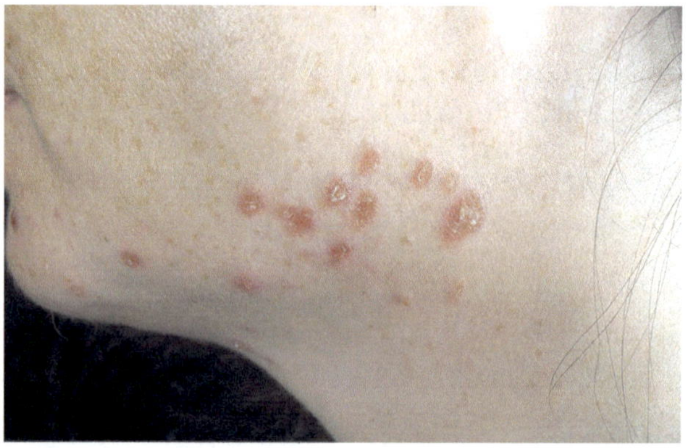

Figure 9.5. Cutaneous sarcoidosis.

Source: https://upload.wikimedia.org/wikipedia/commons/f/f9/Cutaneous_findings_in_systemic_sarcoidosis.JPEG.

9.1.9. Challenges in Understanding the Pathophysiology

It is hard to understand the pathophysiology of sarcoidosis and other granulomatous dermatoses with such a complex interaction between environmental stimuli and immune response. The clinical heterogeneity typically conceals the mechanisms in a variety of misdiagnoses. For instance, overlapping symptoms can be derived from heterogeneous conditions and thereby become difficult to diagnose and treat. Moreover, as in cases like allergic bronchopulmonary aspergillosis (ABPA), disagreement regarding the diagnostic criteria also cripples early intervention and early management (Leonardi et al., 2016). In the same vein, the absence of broad studies and uniform protocols can lead to variable interpretations of clinical presentations, making it cumbersome for researchers to characterize specific pathophysiological processes. Additionally, the multifactorial pathogenesis of such diseases typically leaves behind information gaps regarding particular biomarkers and immune responses engaged, thereby inhibiting therapeutic development and the application of standardized treatment protocols (Ralli et al., 2018).

9.2. Clinical Manifestations of Sarcoidosis

Learning Outcome

1. Understand Common Symptoms of Sarcoidosis;
2. Explain Skin Manifestations of Sarcoidosis;
3. Focus on Pulmonary Involvement;
4. Describe Ocular Complications;
5. Learn Cardiac Involvement;
6. Discuss Neurological Symptoms;
7. Know Musculoskeletal Symptoms;
8. Understand Variability in Presentation;
9. Explain the Importance of Early Detection.

Sarcoidosis is incredibly variable, which tends to confuse clinicians in diagnosing it. The patients may have different symptoms because the disease is multi-systemic, i.e., it affects organs like the lungs, skin, lymph nodes, and others. Cutaneous presentation is most commonly encountered in the form of erythema nodosum, lupus pernio, and granulomatous lesions, which are crucially diagnostic because they may precede pulmonary presentation (Grozdic Milojevic et al., 2019). Sarcoidosis also leads to severe complications in immunocompromised hosts such as HIV-positive individuals, where the disease makes the underlying condition worse and leads to undue delay in appropriate management (Mencarini et al., 2016). The heterogeneity in clinical presentations demands watchful differentiation from other conditions, with a focus on detailed evaluations, including imaging and serum biomarkers, to direct management modalities appropriately. Clarification of such presentations is pivotal for optimizing patient outcomes in the treatment of sarcoidosis.

9.2.1. Common Symptoms of Sarcoidosis

Sarcoidosis is characterized by its polymorphic spectrum of symptoms that may be quite disparate between patients, rendering diagnosis difficult. Pulmonary manifestations are common and are caused by the granulomatous inflammation in the lungs, presenting with chronic cough, dyspnea, and chest pain. Cutaneous manifestations, such as erythema nodosum and lupus pernio, are of particular importance in dermatological settings since they can be presenting signs of the disease in addition to the systemic symptoms of fatigue, weight loss, and fever. Most importantly, the occurrence of sarcoidosis alongside other conditions such as tuberculosis complicates clinical presentation, particularly among immunocompromised patients, as noted in recent studies (Mencarini et al., 2016). Furthermore, granulomatous lesions can also occur in the head and neck regions, stressing the need for comprehensive imaging modalities like FDG PET/CT in ascertaining the severity of the disease and for treatment (Grozdic Milojevic et al., 2019). This heterogeneity is a reflection of the necessity for a cautious approach to diagnosis and treatment in patients with suspected sarcoidosis (Figure 9.6).

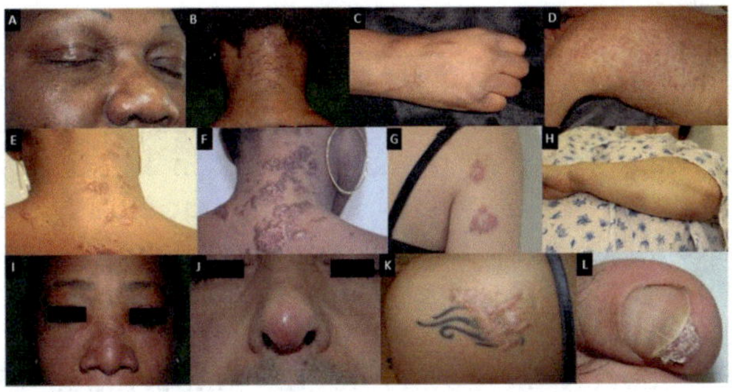

Figure 9.6. Sarcoidosis is characterized by a diverse range of symptoms that can vary significantly among patients, complicating its diagnosis.

Source: https://www.mdpi.com/cells/cells-10-00766/article_deploy/html/images/cells-10-00766-g005.png.

9.2.2. Skin Manifestations of Sarcoidosis

Cutaneous presentations of sarcoidosis are a significant presentation of this complex granulomatous disease, which presents in approximately 25% of patients with sarcoidosis. These presentations can be extremely variable, varying from erythema nodosum, lupus pernio, and plaques, and can be one of the first signs of systemic disease. These lesions not only contribute to the diagnostic process, but their symptoms of pain and discomfort can complicate management. Significantly, studies such as those characterizing head and neck sarcoidosis have showcased the importance of imaging modalities like FDG PET/CT in defining disease localization and response to treatment. Additionally, it is critical to differentiate sarcoidosis from other granulomatous diseases such as tertiary syphilis presenting with similar cutaneous manifestations, hence emphasizing the need for accurate diagnosis and treatment towards improving patient outcome (Solis et al., 2018; Grozdic Milojevic et al., 2019).

9.2.3. Pulmonary Involvement

Pulmonary involvement is one of the hallmark characteristics of this complex disease, often surpassing other organ systems in frequency and impact. Between 90% of patients with sarcoidosis demonstrate pulmonary involvement, ranging from asymptomatic infiltrates to severely disabling respiratory insufficiency. The spectrum points to the importance of early diagnosis and ongoing surveillance, as deteriorating pulmonary function can lead to significant morbidity. Recent research has proved that newer imaging modalities, such as FDG PET/CT, are crucial in assessing pulmonary disease activity and response to treatment, characterizing well the patterns of granulomatous inflammation (Grozdic Milojevic et al., 2019). Sarcoidosis also has a strong association with cutaneous manifestations, occupying approximately 25%–30% of the patients, which sometimes can serve as strong diagnostic pointers. It is essential to understand the complicated interaction between pulmonary and cutaneous manifestations (Figure 9.7).

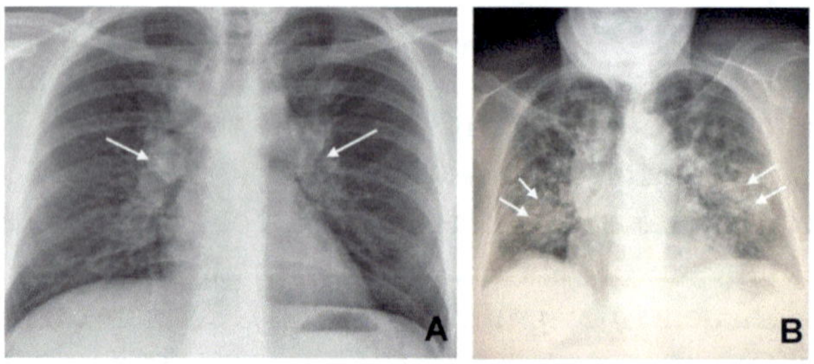

Figure 9.7. Pulmonary involvement in sarcoidosis is one of the hallmark manifestations of this complex disease, often surpassing other organ systems in frequency and significance.

Source: https://www.mdpi.com/jcm/jcm-09-03028/article_deploy/html/images/jcm-09-03028-g001.png.

9.2.4. Ocular Complications

Ocular complications are a concerning problem in sarcoidosis patients, appearing in as many as 79% of disease patients. The most frequent manifestation is uveitis, a chronic intraocular inflammation that significantly impacts visual acuity and quality of life.

A few studies indicate that the pattern and prevalence of ocular sarcoidosis can be rather dissimilar; a recent retrospective study, for instance, found that 43.9% of patients diagnosed with definite or presumed ocular sarcoidosis presented with the eye as their only primary involved organ, highlighting the differences in early diagnosis and treatment (Zur Bonsen et al., 2021). The diagnosis is often made on the basis of International Workshop on Ocular Sarcoidosis criteria, with supporting laboratory evidence such as elevations of soluble interleukin-2 receptor and angiotensin-converting enzyme (Zur Bonsen et al., 2021). As ocular involvement can sometimes present in other organs, it is important to familiarize oneself with these ocular complications for overall patient care in treating sarcoidosis.

9.2.5. Cardiac Involvement

Sarcoidosis-induced cardiac involvement is a dangerous issue since it can lead to severe outcomes. Cardiac sarcoidosis can lead to arrhythmias, heart failure, and sudden death, making it important to be diagnosed and treated early. It is important to note that patients with abnormal electrocardiogram (ECG) are much more likely to develop cardiac sarcoidosis (CS) compared to patients with normal ECGs, especially if they present with symptoms attributed to the heart (Darlington, 2013). In addition, studies indicate that non-Löfgren's syndrome (non-LS) patients are most vulnerable to CS, highlighting the heterogeneity of sarcoidosis presentation (Nunes et al., 2007). The pathophysiologic basis remains obscure, even with the argument that an overactive immune response to undetected antigens plays a central role. Because of the heterogeneity of clinical presentation and the possibility of life-threatening complications, careful monitoring and tailored therapeutic strategies are essential in the management of cardiac involvement in sarcoidosis patients (Figure 9.8).

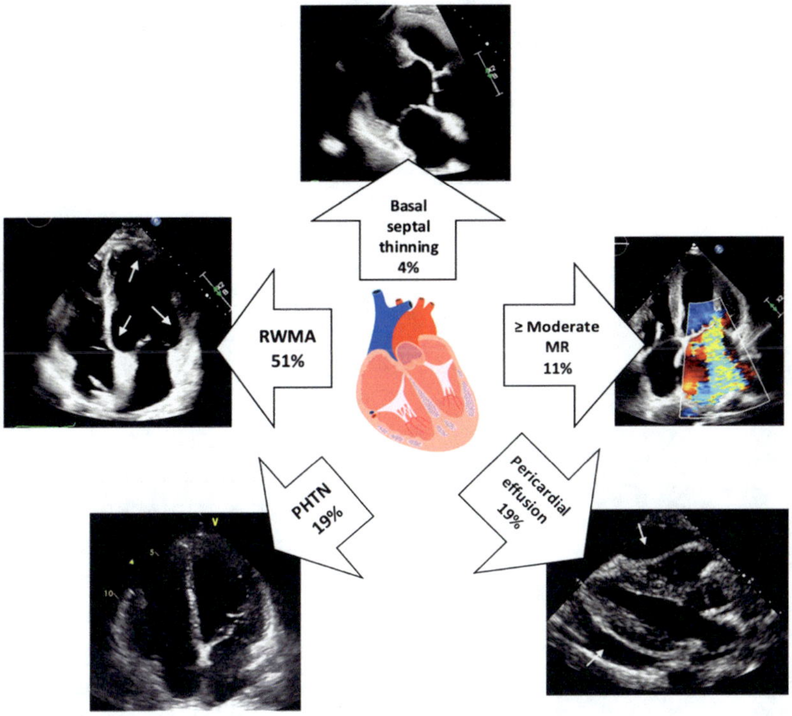

Figure 9.8. Cardiac involvement in sarcoidosis represents a significant concern due to its potential for severe complications.

Source: https://pub.mdpi-res.com/life/life-13-01653/article_deploy/html/images/life-13-01653-g001.png?1690607123.

9.2.6. Neurological Symptoms

Sarcoidosis, being a systemic granulomatous illness, usually presents with a wide range of neurological symptoms that depends on its multifarious effects on the body. Neurological involvement can be seen in about 5%–10% of patients, where it may present as a range of cognitive impairments, memory loss, and peripheral neuropathies. The granulomatous inflammation can extend to the central and peripheral nervous systems with complications from encephalopathy, seizures, and even hearing loss, which can take the form of immune-mediated inner ear disease. According to recent studies, sensorineural hearing loss associated with systemic autoimmune diseases is not uncommon, with early corticosteroid treatment effective in managing symptoms and reclaiming recovery (Ralli et al., 2018). Also, imaging techniques like FDG PET/CT have been used to detect neurological sarcoidosis, which helps in the planning of appropriate treatment measures for the affected individuals (Grozdic Milojevic et al., 2019). This complexity indicates the need for heightened awareness and directed research in order to improve treatment for individuals experiencing these incapacitating symptoms.

9.2.7. Musculoskeletal Symptoms

Musculoskeletal symptoms are one of the most described complications in sarcoidosis patients and often present with arthralgia or arthritis that has an important effect on quality of life. The symptoms are a result of the immune-mediated mechanisms of sarcoidosis, which are capable of causing inflammation of joints and surrounding tissues.

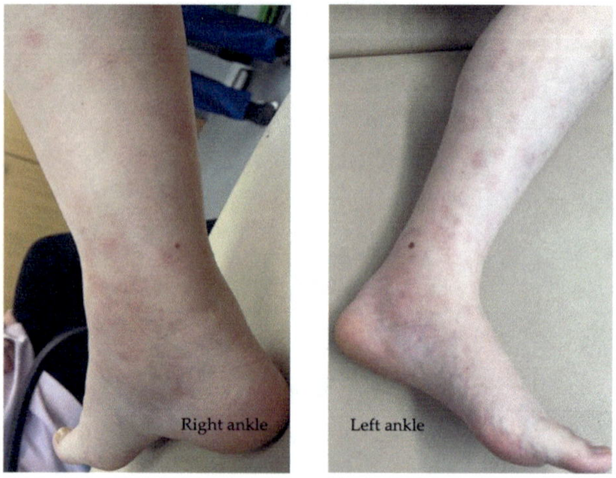

Figure 9.9. Musculoskeletal symptoms are a frequently noted complication in patients with sarcoidosis, often presenting as arthralgia or arthritis that can significantly affect quality of life.

Source: https://www.mdpi.com/diagnostics/diagnostics-14-02842/article_deploy/html/images/diagnostics-14-02842-g003.png.

The presentation of musculoskeletal symptoms is variable and goes from very mild discomfort to aggravating severe joint pain, so it is essential to apply efficient management techniques. With the evolution of the condition, patients may also experience muscle weakness and fatigue, further contributing to their physical disability. Moreover, the coexistence of sarcoidosis with other systemic autoimmune conditions makes the clinical scenario more confusing, thus leading to misdiagnoses and improper treatment. Such musculoskeletal manifestations being recognized are crucial in the achievement of timely and proper intervention and thus better patient outcomes for this intricate dance of granulomatous diseases and immune dysfunctions (Puzanov et al., 2017; Ralli et al., 2018) (Figure 9.9).

9.2.8. Variability in Presentation

Heterogeneity in presentation is a hallmark feature of both sarcoidosis and the granulomatous skin lesions, often making diagnosis and management more challenging. The clinical manifestations are as varied as erythema nodosum, a tender reddish nodule predominantly on the shins, and the more inconspicuous lesions, such as lupus Pernio, which are violaceous plaques typically on the face. The range in skin presentation is a reflection of the underlying complexity of the disease, where individual immune responses and hereditary predispositions are accountable for variable clinical presentations. Along with this, the variation can often lead to misdiagnosis because presentation would cross-react with other cutaneous disorders, making it necessary for more clinical suspicion and a proper evaluation. A sharp sense of these presentations is required, particularly because they would suggest systemic involvement of sarcoidosis, and as such, identification of such variation in the practice becomes paramount (Ralli et al., 2018; Hu et al., 2020).

9.2.9. Importance of Early Detection

The necessity for early diagnosis when it comes to sarcoidosis and granulomatous dermatoses cannot be overstated. Early detection makes early intervention possible, which is vital in avoiding complications in the long run and improving outcomes for the patient. For instance, oral manifestations of Crohn's disease may be predictive of impending gastrointestinal involvement, illustrating the use of early symptoms in providing useful information about the patient's overall health status (Woo, 2015). Moreover, advancements in diagnostic tools, such as second-harmonic generation microscopy, have enabled us to easily distinguish between granulomatous diseases with similar features, e.g., sarcoidosis and tuberculoid leprosy. This technique allows for clearer interpretation of collagen structure in infected tissues, thereby allowing for more accurate diagnoses (Utino et al., 2020). Hence, the integration of early detection methods with new diagnostic technologies is essential in treating sarcoidosis and other granulomatous illnesses efficiently, resulting in improved patient care (Figure 9.10).

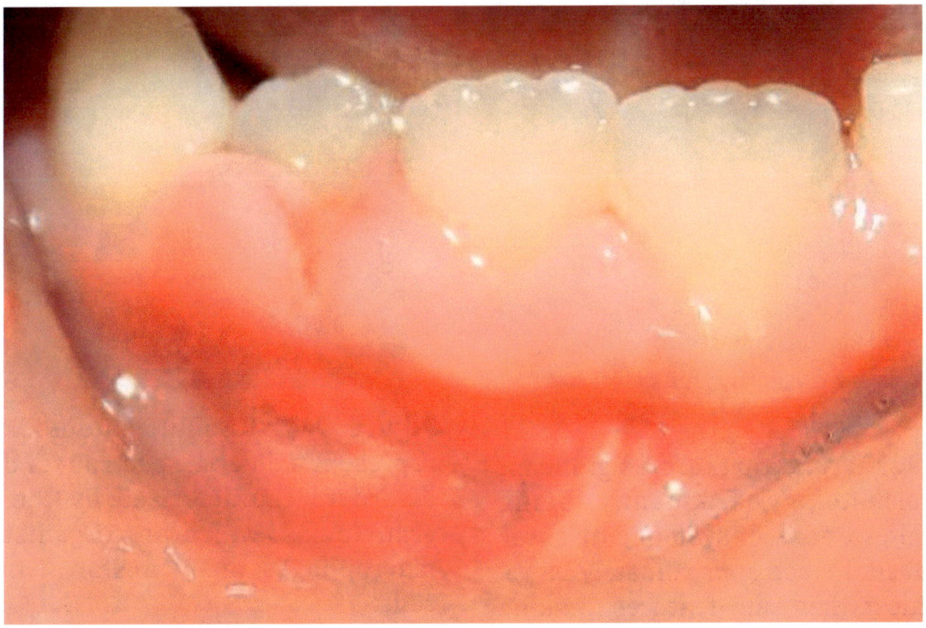

Figure 9.10. The oral manifestations of Crohn's disease can serve as precursors to gastrointestinal involvement, highlighting how early symptoms can provide valuable insight into the patient's overall health status.

Source: https://onlinelibrary.wiley.com/cms/asset/250f9614-0c07-4107-b8e9-04a21d8d9a49/crid830472-fig-0003-m.jpg.

Test Your Knowledge

1. What is the clinical significance of erythema nodosum in sarcoidosis?
2. How does sarcoidosis present in the eyes?

9.3. Granulomatous Skin Conditions

Learning Outcome

1. Understand Definition and Types of Granulomatous Skin Conditions;
2. Explain Common Granulomatous Diseases;
3. Focus on Pathophysiology of Granulomatous Skin Conditions;
4. Describe Clinical Features of Granulomatous Skin Conditions;
5. Learn Diagnostic Approaches for Granulomatous Skin Conditions;
6. Discuss Treatment Options for Granulomatous Skin Conditions;
7. Know the Differential Diagnosis of Granulomatous Skin Conditions;
8. Understand Prognosis and Outcomes.

Granulomatous skin conditions are a significant branch of dermatology, frequently being cutaneous manifestations of systemic diseases such as sarcoidosis. In fact, approximately 25%–30% of sarcoidosis has skin features, making the recognition of these dermatological findings crucial for early diagnosis and management. Psoriasiform sarcoidosis is one such very interesting presentation that can mimic chronic plaque psoriasis and be perplexing from a diagnostic aspect. The resultant clinical overlap highlights the importance of close assessment, especially in high-risk groups, such as pregnant patients, where systemic treatments are a challenge due to the need for close management of maternal and fetal health (Albornoz et al., 2018). Treatment of such granulomatous illnesses not only requires an understanding of their pathological foundation but also an awareness of the more general ramifications for patient management and therapy, thus demonstrating the intertwined intersection of dermatology with systemic disease.

9.3.1. Definition and Types of Granulomatous Skin Conditions

Granulomatous skin disorders form a heterogeneous collection of skin diseases characterized by the occurrence of granulomas, which are collections of organized macrophages that evolve into epithelioid cells.

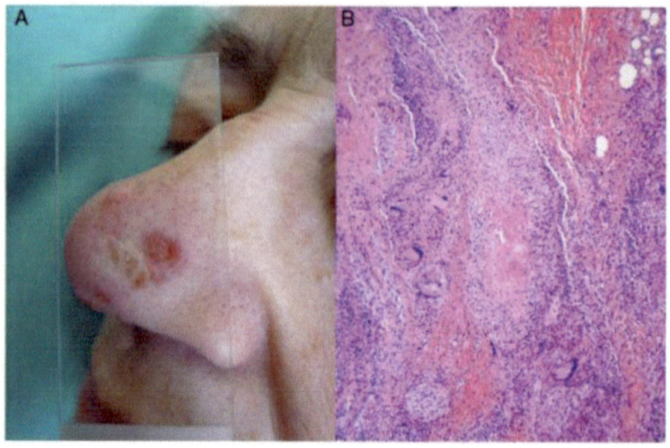

Figure 9.11. Granulomatous skin conditions represent a diverse spectrum of dermatological disorders characterized by the formation of granulomas, which are organized clusters of macrophages that transform into epithelioid cells.

Source: https://ars.els-cdn.com/content/image/1-s2.0-S1578219021002109-gr14.jpg.

They include sarcoidosis, granuloma annulare, and foreign body granulomas, among others, with different etiologies and clinical presentations. Sarcoidosis, on the other hand, is often systemic and can lead to significant complications, with cutaneous sarcoidosis seen in up to one-third of patients, noted in clinical discussion regarding the disease (Bindu & Joshi, 2014). Likewise, granuloma annulare typically presents as asymptomatic, ring-shaped lesions and is traditionally self-limiting. An understanding of the fundamental mechanisms and diverse morphology of these granulomatous diseases is crucial to specific diagnosis and therapy. Moreover, increased awareness is also needed to differentiate these conditions from other dermatologic disorders, thus the call for continued research in this area (Piccinini et al., 2015) (Figure 9.11).

9.3.2. Common Granulomatous Diseases (e.g., Granuloma Annulare)

Granulomatous skin disorders such as granuloma annulare constitute a heterogeneous collection of conditions characterized by granulomas, collections of inflammatory cells formed during inflammation. Granuloma annulare, in particular, is well-known to be benign and self-limiting, occurring typically as an annular lesion with a raised border, and most frequently seen in youth. Even though the etiology is still unclear, its association with systemic diseases, like sarcoidosis, should be dealt with in a similar careful approach. Sarcoidosis is a multi-system disorder that can occur in multiple organs, including the skin, in approximately 25%–30% of patients. Moreover, tuberculoid granulomas are the most frequent presentation found in dermatopathology, as revealed by a retrospective study, which goes on to emphasize the critical role played by histopathological examination in diagnosing these conditions (Almutairi & Al-Sabah, 2023). Identification of the clinical and histologic characteristics of granulomatous diseases is essential to successful treatment and management.

9.3.3. Pathophysiology of Granulomatous Skin Conditions

The pathophysiology of granulomatous cutaneous diseases, such as in sarcoidosis, is a multi-factorial complex of immune responses and chronic inflammation.

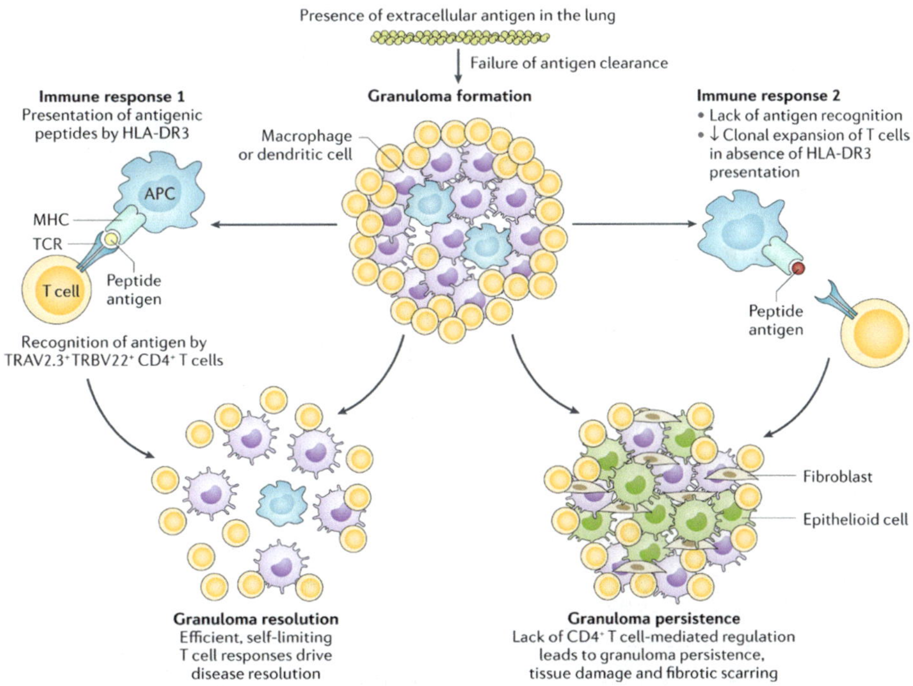

Figure 9.12. The pathophysiology of granulomatous skin conditions.

Source: https://media.springernature.com/lw1200/springer-static/image/art%3A10.1038%2Fs41572-019-0096-x/MediaObjects/41572_2019_96_Fig5_HTML.png.

In sarcoidosis, the formation of non-caseating granulomas is a dysregulated immune response to an unidentified antigen, which leads to an accumulation of macrophages and T-cells within the involved tissue. Such granulomatous inflammation can culminate in very severe cutaneous manifestations of erythema nodosum and lupus pernio that denote systemic disease. The pathogenetic role of impaired phagocytic function in the disease of chronic granulomatous disease (CGD) also underscores the pathology because CGD results from mutations that repress the NADPH oxidase complex for microbial killing and subsequent granuloma formation (Van den Berg et al., 2009). These interactions highlight the intricate mechanisms driving the evolution and severity of granulomatous dermatoses, necessitating targeted therapeutic maneuvers to suppress inflammation and promote healing (Ralli et al., 2018) (Figure 9.12).

9.3.4. Clinical Features of Granulomatous Skin Conditions

Granulomatous dermatoses, which are typically seen in diseases like sarcoidosis, exhibit a variety of clinical features that complicate diagnosis and management. The most important presentations are lupus pernio, erythema nodosum, and papular lesions that may be extremely variable in appearance and potentially confused with other dermatological diseases. Systemic involvement of such cutaneous lesions is also important as they could indicate the presence of underlying granulomatous inflammation elsewhere in the body, particularly the lungs, as seen in evidence of raised serum angiotensin-converting enzyme (ACE) levels in patients with sarcoidosis (Iio et al., 2010). Moreover, more modern imaging technologies like FDG PET/CT are becoming increasingly useful in the detection of granulomatous disease in head and neck sarcoidosis, providing improved therapeutic intervention and follow-up (Grozdic Milojevic et al., 2019). The clinicians need to be aware of such clinical presentations to render proper and timely diagnosis, which is necessary for proper patient management.

9.3.5. Diagnostic Approaches for Granulomatous Skin Conditions

The diagnosis of granulomatous dermatoses, and indeed sarcoidosis, involves a multi-disciplinary process incorporating clinical evaluation, histopathological inspection, and imaging. Initial assessments are often undertaken by history and examination to record the characteristic skin lesions, usually as papules, plaques, or nodules.

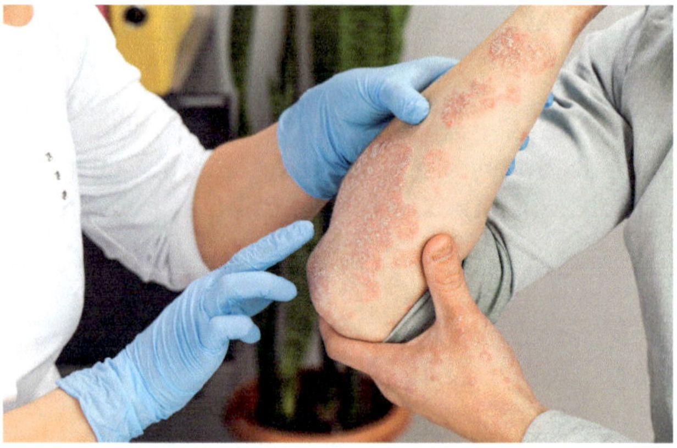

Figure 9.13. Initial assessments often include a thorough patient history and physical examination to identify characteristic skin lesions, which can appear as papules, plaques, or nodules.

Source: https://www.practicenursing.com/media/mqkn5fnt/adobestock_393573411.jpeg.

Histological inspection of skin biopsy is commonly necessary to make the ultimate diagnosis in such conditions as sarcoidosis, where noncaseating granulomas are found. The role of other laboratory studies, such as serum angiotensin-converting enzyme (ACE) levels and imaging techniques like chest X-rays or computed tomography scans, cannot be overstated, as they assist in the delineation of systemic involvement and guiding treatment strategies. Furthermore, the probability of overlap with other autoimmune disorders must be rigorously evaluated to prevent misdiagnosis and proper management. Knowledge of the variable presentation of granulomatous diseases is important for effective diagnostic outcomes (Ralli et al., 2018) (Figure 9.13).

9.3.6. Treatment Options for Granulomatous Skin Conditions

Treatment of granulomatous skin diseases, including sarcoidosis, is mainly based on the severity of symptoms and cutaneous involvement. Corticosteroids are generally the first line of treatment and can successfully diminish inflammation and related symptoms. In failing corticosteroid therapy patients, second-line immunosuppressive agents including methotrexate, azathioprine, or mycophenolate mofetil can be used, which provide an invaluable therapeutic option, especially in systemic or chronic lesions. In certain cases, also beneficial are drugs such as biologics, particularly those that are targeted at inflammatory pathways. Also, the recent findings on the immunological underpinning of granulomatous disease reveal the potential of individualized therapies aimed at specific disease progression patterns in every patient. Thus, widening the range of treatments mirrors the need for a customized treatment of granulomatous dermatoses with both old and novel approaches (Ralli et al., 2018; Kim et al., 2019).

9.3.7. Differential Diagnosis of Granulomatous Skin Conditions

In the differential diagnosis of granulomatous dermatoses, one needs to consider systematically several possible etiologies for sarcoidosis mimicking conditions. Tuberculosis, histoplasmosis, and leprosy are such conditions that need consideration because of the shared clinical presentations. Tuberculosis, especially reactivated types, may present with the same skin involvement, it is important to exclude it prior to diagnosing sarcoidosis (Mencarini et al., 2016). Besides, the atypical presentation of granulomatous infections in immunocompromised hosts complicates diagnosis, e.g., in HIV patients, where there is a diagnostic impasse due to the association of opportunistic disease with granulomatous disease (Mencarini et al., 2016). Another immunologically significant condition is granuloma annulare, which is benign in the majority of cases but must be distinguished from serious conditions like sarcoidosis, which in 25%–30% of cutaneous patients. This comprehensive strategy can substantially improve diagnosis and patient management accuracy (Figure 9.14).

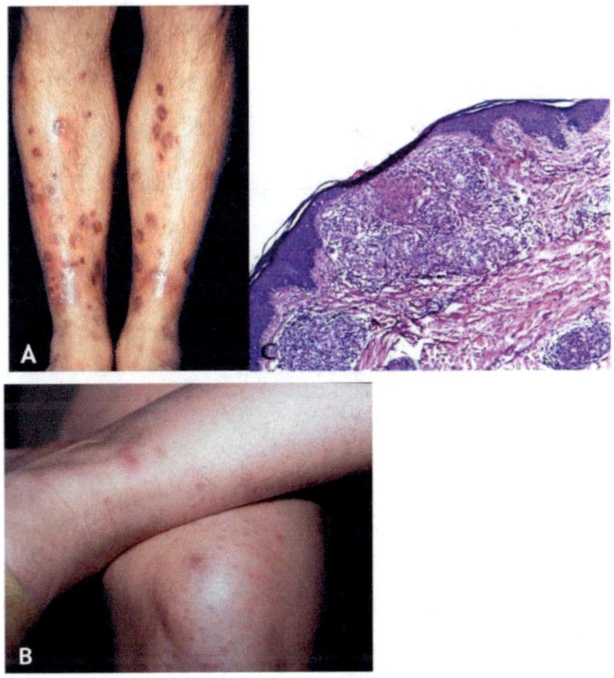

Figure 9.14. Tuberculosis, particularly in reactivated forms, can present with similar skin manifestations, making it crucial to rule out before confirming sarcoidosis.

Source: https://ars.els-cdn.com/content/image/1-s2.0-S0365059621003019-gr8.jpg.

9.3.8. Prognosis and Outcomes

The outcome of sarcoidosis patients, particularly when it affects the skin, largely rests on the extent of organ involvement and the overall well-being of the patients. As much as cutaneous sarcoidosis accounts for 25%–30% of patients, most of the incidences are benign and clear up spontaneously without aggressive intervention. However, pulmonary or any other system complication may complicate the prognosis. Studies have shown that patients with more advanced disease may have worse outcomes, especially if the sarcoidosis is complicated by lung disease or extreme morbidity (Yeşiltaş et al., 2018). Due to heterogeneity in presentation and responses to treatment, early monitoring and individualized management approaches are essential for optimizing outcomes. Thus, while local skin manifestations have an excellent prognosis, an overall knowledge of the patient's status is essential for effective long-term management.

Test Your Knowledge

1. Name infectious causes of granulomatous skin inflammation.
2. What is the histological hallmark of leprosy?

9.4. Diagnosis and Management of Sarcoidosis

Learning Outcome

1. Understand Diagnostic Imaging Techniques;
2. Explain Laboratory Tests for Sarcoidosis;
3. Focus on Biopsy and Histopathological Examination;
4. Describe Treatment Options for Sarcoidosis;
5. Learn Role of Corticosteroids;
6. Discuss Monitoring Disease Progression;
7. Know Multidisciplinary Approach to Management;
8. Understand Patient Education and Support.

Diagnosis and management of sarcoidosis, particularly in instances involving granulomatous cutaneous lesions, need a multidisciplinary approach. Sarcoidosis is characterized by a range of cutaneous lesions in 25%–30% of patients, posing difficulties in diagnosis and management. Cutaneous lesions can be rather varied, like erythema nodosum, lupus pernio, and other forms of granulomatous reactions, and may necessitate dermatological evaluation for proper diagnosis. While clinical assessment is of greatest significance, additional studies like chest X-rays, biopsy of lesions if the lesions are suspicious, and serological tests are required in the diagnosis and assessment of disease extent.

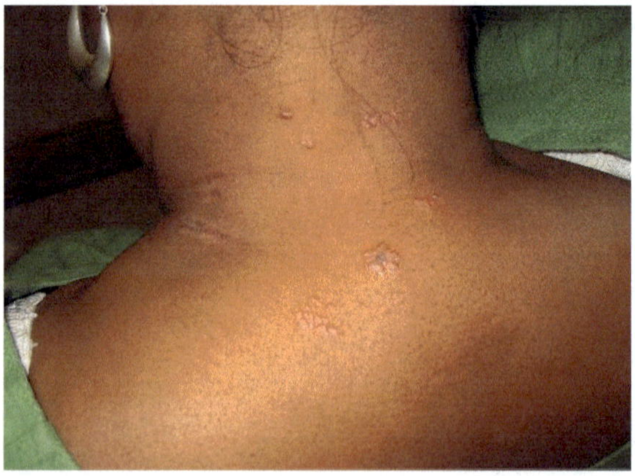

Figure 9.15. Management typically hinges on the severity of symptoms, with corticosteroids being the primary treatment for those with significant dermatological involvement or systemic symptoms.

Source: https://www.dermatologyadvisor.com/wp-content/uploads/sites/20/2019/03/ch1407.fig10.jpg.

Treatment is usually based on symptom severity, but the primary treatment in cases of extensive dermatologic disease or systemic features is corticosteroids. Also, ICD knowledge of the disease variable course allows for individualized treatment strategies, enhancing the patient's outcome and limiting the risk of progression (Van den Berg et al., 2009) (Figure 9.15).

9.4.1. Diagnostic Imaging Techniques

Diagnostic imaging techniques form the backbone of the diagnosis and treatment of sarcoidosis and granulomatous cutaneous diseases and are used to gain visual information, which can be utilized to gauge the pattern of disease. Of these techniques, fluorodeoxyglucose positron emission tomography-computed tomography (FDG PET/CT) has emerged as a reliable tool, enabling clinicians to delineate active sarcoidosis in varied regions of the body, including the head and neck. A study revealed that FDG PET/CT successfully altered the treatment plan of many patients based on its findings, emphasizing its role in therapy choice (Grozdic Milojevic et al., 2019). Imaging techniques also help differentiate between sarcoidosis-induced granulomatous lesions and other skin conditions, which is of the greatest value for accurate diagnosis. Utilization of advanced imaging modalities enhances the ability of the clinician to monitor treatment responses and identify potential complications, thus enhancing the outcomes of patients in such complex conditions (Piccinini et al., 2015).

9.4.2. Laboratory Tests for Sarcoidosis

Diagnosis of sarcoidosis, particularly if cutaneous presentation is in question, demands a comprehensive approach involving the use of several laboratory tests. Increased serum concentrations of the angiotensin-converting enzyme (ACE) are commonly observed in sarcoidosis and can be a helpful diagnostic criterion; however, this increase can also occur with other diseases, so that specificity is lost. Furthermore, demonstration of the noncaseating granulomas, histopathological characteristics of sarcoidosis, must be confirmed by tissue biopsy, usually obtained from cutaneous or lymph node lesions. Other laboratory investigations, such as pulmonary function tests and serum calcium levels, also aid in the determination of the severity of organ involvement and risk of hypercalcemia, which aggravates the course of the disease. Since sarcoidosis is a disease with a systemic process affecting organs like the nervous system in neurosarcoidosis, thorough laboratory evaluation is highly essential to make an appropriate diagnosis and treatment (Figure 9.16).

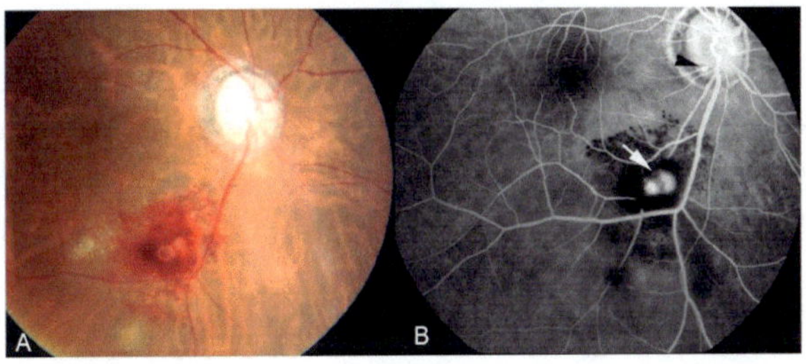

Figure 9.16. Elevated serum angiotensin-converting enzyme (ACE) levels are often associated with sarcoidosis and can serve as a supportive diagnostic marker; however, these levels may also be increased in other conditions, thereby limiting specificity.

Source: https://www.mdpi.com/diagnostics/diagnostics-11-00608/article_deploy/html/images/diagnostics-11-00608-g004.png.

9.4.3. Biopsy and Histopathological Examination

Biopsy and histopathological examination are critical in the diagnosis of sarcoidosis, particularly in the presence of cutaneous manifestations. These skin lesions, found in up to one-third of patients with systemic disease, appear as non-caseating epithelioid cell granulomas that are challenging for dermatopathologists to diagnose due to their varied presentation (Bindu & Joshi, 2014). A biopsy provides a tissue specimen for microscopy that enables clinicians to establish these diagnoses as well as rule out infectious disorders that may clinically and histologically simulate sarcoidosis. Histopathologic observations must correlate with the patient's clinical presentation and radiologic results, as skin lesions can precede systemic manifestations in some situations. Therefore, an integrated approach including biopsy results and clinical acumen is required for diagnosis and appropriate management as well, underlining the position of pathology in the interpretation of sarcoidosis as well as its granulomatous cutaneous lesions.

9.4.4. Treatment Options for Sarcoidosis

Treatment of sarcoidosis is most often needed to be multifocal, particularly when dealing with therapy in patients having multiple systemic involvement. Therapy for most begins with pharmacologic therapy with steroids, which can then offer relief of inflammation and symptoms in the majority of patients. Those with a nonresponse to steroids are more often need to add immunosuppressive therapy to achieve increased control of disease activity. This is particularly pertinent in neurosarcoidosis, where high-dose steroids may yield little benefit, thereby indicating therapies aimed against some inflammatory mechanisms. Infliximab, for instance, has been found to be a possible option, especially for its ability to inhibit TNF-alpha activity, thereby downregulating the overexpression of the Th1 response seen in these patients. Additionally, an awareness of corticosteroids not being equally effective encourages clinicians to investigate different therapeutic strategies intended to address the specific patient presentations, thus achieving improved management of this problematic condition (Ralli et al., 2018).

9.4.5. Role of Corticosteroids

The role of corticosteroids is pivotal in the management of sarcoidosis and associated granulomatous dermatoses primarily due to their potent anti-inflammatory properties.

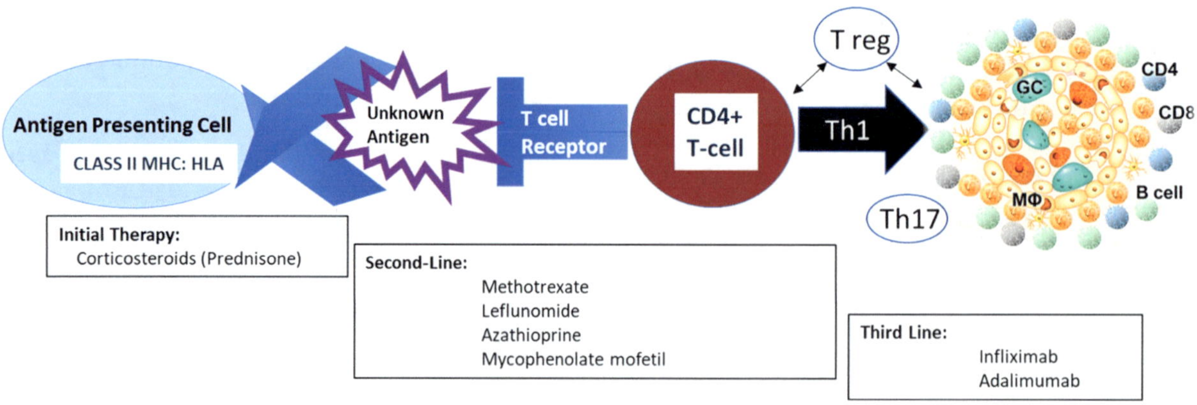

Figure 9.17. Corticosteroids play a pivotal role in managing sarcoidosis and associated granulomatous skin conditions, primarily due to their potent anti-inflammatory properties.

Source: https://www.mdpi.com/jcm/jcm-13-00738/article_deploy/html/images/jcm-13-00738-g001.png.

In severe dermatologic expressions in patients, corticosteroids reduce symptoms such as erythema and lesions, improving overall skin well-being. They are outweighed by the natural immunosuppressive properties, in which, in the case of pre-existing diseases like HIV, it is challenging to control disorders due to potential drug interactions and vulnerability to infection (Mencarini et al., 2016). Furthermore, with the need for systemic therapy during certain situations, the variation in strategies of treatment, particularly during periods of vulnerability like pregnancy, demands careful weighing of the hazards and advantages of corticosteroid therapy (Albornoz et al., 2018). Therefore, while corticosteroids are still a cornerstone of the therapy of sarcoidosis, while maintaining caution, clinicians have to weigh their therapeutic advantage over complications in patients with diverse clinical settings (Figure 9.17).

9.4.6. Monitoring Disease Progression

Following disease progression in sarcoidosis, particularly when occurring in granulomatous skin disorders, is crucial in efficacious patient management and therapeutic decision-making. Advanced imaging techniques, such as FDG PET/CT, have emerged as valuable tools for assessing the extent of internal organ involvement in patients with sarcoidosis.

According to recent data, active disease was identified in a large percentage of patients undergoing this imaging modality, and this highlights its value in determining disease activity and the presence of conditions such as head and neck sarcoidosis (HNS) (Grozdic Milojevic et al., 2019). Moreover, while not unusual in systemic autoimmune conditions are otologic and vestibular complications, their identification and treatment remain a challenge due to their multi-modal presentations. Therefore, it becomes necessary to recognize the whole spectrum of symptoms of sarcoidosis, including immune-mediated organ involvement, to individualize treatment modalities and track therapeutic effects (Ralli et al., 2018).

9.4.7. Multidisciplinary Approach to Management

Multidisciplinary management is essential in managing the complexity of sarcoidosis and associated granulomatous skin conditions. Owing to the multifaceted nature of the diseases, it is rather common that it necessitates coordination of dermatologists, pulmonologists, and rheumatologists, among other specialists, to put in place holistic treatment regimens.

This communication not only enhances the accuracy of diagnosis by combining various clinical perspectives but also ensures that treatment regimens are adequately tailored to each individual patient's presentation and needs. Immunotherapy advances highlight the importance of this teamwork, since immune-related adverse events can prove challenging to manage; hence, early detection and intervention are entirely necessary to patient care (Puzanov et al., 2017).

Secondly, the complex systemic nature of sarcoidosis indicates the importance of coordinating activities while treating, since successful management depends considerably on dissimilarities between various organ systems (Śpiołek et al., 2024). In summary, a multidisciplinary approach leads to improved patient outcomes and improved quality of life for patients with such complex illnesses.

9.4.8. Patient Education and Support

Effective patient education and counseling are important aspects in the treatment and management of sarcoidosis and granulomatous skin diseases, as they allow patients to be actively involved in their care and management. A comprehensive style of education addresses the complexities of sarcoidosis, including its potential symptoms and complications, hence enhancing patient knowledge and compliance. For instance, the awareness of risks associated with granulomatous diseases can assist patients in receiving due medical treatment on time and avoiding complications, for instance, infections in granuloma formation of diseases like CGD, leading to serious health issues (Van den Berg et al., 2009).

Besides that, due to the growing popularity of tattoos and permanent make-up, patients should be informed of the possible negative effects these have on their illnesses, e.g., chronic inflammatory reactions (Piccinini et al., 2015). Finally, developing an informed population of patients not only enhances health outcomes for individuals but also helps develop general public health consciousness of granulomatous illnesses (Figure 9.18).

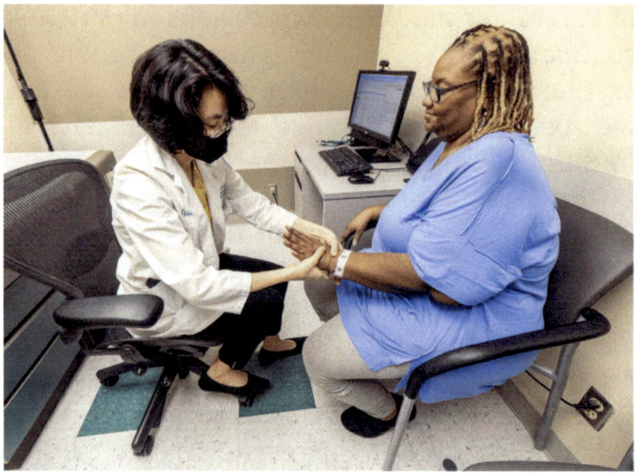

Figure 9.18. Effective patient education and support are crucial components in managing sarcoidosis and granulomatous skin conditions, as they empower patients to actively participate in their treatment and care.

Source: https://umc.edu/news/News_Articles/2023/08/images/Deborah-Norris_07.png.

Test Your Knowledge

1. What are the indications for systemic treatment in sarcoidosis?
2. What is the first-line therapy for pulmonary sarcoidosis?

SUMMARY

Learning about sarcoidosis and its associated granulomatous skin diseases is integral to improving diagnosis and patient outcomes. As seen by the evidence, cutaneous involvement occurs in 25%–30% of sarcoidosis patients, describing a strong overlap between skin and systemic disease processes. The occurrence of non-caseating epithelioid cell granulomas within the skin tends to make diagnosis challenging with its multimodal presentations, such that detailed clinical assessments and exclusion of infections are essential (Bindu & Joshi, 2014). Additionally, recognition of cutaneous lesions as a marker of systemic sarcoidosis emphasizes the necessity of ongoing monitoring and intervention. As researchers learn more about the nuances of this complicated disease, heightened awareness among medical personnel is paramount, with early and successful management interventions employed to maximize quality of life for patients and prevent potential systemic manifestations. Therefore, integrative management of skin as well as systemic findings of sarcoidosis remains crucial in clinical practice.

Research into sarcoidosis and granulomatous dermatoses finds some important aspects that point out the intricacies of diagnosis as well as treatment. Sarcoidosis presents dermatologic manifestations as papules and nodules, which can mimic other cutaneous conditions, thus posing difficulties in clinical assessment. The establishment of permanent makeup legislation and tattoos has raised controversy regarding the potential harmful impact on health, particularly when it comes to allergic reactions and autoimmune disorders, necessitating legislation like that grounded on the Council of Europe Resolution on tattoo safety (Piccinini et al., 2015). Second, the immunologic consequences of interventions such as the Bacillus Calmette-Guérin (BCG) vaccine similarly ask for consideration of granulomatous structures, proving its preventive and potential autoimmune complication functions (Bernini et al., 2015). In total, these points stress possessing an informed, multidimensional approach in managing sarcoidosis and conditions like it regarding patient safety and treatment efficacy.

KEY TERMS FROM THIS CHAPTER

- Sarcoidosis
- Granulomas
- Crohn's disease
- Immune cells
- Lymphatic system
- Skin lesions
- Vitamin D metabolism abnormalities
- Pulmonary hypertension
- Granulomatous skin illnesses
- Concomitant disorders
- Symptomatology
- Lungs
- Chronic cough
- Erythema nodosum
- Hypercalcemia
- Targeted therapy

CRITICAL THINKING QUESTIONS

1. **Which of the following is the hallmark histopathological finding in sarcoidosis?**
   a. Caseating granulomas
   b. Non-caseating granulomas
   c. Suppurative granulomas
   d. Foreign body granulomas
2. **Lupus pernio is most commonly associated with which systemic condition?**
   a. Tuberculosis
   b. Leprosy
   c. Sarcoidosis
   d. Fungal infection
3. **Which of the following investigations is most specific for diagnosing sarcoidosis?**
   a. Elevated serum calcium
   b. Chest X-ray
   c. Serum ACE level
   d. Biopsy showing non-caseating granulomas
4. **Which of the following is NOT a granulomatous skin disease?**
   a. Sarcoidosis
   b. Tuberculosis
   c. Psoriasis
   d. Leprosy
5. **What type of granulomas are typically seen in tuberculosis?**
   a. Non-caseating granulomas
   b. Suppurative granulomas
   c. Caseating granulomas
   d. Sarcoidal granulomas

Short Answer Questions

1. What is the proposed immunological mechanism behind granuloma formation in sarcoidosis?
2. Which cytokines play a central role in sarcoidosis pathogenesis?
3. What are the most common presenting symptoms of sarcoidosis?
4. Describe the typical pulmonary manifestations of sarcoidosis.
5. What are granulomatous skin conditions, and how are they classified?
6. How does cutaneous sarcoidosis typically present?
7. What are the diagnostic criteria for sarcoidosis?
8. What imaging modality is most useful in evaluating pulmonary sarcoidosis?

Answers to Critical Thinking Questions

1. (b); 2. (c); 3. (d); 4. (c); 5. (c)

REFERENCES

1. Puzanov, I., Diab, A., Abdallah, K., Bingham, C. O., 3rd, Brogdon, C., Dadu, R., Hamad, L., Kim, S., Lacouture, M. E., LeBoeuf, N. R., Lenihan, D., Onofrei, C., Shannon, V., Sharma, R., Silk, A. W., Skondra, D., Suarez-Almazor, M. E., Wang, Y., Wiley, K., Kaufman, H. L., ... Society for Immunotherapy of Cancer Toxicity Management Working Group (2017). Managing toxicities associated with immune checkpoint inhibitors: consensus recommendations from the Society for Immunotherapy of Cancer (SITC) Toxicity Management Working Group. *Journal for immunotherapy of cancer*, *5*(1), 95. https://doi.org/10.1186/s40425-017-0300-z (accessed on 23rd July 2025).

2. van den Berg, J. M., van Koppen, E., Ahlin, A., Belohradsky, B. H., Bernatowska, E., Corbeel, L., Español, T., Fischer, A., Kurenko-Deptuch, M., Mouy, R., Petropoulou, T., Roesler, J., Seger, R., Stasia, M. J., Valerius, N. H., Weening, R. S., Wolach, B., Roos, D., & Kuijpers, T. W. (2009). Chronic granulomatous disease: the European experience. *PloS one*, *4*(4), e5234. https://doi.org/10.1371/journal.pone.0005234(accessed on 23rd July 2025).

3. Albornoz CA, Wang JV, Keller M (2018) Psoriasiform Sarcoidosis Presenting in Pregnancy and Treatment Considerations. J Dermatol Res Ther 4:057. doi.org/10.23937/2469-5750/1510057(accessed on 23rd July 2025).

4. Almutairi, R., & Al-Sabah, H. (2023). A retrospective histopathological study of cutaneous granulomatous diseases at a tertiary dermatology center in Kuwait. https://core.ac.uk/download/587419173.pdf (accessed on 23rd July 2025).

5. Grozdic Milojevic I, Tadic M, Sobic-Saranovic D, Saponjski J, Artiko VM. Hybrid Imaging in Head and Neck Sarcoidosis. *J Clin Med.* 2019;8(6):803. Published 2019 Jun 5. doi:10.3390/jcm8060803(accessed on 23rd July 2025).

6. Mencarini, P., Bellagamba, R., Oliva, A., Ghirga, P., Giancola, M. L., Corpolongo, A., Ascoli Bartoli, T., De Nardo, P., Baiocchini, A., Del Nonno, F., Narciso, P., & Nicastri, E. (2016). Pulmonary tuberculosis followed by sarcoidosis in an HIV-infected patient: A case report and a simplified diagnostic flowchart for diagnosis and treatment of sarcoidosis. *Respiratory medicine case reports*, *19*, 150–154. https://doi.org/10.1016/j.rmcr.2016.09.006 (accessed on 23rd July 2025).

7. Baughman, R. P. (2007). Pulmonary hypertension associated with sarcoidosis. https://core.ac.uk/download/pdf/7779654.pdf (accessed on 23rd July 2025).

8. Bernini, L., Manzini, C.U. and Ferri, C. (2015). BCG and Autoimmunity. In Vaccines and Autoimmunity (eds Y. Shoenfeld, N. Agmon-Levin and L. Tomljenovic). https://doi.org/10.1002/9781118663721.ch21(accessed on 23rd July 2025).

9. Paola, P., Ivana, B., Sazan, P., & Chiara, S. (2015). Safety of tattoos and permanent make-up: Compilation of information on legislative framework and analytical methods.https://core.ac.uk/download/81685083.pdf (accessed on 23rd July 2025).

10. Kim, S. J., Peluso, M. J., Wang, Y., Bikle, D., Shoback, D., & Kim, S. (2018). Rapid onset of hypercalcemia from high-grade lymphoma in the setting of HIV-related immune reconstitution inflammatory syndrome. *Bone reports*, *10*, 100194. https://doi.org/10.1016/j.bonr.2018.100194(accessed on 23rd July 2025).

11. Bindu, S. M., & Joshi, S. (2014). Cutaneous sarcoidosis: A rare case report. Int J Med Res Helath Sci. 2014;3(3):779-781. https://core.ac.uk/download/pdf/27194343.pdf (accessed on 23rd July 2025).

12. Nunes, H., Bouvry, D., Soler, P. *et al.* Sarcoidosis. *Orphanet J Rare Dis* **2**, 46 (2007). https://doi.org/10.1186/1750-1172-2-46(accessed on 23rd July 2025).

13. Utino, F. L., Garcia, M., Velho, P. E. N. F., França, A. F. E. D. C., Stelini, R. F., Pelegati, V. B., Cesar, C. L., de Souza, E. M., Cintra, M. L., & Damiani, G. V. (2018). Second-harmonic generation imaging analysis can help distinguish sarcoidosis from tuberculoid leprosy. *Journal of biomedical optics*, *23*(12), 1–7. https://doi.org/10.1117/1.JBO.23.12.126001(accessed on 23rd July 2025).

14. Chang, A. L. S., Chen, J., Eriksson, N. K., Hinds, D. A., Gillett, C. P., et al. (2015). Assessment of the genetic basis of rosacea by genome-wide association study. https://core.ac.uk/download/286362504.pdf (accessed on 23rd July 2025).

15. Leonardi L, Cinicola BL, Laitano R, Duse M (2016) Allergic Bronchopulmonary Aspergillosis: Diagnostic and Treatment Challenges. J Pulm Respir Med 6: 361. doi: 1 0.4172/2161-105X.1000361(accessed on 23rd July 2025).

16. Ralli, M., D'Aguanno, V., Di Stadio, A., De Virgilio, A., Croce, A., Longo, L., Greco, A., & de Vincentiis, M. (2018). Audiovestibular Symptoms in Systemic Autoimmune Diseases. *Journal of immunology research*, *2018*, 5798103. https://doi.org/10.1155/2018/5798103(accessed on 23rd July 2025).

17. Darlington, P. (2013). *Studies of Different Clinical Manifestations of Sarcoidosis and The Role of Genetic Factors*. https://core.ac.uk/download/70340776.pdf (accessed on 23rd July 2025).

18. Hu, M. K., Mathur, A., & Dempsey, O. J. (2020). Pulmonary sarcoidosis: a clinical update. *The journal of the Royal College of Physicians of Edinburgh*, *50*(3), 322–329. https://doi.org/10.4997/JRCPE.2020.324 (accessed on 23rd July 2025).

19. Yeşiltaş, Y. S., Gündüz, A. K., Erden, E., & Shields, C. L. (2018). Lacrimal gland tumors in Turkey: types, frequency, and outcomes. *International journal of ophthalmology*, *11*(8), 1296–1302. https://doi.org/10.18240/ijo.2018.08.08(accessed on 23rd July 2025).

20. Śpiołek, O., Siwiec, J., Słowikowska, A., Teofilak, M., Szatkowska, J., Smyl, N., ... Fabian, D. (2024). A Comprehensive Review of Sarcoidosis: From Clinical Manifestations to Management Strategies. *Journal of Education, Health and Sport*, *75*, 56452. https://doi.org/10.12775/JEHS.2024.75.56452(accessed on 23rd July 2025).

21. Solis, R. N., Kuhn, B. T., & Farwell, D. G. (2018). An Unusual Case of Tertiary Syphilis Behaving Like Tongue Squamous Cell Carcinoma. *Journal of investigative medicine high impact case reports*, *6*, 2324709618820355. https://doi.org/10.1177/2324709618820355(accessed on 23rd July 2025).

22. Iio, K., Iio, T. U., Okui, Y., Ichikawa, H., Tanimoto, Y., Miyahara, N., Kanehiro, A., Tanimoto, M., Nakata, Y., & Kataoka, M. (2010). Experimental pulmonary granuloma mimicking sarcoidosis induced by Propionibacterium acnes in mice. *Acta medica Okayama*, *64*(2), 75–83. https://doi.org/10.18926/AMO/32852 (accessed on 23rd July 2025).

23. Rossides, M. (2021). *Epidemiological Aspects of Sarcoidosis: Risk Factors and Long-Term Consequences*. https://core.ac.uk/download/389617008.pdf (accessed on 23rd July 2025).

24. Woo, V. L. (2015). Oral manifestations of Crohn's disease: A case report and review of the literature. https://core.ac.uk/download/85003680.pdf (accessed on 23rd July 2025).

25. Zur Bonsen, L. S., Pohlmann, D., Rübsam, A., & Pleyer, U. (2021). Findings and Graduation of Sarcoidosis-Related Uveitis: A Single-Center Study. *Cells, 11*(1), 89. https://doi.org/10.3390/cells11010089(accessed on 23rd July 2025).

GENETIC SKIN DISORDERS

10

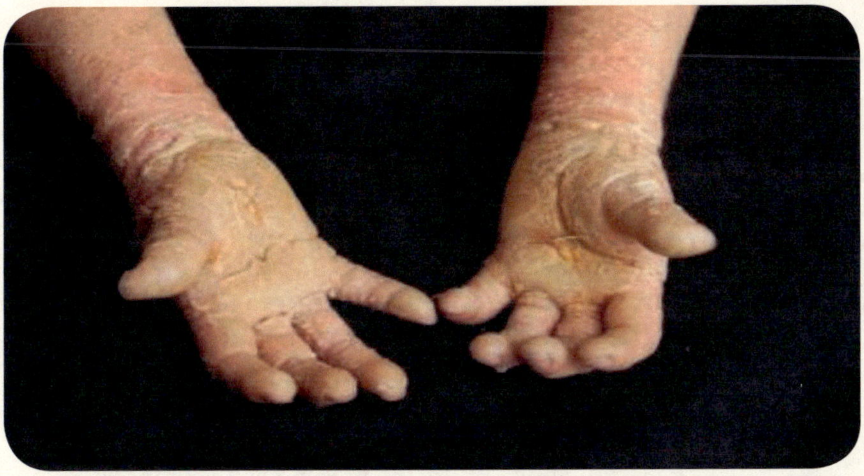

LEARNING OBJECTIVES

After studying this chapter, you will be able to:

1. Understand Ichthyosis;
2. Explain Epidermolysis Bullosa;
3. Describe Societal and Ethical Considerations.

Introduction

Genetic dermatological disorders, such as ichthyosis and epidermolysis bullosa (EB), are characterized by profound phenotypic heterogeneity and severe morbidity for affected individuals. These disorders are caused by gene mutations that disrupt skin architecture and function, with clinical signs that vary from mild dryness to rare, disabling blistering. Ichthyosis appears as abnormal thickening and scaling of the skin, whereas EB is truly defined by the fragility of the skin with blistering. Recent advances in genetic research have elucidated some underlying mechanisms, including revertant mosaicism, that have redefined disease pathology and potential therapies (Van den Akker et al., 2022). The interaction between the genetic mutations and clinical phenotype offers a basis for precise genetic diagnosis, a consideration of paramount importance not only for treatment but also for advising families and patients regarding inheritance and prognosis. As practice continues, integration of these findings into patient care remains essential to improve patient outcomes (Leeb et al., 2022).

10.1. Ichthyosis

Learning Outcome

1. Understand Definition and Types of Ichthyosis;
2. Explain Genetic Mutations associated with Ichthyosis;
3. Focus on Symptoms and Clinical Presentation;
4. Describe Diagnosis and Testing Methods;
5. Learn Treatment Options and Management Strategies;
6. Discuss Psychological and Social Implications.

Ichthyosis is a genetically diverse group of dermatoses characterized by overproduction and dyscrasia of shedding of the skin, leading to characteristic dryness and scaling of the epidermal surface. Ichthyosis is caused by many genetic mutations that affect keratinocyte differentiation and function, highlighting the complex interaction between genetics and cutaneous health.

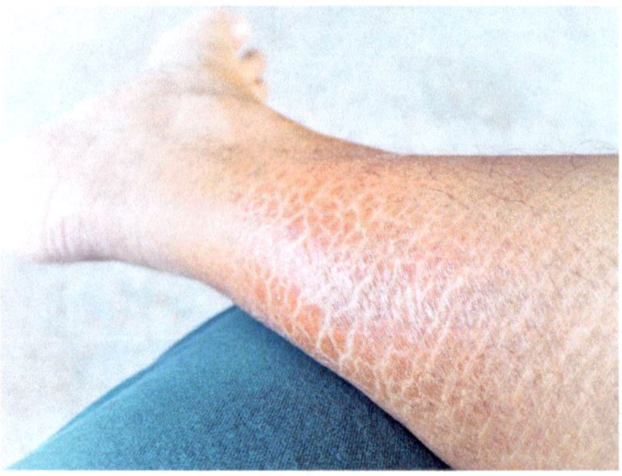

Figure 10.1. Ichthyosis.

Source: https://balmonds.co.uk/cdn/shop/articles/ichthyosis-3.jpg?v=1593683639.

Ichthyosis patients are not only physically uncomfortable but also socially and psychologically challenged since external signs have a profound impact on self-esteem and quality of life. The skin performs a multitude of functions, among which is its role in being a barrier to infection, protecting internal organs, and regulating general homeostasis, hence the significance of examining ichthyosis within the context of overall skin diseases (Campbell & Banta-Wright, 2000). The most recent study on revertant mosaicism promises new treatments, which might expand the range of possibilities for reversing ichthyosis appearance through the use of genetic correction methods (Van den Akker et al., 2022). Ichorosis is thus the intersection of genetics, dermatology, and new therapeutic research (Figure 10.1).

10.1.1. Definition and Types of Ichthyosis

Ichthyosis represents a heterogeneous collection of genetic skin disorders with abnormal cornification and impaired epidermal barrier function leading to a range of clinical manifestations. They may be inherited or acquired and present as scaling skin ranging from mild dryness to diffuse thickening and desquamation. The defective differentiation of keratinocytes results in characteristic symptoms such as itching, frequent infection, and heat intolerance, as well as potential ocular, auditory, and nutritional issues that need to be monitored regularly (Gutiérrez-Cerrajero et al., 2023). There are many varying types of ichthyosis, such as lamellar ichthyosis, epidermolytic ichthyosis, and ichthyosis vulgaris, which are each characterized by some genetic mutations (Ballout, 2015). While ichthyosis markedly disables patient quality of life, available treatments are mostly symptomatic relief-based, with no requirement for increased insight into the underlying molecular mechanisms for more effective therapy.

10.1.2. Genetic Mutations associated with Ichthyosis

Understanding genetic mutations of ichthyosis is valuable in delineating the pathophysiology of the disease, which includes impairment of skin barrier function and integrity. Ichthyosis is a heterogenous collection of genetic disorders of dry, scaly skin caused by numerous mutations, specifically within KRT1, KRT10, and KRT17 keratin genes. These genetic variations disrupt normal keratinization and lead to clinical presentations of ichthyosis. Genetic advances in recent times explained the phenomenon of revertant mosaicism (RM), wherein spontaneous genetic healing diminishes the severity of the disease.

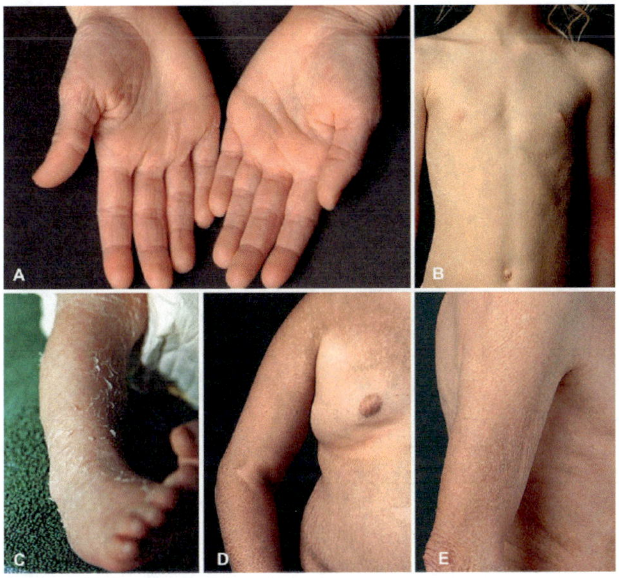

Figure 10.2. Ichthyosis encompasses a diverse group of genetic conditions characterized by dry, scaly skin resulting from various mutations, most notably in keratin genes such as KRT1, KRT10, and KRT17.

Source: https://www.researchgate.net/publication/45274663/figure/fig1/AS:276845959368717@1443016628754/Clinical-examples-of-common-ichthyosis-accentuated-palmoplantar-markings-of-ichthyosis.png.

This process, previously described in epidermolysis bullosa, would suggest the potential for a treatment strategy in ichthyosis as well, and this research initiates a paradigm shift in the perception of what genetic dermatological diseases are. Also, the sophisticated interaction between cutaneous physiology and ichthyosis makes it imperative to explore nursing management and skin care interventions to enhance patient quality of life, thus making these disorders even more complex (Campbell & Banta-Wright, 2000; Van den Akker et al., 2022) (Figure 10.2).

10.1.3. Symptoms and Clinical Presentation

The clinical presentation and signs of genetic skin conditions such as ichthyosis and epidermolysis bullosa provide serious indications regarding their pathophysiology and the impact on the affected patients. Ichthyosis, which is dry, scaly skin, comes in several forms of varying severity, affecting mobility and mood (Campbell & Banta-Wright, 2000). Alternatively, epidermolysis bullosa presents with extremely friable skin that blisters and peels after trivial trauma, leading to excruciating wounds and potential complications such as infection (Kiener, 2025). These visible signs not only indicate the resultant genetic mutations that cause keratinization and epidermal dysfunction but also mark the larger effect on patients' quality of life. Recognition of these signs is critical for early diagnosis and effective management, underlining the necessity of continued research into targeted treatment therapies that can minimize the weight of such disabling genetic conditions.

10.1.4. Diagnosis and Testing Methods

Genetic skin illnesses such as ichthyosis and epidermolysis bullosa are widely diagnosed using advanced testing methods, including genetic sequencing and histopathologic analysis. Genetic analysis plays a significant role in the detection of individual mutations responsible for these diseases, that allow for individualized diagnosis and treatment protocols. For instance, linkage analysis in lamellar ichthyosis has mapped two large loci at 14q11 and 2q33–35, which have given insight into the hereditary nature of the disorder (Bichakjian et al., 1998). Such insight is imperative because modern genetic technology, including whole genome sequencing, further enhances our ability to diagnose complex genodermatoses, as is evident from ongoing studies (Leeb et al., 2022). Also, these diagnostic advances not only clarify the direction and outcome of such diseases but also assist with responsible genetic counseling, ultimately influencing family planning and management plans for patients in dermatology (Figure 10.3).

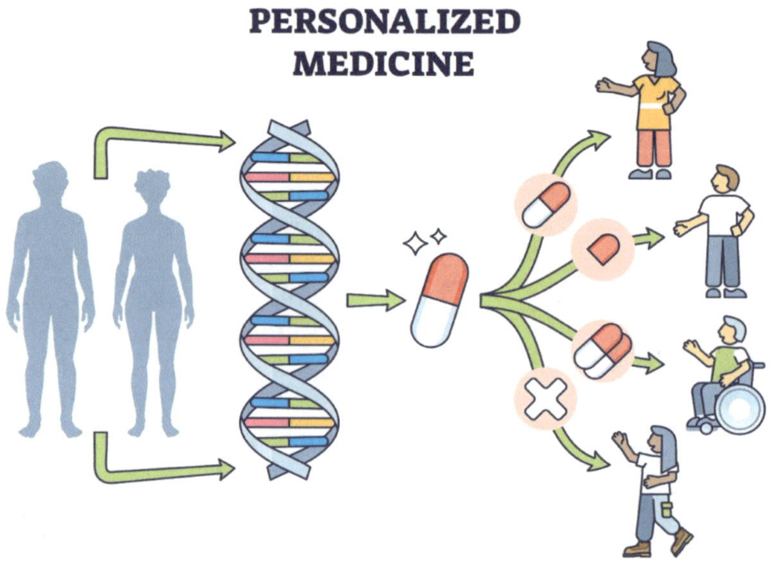

Figure 10.3. Genetic testing plays a crucial role in identifying specific mutations associated with these conditions, allowing for personalized diagnosis and treatment plans.

Source: https://www.medznat.ru/uploads/images/post_content/7182/image_3/1690458980image_3.webp.

10.1.5. Treatment Options and Management Strategies

The management of individuals with genetic skin disorders such as ichthyosis and epidermolysis bullosa demands a strategy that addresses both relief from symptoms and enhancing quality of life. Frequent use of emollients and moisturizers in the management of dryness and scaling is an important aspect of care, as for ichthyosis, where keratin protein mutation leads to excessive hardening and thickening of the skin. Additionally, psychosocial care and learning are crucial in the control of the physical and emotional needs of these illnesses, as highlighted by studies identifying a significant rate of epidermolytic ichthyosis patients experiencing severe pain and restricted daily activities (Frommherz et al., 2025). Moreover, the inclusion of expanded carrier screening gives individuals and families a valuable means of making well-informed reproductive choices that are relevant to them, and this highlights the role of full genetic counseling in directing management plans (Mastantuoni et al., 2018). Overall, these interventions aim to optimize physical health as well as psychosocial well-being for those with these disorders.

10.1.6. Psychological and Social Implications

The psychological and social impact of genetic skin conditions such as ichthyosis and epidermolysis bullosa is profound and multifaceted. The victims experience significant emotional suffering, brought about by apparent and quite painful symptoms that can render them socially isolated and stigmatized. Research has indicated that the majority of patients experience insufficiencies in the medical care and a lack of psychological support, increasing their emotional burden (Hewitt, 2025). In addition, psychological effects may influence functioning and social interactions on a day-to-day basis, leading to reduced quality of life. This points to the importance of integrated care models that include psychological support as a fundamental element of care. Interventions that use digital technology to provide emotional, information, and peer support are under development to address these needs, evidence of the worth of patient autonomy and integrative care to address the psychological needs of these disabling skin conditions (Zamiri, 2010) (Figure 10.4).

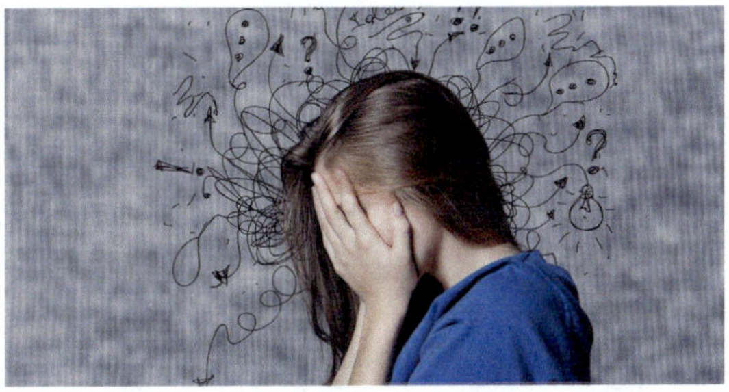

Figure 10.4. Individuals affected by these conditions often face significant emotional distress, stemming from visible and sometimes painful symptoms that can lead to social isolation and stigmatization.

Source: https://www.apexhospitals.com/_next/image?url=https%3A%2F%2Fbed.apexhospitals.com%2Fuploads%2Fmental_health2_4b39720bf5.jpg&w=1920&q=75.

Test Your Knowledge

1. What systemic diseases can be associated with acquired ichthyosis?
2. How is ichthyosis diagnosed (clinical, histopathology, genetic testing)?

10.2. Epidermolysis Bullosa

Learning Outcome

1. Understand the Definition and Classification of Epidermolysis Bullosa;
2. Explain Genetic Mutations Linked to Epidermolysis Bullosa;
3. Focus on Symptoms and Clinical Manifestations;
4. Describe Diagnosis and Assessment Techniques;
5. Learn Treatment Options and Care Management;
6. Discuss Impact on Daily Living and Mental Health;
7. Know Future Perspectives in Epidermolysis Bullosa Treatment.

Epidermolysis bullosa (EB) is a group of genetic skin disorders that are linked to extremely fragile skin, blistering, and wound formation with minimal friction or trauma. The pathology underlying EB is attributed to mutations in genes encoding structural proteins, such as laminin, which plays a critical role in maintaining the integrity of skins basement membrane (Reynolds, 2012). Recent research has unveiled the significance of revertant mosaicism (RM), wherein spontaneous correction of genetic mutations can, in certain instances, reverse to normal skin function, promising a hope for future therapy (Van den Akker et al., 2022). Such a scenario enhances the understanding of potential therapeutic approaches aimed at correcting the underlying genetic flaws in EB patients. Consequently, while treatments currently used are often symptomatic, research into mechanisms of RM might usher in novel strategies in the management of this incapacitating condition in the broader perspective of genetic skin disease.

10.2.1. Definition and Classification of Epidermolysis Bullosa

Epidermolysis bullosa (EB) is a rare collection of inherited skin disorders characterized by extreme fragility of skin with resulting blistering and erosions following minimal trauma. The severity of EB is largely based on the extent of the skin in the presence of abnormality, which is further divided into four primary forms: EB simplex, junctional EB, dystrophic EB, and kindler syndrome. All these are due to mutations in single genes that play a role in the structural integrity of the skin and also reflect the severity and pattern of presentation (Bauer, 2018). Aside from the genetic etiology of such disorders, their classification may also encompass associated phenotypic characteristics in addition to pathways of skin development such as keratins and cadherins, yielding a holistic view which is informed by both clinical observations and molecular diagnoses (Wright et al., 2019). This integrated system of classification therefore, facilitates individualization of management approaches for the individuals involved (Figure 10.5).

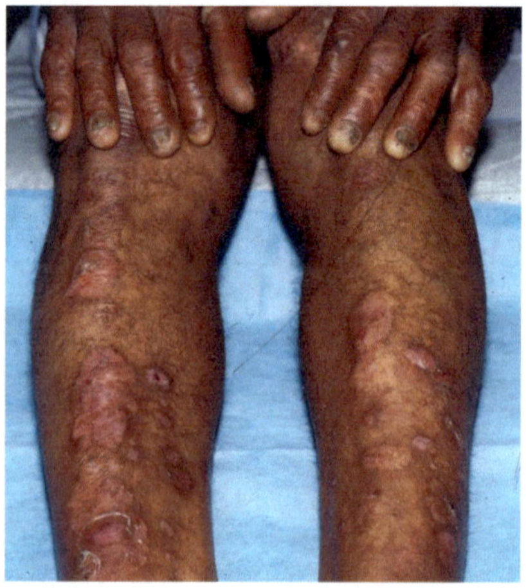

Figure 10.5. Epidermolysis bullosa (EB) is a group of rare genetic skin disorders characterized by extreme fragility of the skin, leading to blistering and wounds resulting from minimal trauma.

Source: https://media.springernature.com/lw685/springer-static/image/art%3A10.1186%2F1750-1172-5-12/MediaObjects/13023_2009_Article_175_Fig8_HTML.jpg.

10.2.2. Genetic Mutations Linked to Epidermolysis Bullosa

Epidermolysis bullosa (EB) is a group of rare hereditary skin disorders with severe skin fragility and formation of blisters due to minor mechanical trauma. The disease results from mutations in genes coding for the synthesis of proteins crucial for the integrity and structure of the skin, such as keratins and collagen. The mutations lead to varying levels of severity; for instance, in junctional EB, laminin gene mutations interfere with the attachment of the epidermis to the dermis, and this results in widespread blistering and scarring (Mastantuoni et al., 2018). Understanding the genetic disparities involved in EB not only helps in diagnosis but also opens the door to targeted treatment and personalized medicine. Moreover, the place of genetic counseling and expanded carrier screening for prospective parents cannot be overlooked, as it provides crucial information about the genetic risks of prospective offspring (Bichakjian et al., 1998). Hence, the evolution of knowledge about these genetic mutations is likely to improve patient outcomes in EB.

10.2.3. Symptoms and Clinical Manifestations

Symptoms and clinical presentations of genetic skin conditions such as ichthyosis and epidermolysis bullosa (EB) are diverse and significantly influence individuals quality of life. In epidermolytic ichthyosis, among others, patients usually have extensive skin involvement, which is differentiated as localized, intermediate, and severe based on clinical presentation and severity scoring like the modified Ichthyosis Area Severity Index (mIASI) (Frommherz et al., 2025). Manifestations of symptoms include intense itching and discomfort, present in nearly half of the patients, which restricts activity and leads to overall poor quality of life. Similarly, EB shows a range of manifestations, e.g., blistering and skin fragility, with attendant complications such as infection and scarring. Revertant mosaicism in EB illustrates increased appreciation of clinical presentations and potential avenues for new therapies, exemplifying the complexities in these genetic diseases (Van den Akker et al., 2022) (Figure 10.6).

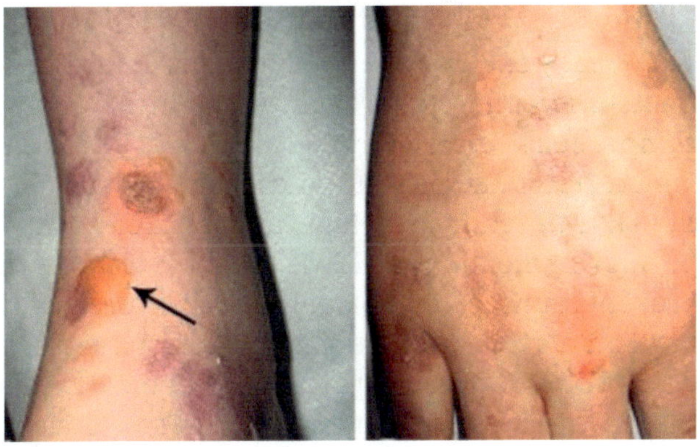

Figure 10.6. Common symptoms include intense itching and severe pain, affecting nearly half of the patients, which contributes to daily restrictions in activities and an overall diminished quality of life.

Source: https://images.ctfassets.net/1ny4yoiyrqia/6ll643z64Ylqfanei1vtbj/c352f4bd808dea48cc20168dbee6d53d/epidermolysis-bullosa-acquista.jpg.

10.2.4. Diagnosis and Assessment Techniques

Effective diagnosis and assessment methods are essential for the correct identification and treatment of genetic skin disorders such as ichthyosis and epidermolysis bullosa. They all need a multidisciplinary strategy that integrates clinical evaluation, family history, and expert molecular genetic testing. Clinically, the practitioner must be sensitive to the usual presentations of these disorders, such as for example, the thickened skin in ichthyosis or weakened, blistering skin in epidermolysis bullosa. In addition, advancements in next-generation sequencing technology have significantly enhanced diagnostic accuracy by uncovering specific genetic variants causing such conditions, as noted in a study examining inherited skin diseases (Kiener, 2025). Awareness of the pathomechanisms behind such conditions is critical for building patient-specific management plans that optimize outcomes, highlighting the need for careful diagnostic approaches to address genetic skin disorders' (Campbell & Banta-Wright, 2000) complexity.

10.2.5. Treatment Options and Care Management

The treatment of genetic skin disorders like ichthyosis and epidermolysis bullosa (EB) needs a multi-disciplinary approach, which involves treatment options as well as a careful consideration of comprehensive care strategies. Effective treatment is typically done with topical therapy, including moisturizers and keratolytics, which play significant roles in managing dryness and scaling of the skin in ichthyosis. Pain management and wound care are crucial in preventing infection and promoting healing in EB. A recent observational study also identifies the heterogeneous clinical presentations of epidermolytic ichthyosis, which have shown that close to 50% of the affected patients develop severe pain and pruritus that negatively affects their quality of life (Frommherz et al., 2025). Given the psychological burden that these disorders place on a person, combined with the need for continuous management, genetic counseling and psychosocial support are essential components of management, especially as expanding carrier screening identifies new instances (Mastantuoni et al., 2018). Care plans are thus needed to be tailored to properly treat the unique needs of each patient (Figure 10.7).

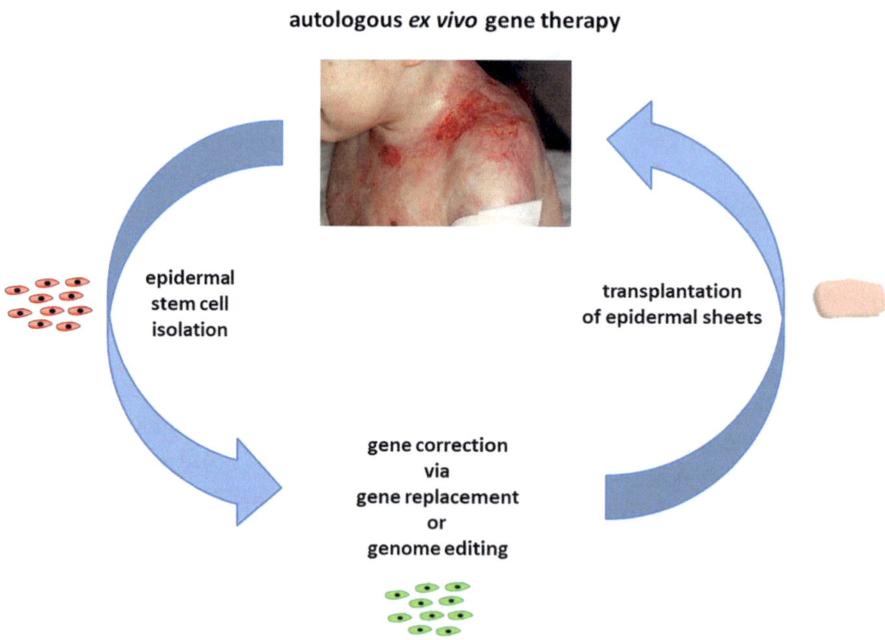

Figure 10.7. The management of genetic skin disorders such as ichthyosis and epidermolysis bullosa (EB) requires a multifaceted approach that incorporates both treatment options and comprehensive care strategies.

Source: https://www.frontiersin.org/files/Articles/658295/fgene-12-658295-HTML/image_m/fgene-12-658295-g001.jpg.

10.2.6. Impact on Daily Living and Mental Health

Genetic skin patients, such as ichthyosis and epidermolysis bullosa, typically have serious issues beyond physical symptoms that impact daily living and mental health. The management of these conditions is usually described in terms of chronic discomfort, ongoing care routines, and social stigmatization, which can significantly restrict daily functioning; for example, studies suggest that approximately 78% of patients indicate the limitation caused by requirements for therapeutic care and skin problems (Frommherz et al., 2025). Moreover, the psychological impact is not to be underestimated, with minimal mental health provision and the biomedical model of treatment serving to devalue such patients' emotional lives (Hewitt, 2025). The need for integrated interventions designed specifically to enhance quality of life is paramount, and with this, there is an urgent need to introduce psychological intervention and self-management techniques into care planning to enable coping with the multifaceted challenges posed by these disabling illnesses.

10.2.7. Future Perspectives in Epidermolysis Bullosa Treatment

Future prospects in epidermolysis bullosa (EB) treatment are illustrated by innovative therapeutic approaches capable of altering patient outcomes at a root level. Developments in gene therapy, especially for severe manifestations such as Recessive Dystrophic Epidermolysis Bullosa (RDEB), represent a futuristic course of treatment by targeting the genetic mutations responsible for the disease. By delivering functional copies of defective genes, researchers aim to substitute the critical proteins that keep skin whole and potentially turn around the blisters' underlying disease processes. Furthermore, the significant role of inflammation in the pathogenesis of EB has been evidenced; therapeutic interventions like apremilast, which aim at inflammatory processes, have exhibited remarkable improvements in the blistering of the skin in patients affected by EB, as supplemented by recent findings of persistent infiltration of inflammatory cells into affected skin (Castela et al., 2018). In total, ongoing research lends even more validity to the need for clinical trials to establish these new treatments and ascertain their long-term efficacy and safety (Raoufinia et al., 2024) (Figure 10.8).

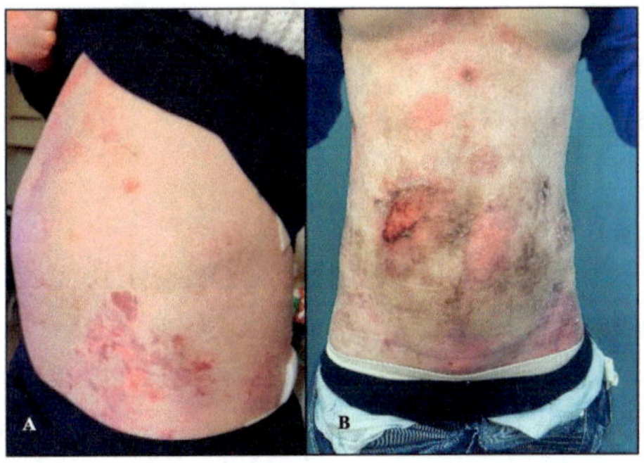

Figure 10.8. Advances in gene therapy, especially for severe subtypes such as Recessive Dystrophic Epidermolysis Bullosa (RDEB), present a forward-thinking approach by targeting the genetic mutations responsible for the disease.

Source: https://www.mdpi.com/diseases/diseases-12-00104/article_deploy/html/images/diseases-12-00104-g001.png.

Test Your Knowledge

1. What is the inheritance pattern of the major EB subtypes?
2. What are the common complications of severe forms of EB?

10.3. Societal and Ethical Considerations

Learning Outcome

1. Understand Stigmatization of Individuals with Skin Disorders;
2. Explain Access to Healthcare and Treatment Disparities;
3. Focus on Ethical Implications of Genetic Testing;
4. Describe Role of Advocacy Groups and Support Networks;
5. Learn Public Awareness Campaigns and Education;
6. Discuss Psychological Support for Affected Individuals;
7. Know Employment and Social Integration Challenges;
8. Understand Insurance Coverage and Financial Burdens;
9. Explain Future Ethical Considerations in Genetic Research.

The research on genetic skin illnesses such as ichthyosis and epidermolysis bullosa puts into prominence pertinent social and ethical concerns that need to be tackled with careful scrutiny. The psychological burden related to these conditions points to the limitations of the current biomedical model that is prone to overlooking psychological support as an integral part of holistic patient treatment (Hewitt, 2025). Moreover, social beliefs regarding visible skin disease may result in stigmatization, influencing the mental health and social interaction of patients. As genomics increases as a science, spurred by behemoth undertakings like the Human Genome Project, which has made it easier to comprehend genetic disease, ethical considerations involving genetic testing and intervention are a concern of utmost importance. Issues such as informed consent, confidentiality, and vulnerability to genetic discrimination must be at the forefront of discussions about modalities of treatment. Resolution of these ethical issues is essential so that treatment and support reach affected individuals fairly in society.

10.3.1. Stigmatization of Individuals with Skin Disorders

Stigmatization of carriers of genetic skin illnesses, such as ichthyosis and epidermolysis bullosa, is highly articulated in social interaction and personal experience and comes to cause profound psychological anguish. Although these conditions are biologically determined, individuals so affected tend to encounter stereotypes and prejudices upholding their exclusion.

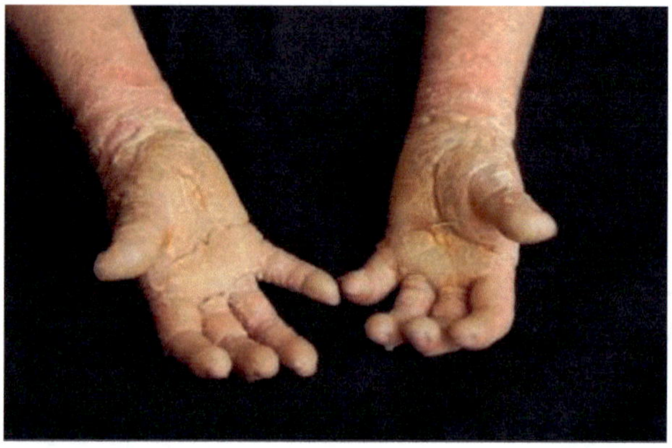

Figure 10.9. The stigmatization of individuals with genetic skin disorders, such as ichthyosis and epidermolysis bullosa, manifests profoundly in societal interactions and personal experiences, ultimately leading to significant psychological distress.

Source: https://img.medscapestatic.com/pi/meds/ckb/79/61679tn.jpg.

The prevailing biomedical model of dermatology is known to overlook the necessity of psychological support in coping with eczema stigma, for example, the necessity for integrative self-management strategies (Hewitt, 2025). In addition, existing intervention is realized to be of minimal effectiveness due to barriers in acceptability and accessibility, necessitating a paradigm shift towards more inclusive models of care (Adaskevich, 2016). This ongoing stigmatization not only exacerbates the emotional and psychological load on the affected individuals but also creates a cycle of discrimination and segregation, underlining the urgent need for heightened public awareness and targeted interventions bridging the gap between medical treatment and psychosocial care (Figure 10.9).

10.3.2. Access to Healthcare and Treatment Disparities

The disparities in care access and treatment experienced by individuals with genetic skin disorders, such as ichthyosis and epidermolysis bullosa, illustrate gigantic inequalities in the care system. These conditions typically carry a heavy psychological burden that continues to remain unmet due to the prevailing biomedical model of care, which focuses on addressing primarily physical symptoms and ignores psychological care (Hewitt, 2025). Consequently, patients may find it challenging to obtain appropriate treatment options and emotional support required to cope with their conditions. Besides, the development of digital interventions, like the MiDerm app, is a viable avenue in addressing self-management challenges; however, as the study reports, psychological support and peer support are not yet sufficient within mainstream healthcare settings (Hewitt, 2025). Moreover, cross-disciplinary research describing human and companion animal disease similarities at the genetic level opens doors to more integrated forms of intervention that would eventually be practiced on both populations.

10.3.3. Ethical Implications of Genetic Testing

The ethical issue of informed consent and susceptibility to discrimination are important factors in the application of genetic testing in the diagnosis of skin diseases such as ichthyosis and epidermolysis bullosa. With improvements in genomic technology, such as next-generation sequencing, the detection of pathogenic variants is becoming better, with the prospect for more accurate diagnosis and targeted treatment (Kiener, 2025). However, these developments also lead to controversial ethical concerns, particularly with genetic information being increasingly accessible. Misuse by insurers or employers of genetic data can potentially lead to concern over discrimination against an individual based on their genetic predisposition to skin diseases or other illness. Furthermore, the question of informed consent is of paramount importance; patients must fully understand the implications of genetic testing, including possible psychological impacts and the social implications of having their genetic information made public or kept on file (Häfliger et al., 2025). Thus, a delicate ethical model must navigate the challenges appropriately (Figure 10.10).

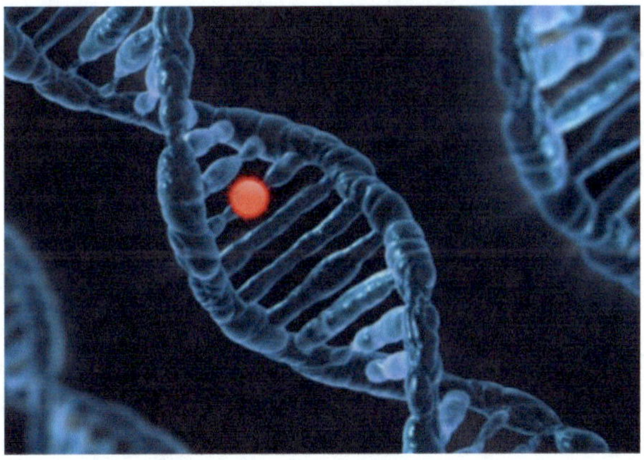

Figure 10.10. With advancements in genomic technologies, such as next-generation sequencing, the ability to identify pathogenic variants has improved, providing opportunities for more accurate diagnoses and targeted therapies.

Source: https://cdn.prod.website-files.com/65b10cf2a9c7f9d23b4bb47d/65b10cf2a9c7f9d23b4bb4db_what-is-ngs-testing-unveiling-the-essentials-of-next-generation-sequencing.jpg.

10.3.4. Role of Advocacy Groups and Support Networks

Support networks and advocacy groups can play a significant role in the treatment and recognition of genetic skin diseases such as ichthyosis and epidermolysis bullosa (EB). They assist in giving necessary resources to patients and their families by filling gaps that enhance emotional care and shared experiences. They may also serve as key conduits in delivering news on the most recent research and available treatments, thereby empowering patients to become proactive participants in their healthcare decisions. They also highlight the place of psychological care in the healthcare system, counteracting the detrimental emotional burden these conditions carry. For instance, it has been shown through research that patients often lack medical care and treatment, bringing forth the need for combined interventions encompassing medical and psychological issues (Hewitt, 2025). Encouraging caregivers' self-efficacy and well-being through enhanced flows of personalized information and support is critical in affecting impacted children indirectly as well (Walsh et al., 2023).

10.3.5. Public Awareness Campaigns and Education

Public education and campaigns are key to advancing the knowledge and compassion for genetic skin diseases such as ichthyosis and epidermolysis bullosa (EB). They assist in de-mystifying the conditions, encourage an understanding and acceptance by communities, and inform patients and caregivers about the treatment and support that is available to them. Patient-centered nonprofits are essential in this context, as they bridge large gaps in research and development, ultimately influencing patient care and quality of life. To illustrate, efforts highlighting the everyday plight of those afflicted by these disorders can be utilized to galvanize community activism and policy change, improving access to effective treatments (Schutz, 2013). Additionally, the integration of educational activities in clinics ensures that medical professionals are better equipped to offer empathetic, evidence-based care, thus promoting the culture of empathy and patient advocacy for patients with ichthyosis and EB (Manley et al., 2018) (Figure 10.11).

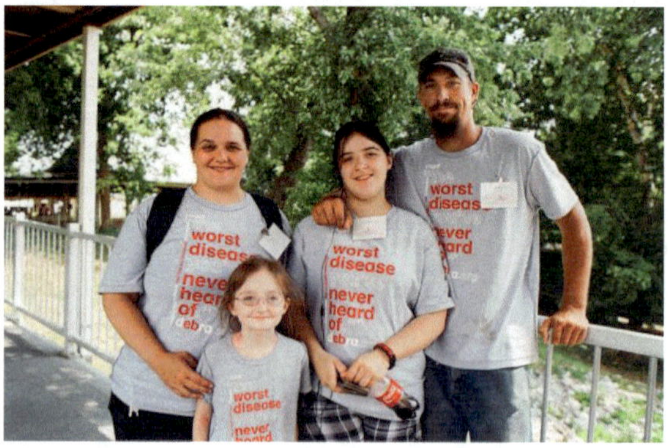

Figure 10.11. Public awareness campaigns and education are vital in advancing the understanding and management of genetic skin disorders such as ichthyosis and epidermolysis bullosa (EB).

Source: https://www.debra.org/sites/default/files/styles/para_text_with_image/public/2023-07/DEBRA_EpidermolysisBullosa_Support5.jpg?itok=tUWMyNP3.

10.3.6. Psychological Support for Affected Individuals

Psychological counseling to patients impacted by genetic skin conditions, such as ichthyosis and epidermolysis bullosa, is of utmost importance in dealing with the compounded problems faced by the affected patients. The physical appearance of the disease generally triggers significant psychosocial distress, impact on self-esteem, and interpersonal relationships. Case studies indicate that continuing psychological treatment and genetic counseling need to be included in management plans; these therapies arm the individual with self-management skills and resilience against the emotional burden of chronic skin disease (Mastantuoni et al., 2018). Furthermore, studies focusing on epidermolytic ichthyosis highlight that patients have significant quality of life impairments, wherein 78% of the patients report limitations in activities of daily living due to treatment needs (Frommherz et al., 2025). Therefore, there is a need to support psychological support networks to not just improve mental health results but additionally the quality of life in individuals coping with the complexities of genetic skin diseases.

10.3.7. Employment and Social Integration Challenges

Patients with congenital skin disorders, such as ichthyosis and epidermolysis bullosa, face serious work-related and social integration issues, mainly because of the overt nature of the diseases.

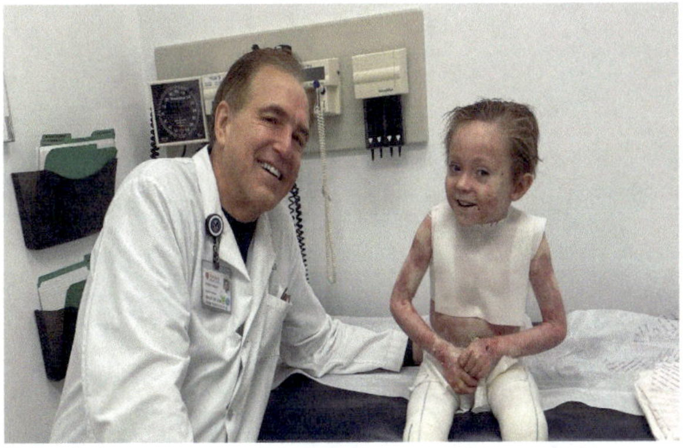

Figure 10.12. Individuals with genetic skin disorders, such as ichthyosis and epidermolysis bullosa, face significant employment and social integration challenges, largely stemming from the visible nature of their conditions.

Source: https://external-preview.redd.it/WShgqohZ90fEpFb4suUCatZgP85T-Fe5GV32_Sdyqms.jpg?auto=webp&s=3eb313043d9d732128635fa91260189a9f1217f6.

The psychological burden of these dermatoses can entail social stigmatization, affecting self-esteem and personal relationships, which in turn complicates workforce engagement. Moreover, recent studies emphasize the deficits in psychological care, corroborating the overwhelming need for interventions that encourage social resilience and skill acquisition (Hewitt, 2025). Moreover, mindfulness interventions have been proven useful in alleviating stress among affected families, suggesting that they would be able to cope better with workplace relations (Hughes, 2025). As such persons seek to merge with workplace environments, barriers such as discrimination and lack of knowledge about their conditions need to be broken so that a culture supportive of diversity and equal opportunities to all is established (Figure 10.12).

10.3.8. Insurance Coverage and Financial Burdens

The costs of treating genetic cutaneous disorders such as ichthyosis and epidermolysis bullosa are far more than the initial cost of treatment; they can put heavy recurring burdens on the families affected. Insurance coverage largely dictates access to necessary treatment, including specialized dermatologic therapies and supportive care. Yet, most insurance policies are likely not to cover the expenses of these rare conditions in any form, causing patients and families to incur devastating out-of-pocket expenses. An example is with epidermolysis bullosa patients who need costly wound care management and supportive devices for living in a quality manner even though such coverage may not be adequate as provided by standard health insurance plans. This lack of coverage further adds to the economic costs to families, demonstrating the imperative for policy enhancement to support ensuring victims of genetic skin disease receive the help they require in order to survive (Carvalho et al., 2019; Ciolfi et al., 2020).

10.3.9. Future Ethical Considerations in Genetic Research

As genetic research moves forward, particularly with disorders such as ichthyosis and epidermolysis bullosa, there are numerous ethical concerns to ponder. The rapidly growing ability to manipulate genetic expressions raises issues of consent, particularly where research is undertaken using vulnerable patients, such as infants with severe disorders like Harlequin Ichthyosis. The implications of identifying mutations, such as in the ABCA12 gene, call for particular attention to the probable psychological impact on families and broader ramifications of genetic testing (Bland, 2016). In addition, research into genetically engineered skin substitutes presents ethical issues regarding the use of animal models and the commodification of human skin (Marques et al., 2017). These issues challenge investigators, clinicians, and ethicists to ensure that follow-up studies both expand the treatment options and uphold the virtues of respect, beneficence, and justice in biomedical research.

Test Your Knowledge

1. Which principle of biomedical ethics emphasizes fair access to dermatologic care for patients with rare skin diseases?
2. What are the ethical concerns surrounding genetic testing in children with inherited skin disorders?

SUMMARY

In research into genetic skin conditions such as ichthyosis and epidermolysis bullosa, one has to acknowledge the marvelous advancements in genetic research and how this has influenced diagnosis and treatment. Identification of disease-causing pathogenic variants not only deepened our understanding of their pathogenesis but also paved the way for more effective therapeutic intervention. As seen, the intersection of next-generation sequencing technology makes it possible to rapidly detect genetic defects with easier diagnosis and personalized treatment plans (Kiener, 2025). Further, initiatives like expanded carrier screening also underscore the importance of early detection and genetic counseling, enabling prospective parents to make a well-informed reproductive choice (Mastantuoni et al., 2018). These advances collectively indicate a universal move towards precision medicine that promises better results for those afflicted with genetic skin diseases and underscores the unity of veterinary and human medicine in the treatment of such formidable diseases.

The studies of genetic skin diseases, particularly ichthyosis and epidermolysis bullosa, provide significant information on their multifactorial etiology as well as treatment planning. Existing research has revealed that ichthyosis exists in various genetic forms, where particular mutations are responsible for different phenotypes, and this indicates the necessity of isolating the genetic basis for proper diagnosis and treatment (Kiener, 2025). Furthermore, epidermolysis bullosa is also characterized by its blistering, which arises from some genetic defects that compromise skin integrity, and existing research is being conducted on emerging therapies like *ex vivo* gene modification (Jayarajan et al., 2021). Taken together, these diseases not only decrease patients' quality of life due to their chronic and severe nature, but also represent a key area of investigation aimed at the development of targeted therapies. The intersections between genetic findings and potential therapeutic advances strengthen the demand for continued research in this area and improve both veterinary and human medicine through consistent knowledge of genetic dermatological illnesses.

KEY TERMS FROM THIS CHAPTER

- Ichthyosis
- Phenotypic heterogeneity
- Skin architecture
- Genetic mutations
- Keratinocyte differentiation
- Lamellar ichthyosis
- Ichthyosis vulgaris
- Epidermolysis bullosa
- Epidermolysis bullosa (EB)
- Gene mutations
- Blistering
- Phenotype
- Genetic correction
- Epidermolytic ichthyosis
- Revertant mosaicism (RM)

CRITICAL THINKING QUESTIONS

1. **Which of the following is a hallmark feature of Neurofibromatosis type 1 (NF1)?**
   a. Ash-leaf macules
   b. Café-au-lait spots
   c. Malar rash
   d. Gottron's papules
2. **The most common form of inherited ichthyosis is:**
   a. Lamellar ichthyosis
   b. X-linked ichthyosis
   c. Ichthyosis vulgaris
   d. Harlequin ichthyosis
3. **Which of the following genetic disorders presents with "ash-leaf spots" and facial angiofibromas?**
   a. Neurofibromatosis type 2
   b. Xeroderma pigmentosum
   c. Tuberous sclerosis
   d. Epidermolysis bullosa
4. **Which skin disorder is due to a defect in melanin synthesis?**
   a. Tuberous sclerosis
   b. Albinism
   c. Vitiligo
   d. Psoriasis
5. **Harlequin ichthyosis is caused by a mutation in which gene?**
   a. ABCA12
   b. COL7A1
   c. FBN1
   d. TSC1

Short Answer Questions

1. What is ichthyosis, and how is it classified?
2. What are the clinical features of ichthyosis vulgaris?
3. What is epidermolysis bullosa, and how is it classified by level of skin cleavage?
4. What are the key features of EB simplex, junctional EB, and dystrophic EB?
5. What are the psychosocial challenges faced by patients with visible genetic skin disorders?
6. How can genetic counseling benefit families of individuals with ichthyosis or EB?

Answers to Critical Thinking Questions

1. (b); 2. (c); 3. (c); 4. (b); 5. (a)

REFERENCES

1. Wright, J. T., Fete, M., Schneider, H., Zinser, M., Koster, M. I., Clarke, A. J., Hadj-Rabia, S., Tadini, G., Pagnan, N., Visinoni, A. F., Bergendal, B., Abbott, B., Fete, T., Stanford, C., Butcher, C., D'Souza, R. N., Sybert, V. P., & Morasso, M. I. (2019). Ectodermal dysplasias: Classification and organization by phenotype, genotype and molecular pathway. *American journal of medical genetics. Part A, 179*(3), 442–447. https://doi.org/10.1002/ajmg.a.61045(accessed on 23rd July 2025).

2. Raoufinia, R., Rahimi, H. R., Keyhanvar, N., Moghbeli, M., Abdyazdani, N., Rostami, M., Naghipoor, K., Forouzanfar, F., Foroudi, S., & Saburi, E. (2024). Advances in Treatments for Epidermolysis Bullosa (EB): Emphasis on Stem Cell-Based Therapy. *Stem cell reviews and reports, 20*(5), 1200–1212. https://doi.org/10.1007/s12015-024-10697-4(accessed on 23rd July 2025).

3. Adaskevich, V. P. (2016). *Skin Diseases and Sexually Transmitted Infections.* https://core.ac.uk/download/80150454.pdf (accessed on 23rd July 2025).

4. Gutiérrez-Cerrajero, C., Sprecher, E., Paller, A. S., Akiyama, M., Mazereeuw-Hautier, J., Hernández-Martín, A., & González-Sarmiento, R. (2023). Ichthyosis. *Nature reviews. Disease primers, 9*(1), 2. https://doi.org/10.1038/s41572-022-00412-3(accessed on 23rd July 2025).

5. Mastantuoni, E., Saccone, G., Al-Kouatly, H. B., Paternoster, M., D'Alessandro, P., Arduino, B., Carbone, L., Esposito, G., Raffone, A., De Vivo, V., Maruotti, G. M., Berghella, V., & Zullo, F. (2018). Expanded carrier screening: A current perspective. *European journal of obstetrics, gynecology, and reproductive biology, 230*, 41–54. https://doi.org/10.1016/j.ejogrb.2018.09.014(accessed on 23rd July 2025).

6. Frommherz, L., Giehl, K., Hofmann, J., Huebner, S., Kiekbusch, K., Sabkova, T., Süßmuth, K., Alter, S., Tantcheva-Poór, I., Ott, H., Fischer, J., & Has, C. (2025). Epidermolytic ichthyosis: Clinical spectrum and burden of disease in a large German cohort. *Journal of the European Academy of Dermatology and Venereology : JEADV, 39*(5), 1028–1037. https://doi.org/10.1111/jdv.20096(accessed on 23rd July 2025).

7. Carvalho, I., Freixo, J.P., Marques, M., Cardoso, M.E., J., Fino, Alves, C., Marques, B., Talkowski, M., H., Correia, Morton, C., Dezső, D., Lepamets, M., Martin-Brevet, S., T.Laisk, -., Podar, Metspalu, A., Lindgren, C.M., S., Jacquemont, Draganski, B., Mägi, R., & Reymond, A. (2018). Abstracts from the 50th European Society of Human Genetics Conference: Posters. *European Journal of Human Genetics*, 1-707.(accessed on 23rd July 2025).

8. Ciolfi, A., Aref-Eshghi, E., Pizzi, S., Pedace, L., Miele, E., Kerkhof, J., Flex, E., Martinelli, S., Radio, F. C., Ruivenkamp, C. A. L., Santen, G. W. E., Bijlsma, E., Barge-Schaapveld, D., Ounap, K., Siu, V. M., Kooy, R. F., Dallapiccola, B., Sadikovic, B., & Tartaglia, M. (2020). Frameshift mutations at the C-terminus of HIST1H1E result in a specific DNA hypomethylation signature. *Clinical epigenetics, 12*(1), 7. https://doi.org/10.1186/s13148-019-0804-0(accessed on 23rd July 2025).

9. Ballout, F. R. (2015). The role of MBTPS2 in epidermal proliferation and differentiation. https://core.ac.uk/download/650463504.pdf (accessed on 23rd July 2025).

10. Campbell, J. M., & Banta-Wright, S. A. (2000). Neonatal skin disorders: a review of selected dermatologic abnormalities. *The Journal of perinatal & neonatal nursing, 14*(1), 63–83. https://doi.org/10.1097/00005237-200006000-00006(accessed on 23rd July 2025). Castela, E., Tulic,

M. K., Rozières, A., Bourrat, E., Nicolas, J. F., Kanitakis, J., Vabres, P., Bessis, D., Mazereeuw, J., Morice-Picard, F., Baty, D., Berard, F., Lacour, J. P., Passeron, T., & Chiaverini, C. (2019). Epidermolysis bullosa simplex generalized severe induces a T helper 17 response and is improved by apremilast treatment. *The British journal of dermatology, 180*(2), 357–364. https://doi.org/10.1111/bjd.16897(accessed on 23rd July 2025).

11. Bauer, Anina Estrella (2018). *Genetic analysis of genodermatoses.* (Thesis). Universität Bern, Bern(accessed on 23rd July 2025).
12. Bichakjian, C. K., Elder, J. T., Goldberg, S., Nair, R. P., Voorhees, J. J., et al. (1998). Prenatal exclusion of lamellar ichthyosis based on identification of two new mutations in the transglutaminase 1 gene. https://core.ac.uk/download/pdf/82176844.pdf (accessed on 23rd July 2025).
13. Bland, P. J. (2016). *The Genetic and Functional Role of ABCA12 in Harlequin ichthyosis.* https://core.ac.uk/download/77040949.pdf (accessed on 23rd July 2025).
14. van den Akker, P. C., Bolling, M. C., & Pasmooij, A. M. G. (2022). Revertant Mosaicism in Genodermatoses: Natural Gene Therapy Right before Your Eyes. *Biomedicines, 10*(9), 2118. https://doi.org/10.3390/biomedicines10092118(accessed on 23rd July 2025).
15. Marques, A. P., Pirraco, R. P., Reis, R. L., & Cerqueira, M. T.., et al. (2017). Skin tissue models. https://core.ac.uk/download/155248219.pdf (accessed on 23rd July 2025).
16. Jayarajan, V., Kounatidou, E., Qasim, W., & Di, W. L. (2021). Ex vivo gene modification therapy for genetic skin diseases-recent advances in gene modification technologies and delivery. *Experimental dermatology, 30*(7), 887–896. https://doi.org/10.1111/exd.14314(accessed on 23rd July 2025).
17. Häfliger, I. M. (2025). *Forward vs. Reverse Genetics: A Bovine Perspective Based on Visible and Hidden Phenotypes of Inherited Disorders.* https://core.ac.uk/download/521342907.pdf (accessed on 23rd July 2025).
18. Hewitt, R. (2025). *The MiDerm App: A Mixed Methods Approach to Developing a Complex Digital Behavior Change Intervention for Adults Living with Skin Conditions.* https://core.ac.uk/download/613173442.pdf (accessed on 23rd July 2025).
19. Hughes, O. (2025). *Mindfulness-Based Online Support for Children and Families Affected by Skin Conditions.* https://core.ac.uk/download/595951183.pdf (accessed on 23rd July 2025).
20. Manley, K., Jackson, C., Martin, A. and Wright, T. 2018. Using participatory, practice development, Delphi and realist research approaches to understand how frontline teams can use the workplace to make sustainable improvements in the quality of their practice.(accessed on 23rd July 2025).
21. Kiener, S. (2025). *Genetic Investigation of Inherited Skin Diseases in Cats and Dogs.* https://core.ac.uk/download/596769902.pdf (accessed on 23rd July 2025).
22. Walsh, C., Leavey, G., & McLaughlin, M. (2023). Information provision to caregivers of children with rare dermatological disorders: an international multimethod qualitative study. *BMJ open, 13*(7), e070840. https://doi.org/10.1136/bmjopen-2022-070840(accessed on 23rd July 2025).
23. Leeb, T., Roosje, P., & Welle, M. (2022). Genetics of inherited skin disorders in dogs. *Veterinary journal (London, England : 1997), 279*, 105782. https://doi.org/10.1016/j.tvjl.2021.105782(accessed on 23rd July 2025).

24. Polis Schutz, J. (2013). *The Contribution of Disease Focused Nonprofits to Biomedical Research and Development.* https://core.ac.uk/download/19879075.pdf (accessed on 23rd July 2025).

25. Reynolds, J. M. (2012). *Analysis of the Effects and Current Treatments of Laminin Deficiency.* https://core.ac.uk/download/58824508.pdf (accessed on 23rd July 2025).

26. Zamiri, M. (2010). *Towards a Comprehensive Resource for Elucidating the Pathogenesis of Inherited Keratodermas.* https://core.ac.uk/download/429730145.pdf (accessed on 23rd July 2025).

PEDIATRIC DERMATOLOGY: COMMON CHILDHOOD SKIN CONDITIONS

11

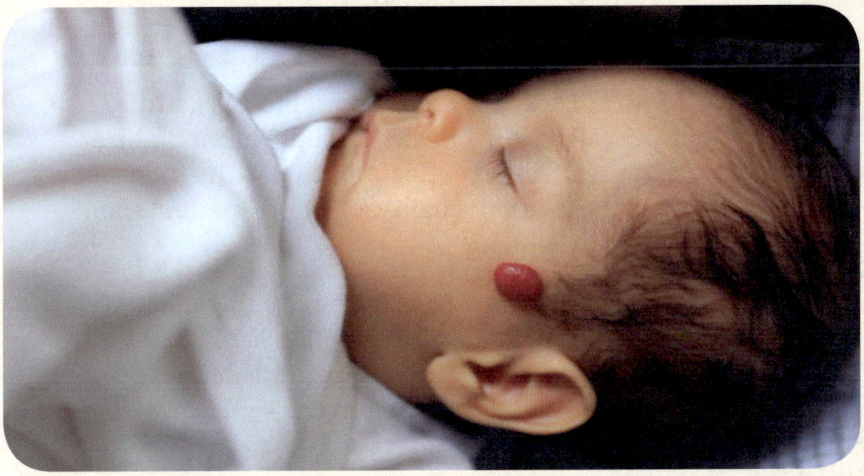

LEARNING OBJECTIVES

After studying this chapter, you will be able to:

1. Understand Eczema;
2. Explain Acne in Adolescents;
3. Describe Psoriasis in Children;
4. Focus on Infectious Skin Conditions.

Introduction

It is important to understand pediatric dermatology because it deals with a variety of skin issues that are frequently seen in children, which may have a considerable influence on their health and lifestyle. Skin illnesses in children are not only common but also of various forms, including benign ones like eczema and acne and infections like fungal infections and other complicated disorders. A study conducted in a pediatric dermatological clinic highlighted that acne, eczema, and naevi were the most frequently observed conditions among children, which justifies the clinical significance of these conditions among pediatric patients (Sciberras & Boffa, 2013). As dermatological conditions are more likely to be associated with psychological distress and social problems, it is necessary to understand the correlation between dermatology and other medical conditions. Conditions such as obsessive-compulsive disorder are bound to complicate skin disorders by way of compulsive rituals, highlighting the need for a multidisciplinary treatment approach (Tampa et al., 2015). Pediatric dermatoses are thus not merely a matter of cosmetics but an essential branch of general pediatrics.

11.1. Eczema (Atopic Dermatitis)

Learning Outcome

1. Understand Definition and Types of Eczema;
2. Explain Symptoms and Signs of Eczema;
3. Focus on Common Triggers for Eczema Flare-ups;
4. Describe Diagnosis Methods for Eczema;
5. Learn Treatment Options for Eczema;
6. Discuss Role of Moisturizers in Management;
7. Know Long-term Management Strategies;
8. Understand Psychological Impact of Eczema on Children;
9. Explain Parental Education and Support Resources.

Eczema, or atopic dermatitis, is a frequent chronic skin condition in children that significantly affects not only the skin but also the overall well-being and quality of life of patients and their families. Characterized by islands of dryness and itching, the condition usually presents in childhood and is concomitant with other atopic illnesses such as asthma and allergies, presenting a vexing challenge for pediatricians and dermatologists. Despite immunotherapy's efficacy in the treatment of pediatric asthma and allergic rhinitis, it is inconclusive with respect to eczema due to differing research outcomes; in fact, allergen avoidance treatment has been found to be poorly effective in eczema treatment (Ginsberg & Eichenfield, 2016). In one clinic-based study of a dermatology clinic, eczema was one of the most common skin conditions, and this underscores the need for special management programs and adequate referrals by general practitioners, who referred a high percentage of patients (Sciberras & Boffa, 2013). Hence, awareness and management of atopic dermatitis are crucial for improving pediatric dermatological care (Figure 11.1).

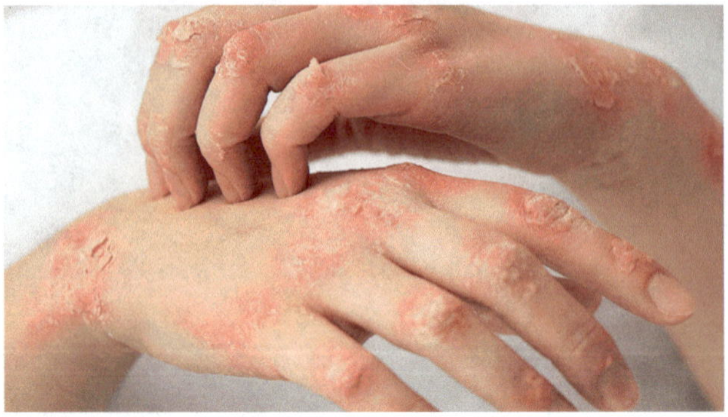

Figure 11.1. Eczema, or atopic dermatitis, is a prevalent chronic skin condition in children that significantly affects not only the skin but also the overall quality of life of patients and their families.

Source: https://www.apexhospitals.com/_next/image?url=https%3A%2F%2Fbed.apexhospitals.com%2Fuploads%2Fatopic_dermatitis_63017e8fbb.png&w=1920&q=75.

11.1.1. Definition and Types of Eczema

Dermatitis, or eczema, is a heterogeneous group of inflammatory cutaneous disorders that are associated with scaling, redness, and itching. The most common form, atopic dermatitis, is frequently linked with allergies and asthma and tends to occur in young children, so its treatment is essential during early childhood development. Contact dermatitis, another frequent eczema type, develops from exposure of the skin to irritants or allergens, causing local inflammation. Seborrheic dermatitis tends to occur as oily scales on the scalp and is also very common in infants, who are usually described as having cradle cap. Lastly, dyshidrotic eczema presents as fluid-filled blisters on the palms and soles, contributing to significant discomfort. Each subtype of eczema requires tailored treatment strategies, highlighting the need for an informed approach to pediatric dermatological care. Good counseling and education can play important roles in boosting these therapies' adherence as directed for these disorders, highlighting the important role of healthcare providers in controlling eczema (Burden-Teh et al., 2016; Giua et al., 2021).

11.1.2. Symptoms and Signs of Eczema

Eczema, or atopic dermatitis, presents with a range of symptoms and signs that can have a significant impact on a child's quality of life. Classical presentations are intense pruritus, frequently leading to scratching and irritation of the skin inflammation.

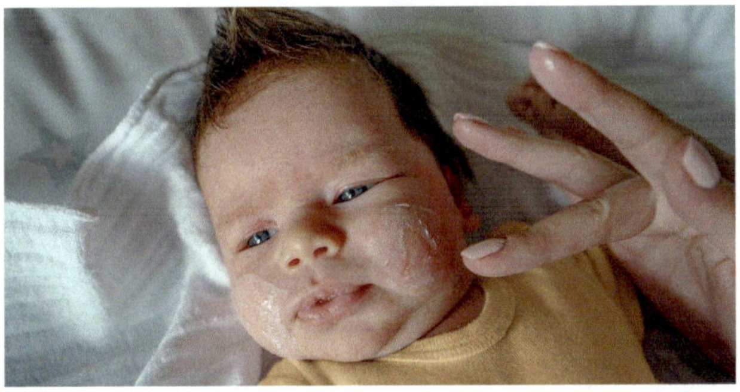

Figure 11.2. In infants, eczema frequently appears on the face and scalp, while older children may develop lesions in the creases of the elbows and knees, a pattern that reflects the evolving nature of the condition.

Source: https://media.post.rvohealth.io/wp-content/uploads/2021/12/eczema-newborn-baby-face-facebook-1200x628.jpg.

In clinical practice, affected areas typically present as reddened, inflamed areas of skin, which later may become scaly and dry. In infants, eczema tends to occur on the face and scalp, while in older children, the lesions in the elbow and knee folds are a frequent evolution, which reflects the evolving nature of the disease. The emotional distress of eczema has been identified to play a role in increasing symptom severity, which emphasizes the complexity of the condition's pediatric patient impact (Burden-Teh et al., 2016). Effective management relies on an integrative approach that fulfills both bodily symptom and emotional status needs, alongside personalized treatment as suggested by the Taiwanese Dermatological Association (Chen et al., 2015) (Figure 11.2).

11.1.3. Common Triggers for Eczema Flare-ups

Eczema, or atopic dermatitis, is susceptible to sudden flare-ups as a result of many extrinsic and intrinsic stimuli. Environmental precipitants commonly found are allergens such as dust mites, pet dander, and pollen that strongly exacerbate the condition, especially in children with a congenital sensitivity. Irritants such as soaps, detergents, and certain fabric types also are capable of triggering skin reactions, leading to extensive itching and inflammation. Climate factors, high and low temperatures, and humidity are also responsible for precipitating flare-ups. Stress has also been identified as a significant factor because psychological distress may worsen symptoms and severity of eczema, which has been indicative of the multifactorial nature of the disease (Burden-Teh et al., 2016). Management of these stimuli is essential to minimize flare-ups as observed in interventions like using individualized written Allergy Action Plans (EAP) that provide caregivers with improved control over their child's eczema (Sena, 2019). Awareness of these triggers ultimately aids in developing effective management plans for children.

11.1.4. Diagnosis Methods for Eczema

Diagnosis of eczema in pediatric patients is a multifaceted process that begins with a general clinical evaluation of the patient's history and physical skin examination. Because eczema may present differently, the dermatologist will need to assess some features, such as pruritus, xerosis, and lesional distribution. Diagnosis typically follows established criteria such as the Investigators Static Global Assessment, which provides classification of the severity of atopic dermatitis (AD) in children. In certain cases, diagnostic methods may involve patch testing for the detection of allergens or skin biopsies to rule out other skin conditions. The combination of therapy regimens, such as crisaborole ointment in mild to moderate AD, was demonstrated to have a significant impact on quality of life among affected individuals and families, emphasizing the importance of precise diagnosis and robust management guidelines within pediatric dermatology (Sciberras & Boffa, 2013; Simpson et al., 2018) (Figure 11.3).

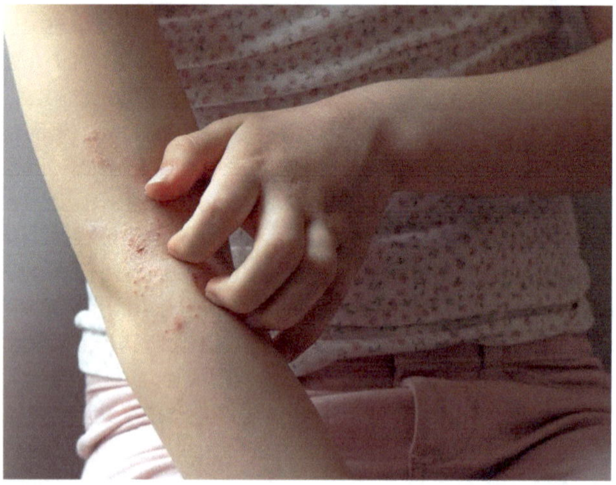

Figure 11.3. Given that eczema can present in varying forms, the dermatologist must assess specific symptoms such as pruritus, xerosis, and the characteristic distribution of lesions.

Source: https://epidermatology.com.sg/wp-content/uploads/2023/06/epi-eczema-children-scaled.jpg.

11.1.5. Treatment Options for Eczema

Eczema, particularly atopic eczema (AE), is a significant issue in pediatric dermatology that needs effective management measures. There are a number of treatment options available, ranging from topical therapies such as corticosteroids and calcineurin inhibitors to systemic drugs such as azathioprine and ciclosporin, proven to be of sufficient efficacy in symptom management and quality of life in affected children (Nankervis et al., 2016). Notwithstanding the multitude of treatment modalities, there are still considerable gaps in the evidence that underpins many common interventions, hence the need for constant research and trials in the clinical setting. Further, new findings on the safety and long-term efficacy of phototherapy raise the necessity to establish standardized treatment protocols to improve outcomes among patients (Vermeulen et al., 2019). This ongoing quest for efficient treatments underscores the evolving art of eczema management, particularly where children as patients will respond differently to treatment. Addressing these differences is critical in providing the best treatment to children suffering from this condition.

11.1.6. Role of Moisturizers in Management

Moisturizers play a critical role in the management of the majority of prevalent skin diseases of childhood, particularly in the relief of atopic dermatitis and eczema symptoms. These humectants work to restore and maintain the skin's natural barrier, lost in involved children and leading to increased transepidermal water loss and irritant permeability. Management with successful treatment using skin-directed therapy is accomplished through frequent use of moisturizers to alleviate dryness, reduce inflammation, and prevent flares of dermatitis. Recent research highlights the importance of individual moisturizer selection, acknowledging the skin type of each child and the allergen content of some moisturizers (Jones, 2024). Also, as therapeutic interventions improve, caregivers and physicians must bring to the fore the pivotal role of moisturization as a preventive intervention against the occurrence of flares in skin conditions like atopic dermatitis, which severely impacts the quality of life of children with the condition (Alqahtani et al., 2023) (Figure 11.4).

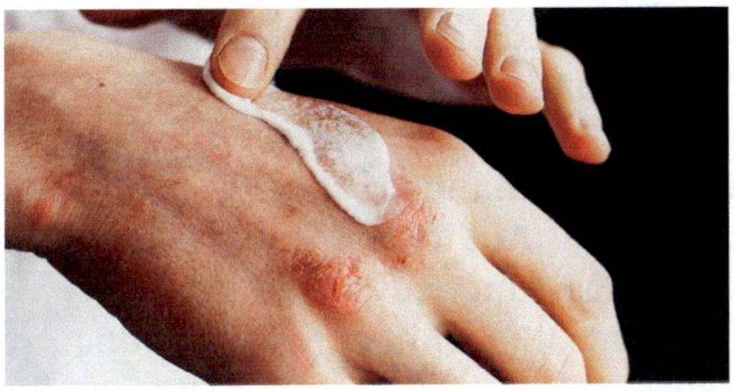

Figure 11.4. Moisturizers play a critical role in the management of common childhood skin conditions, particularly in mitigating symptoms associated with atopic dermatitis and eczema.

Source: https://allergyasthmanetwork.org/wp-content/uploads/2024/10/Eczema-on-hands-1080x567.jpg.

11.1.7. Long-term Management Strategies

Long-term management of children's dermatological conditions involves a holistic approach merging existing dermatology and effective complementary therapy. Chronic illnesses such as eczema, psoriasis, and acne require constant monitoring and personalized treatment strategies to avoid flare-ups and enhance the quality of life in the child. Integrating concepts of Ayurveda, for instance, offers holistic strategies that address fundamental imbalances in the body, as emphasized in the latest literature (Dr. Mohod & Thakare , 2025). Such approaches include the use of herbal remedies like Neem and dietary modification, which play a significant role in skin wellness. In addition, emphasizing lifestyle modifications in the way of stress management by yoga and meditation can provide a complementary advantage in managing skin ailments. Meanwhile, routine dermatological assessment is essential to make treatment protocols so that these remain effective over time without risking potential complications occurring due to prolonged-duration therapy (Suliman et al., 2025). In this way, an integrative strategy permits sustained relief and overall well-being in children with chronic dermatological issues.

11.1.8. Psychological Impact of Eczema on Children

The psychological consequences of eczema, particularly atopic dermatitis, on children are intense and extensive.

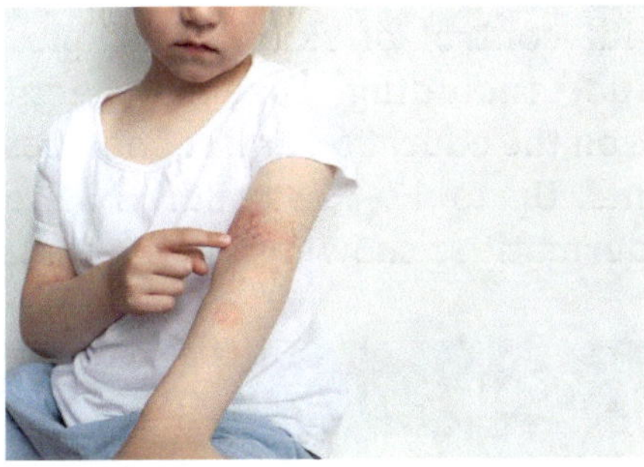

Figure 11.5. Children with severe atopic dermatitis often experience significant psychological distress, which can exacerbate their symptoms and lead to a vicious cycle of worsening skin issues and emotional turmoil.

Source: https://www.news-medical.net/images/news/ImageForNews_756715_16926112514824073.jpg.

A disease of chronic skin consisting of inflammation and intense itching, eczema affects not just physical but also emotional and social well-being. Severely ill children with atopic dermatitis most often experience severe psychological distress, which aggravates their condition and is responsible for the formation of a vicious circle of worsening skin conditions and emotional problems (Burden-Teh et al., 2016). Also, the implications of this disease can extend into adulthood, when people who had severe eczema as children generally report delayed social development and impaired quality of life in subsequent periods of their lives (Brenninkmeijer et al., 2009). This psychological burden emphasizes the importance of comprehensive treatment practices involving not just physical symptoms but also the emotional health of affected children, promoting resilience and coping as key elements of pediatric dermatologic care (Figure 11.5).

11.1.9. Parental Education and Support Resources

Successful control of skin conditions during childhood, including eczema, particularly depends on the education and support resources of parents. Up to 13% of children suffer from atopic dermatitis, showing the importance of caregivers having a complete understanding and competency in the management of this condition (Sena, 2019). Written Eczema Action Plan (EAP) implementation can also empower parents, boosting their self-efficacy and providing structured guidance to treatment protocols. Evidence confirms that these types of plans have a dramatic improvement in eczema severity as well as enhanced caregiver confidence (Sena, 2019). Additionally, the integration of psychological and educational interventions can potentially enhance compliance with conventional therapies, resulting in better outcomes for children. By offering parents tailored resources and actionable strategies, healthcare professionals are able to bridge the communication gap and ensure families feel supported, ultimately optimizing management and satisfaction in pediatric dermatology.

Test Your Knowledge

1. What are common triggers or exacerbating factors in eczema?
2. What is the role of filaggrin gene mutations in the pathogenesis of eczema?

11.2. Acne in Adolescents

Learning Outcome

1. Understand Definition and Types of Acne;
2. Explain Causes of Acne in Adolescents;
3. Focus on Symptoms and Severity Classification;
4. Describe Diagnosis and Assessment of Acne;
5. Learn Treatment Options for Acne;
6. Discuss the Importance of Skincare Routines;
7. Know Psychological Effects of Acne on Teenagers;
8. Understand Myths and Misconceptions About Acne;
9. Explain the Role of Diet and Lifestyle in Acne Management.

Acne in teens is one of the most frequent skin illnesses encountered in pediatric dermatology and has significant effects on both physical self-perception and psychological adjustment. Adolescence is preceded by endocrine changes that trigger sebaceous gland activity and result in increased production of oil, which in turn leads to occlusion of the hair follicles. This pathophysiology not only favors acne-causing bacteria but also triggers inflammatory responses, manifesting as papules, pustules, and sometimes cystic lesions. Epidemiological studies indicate that acne affects as many as 85% of teenagers, with a high prevalence in males due to their greater sebum output (Ayanlowo et al., 2018). Apart from its corporeal expressions, acne may also cause emotional suffering, anxiety, and depression, necessitating multilateral management interventions that involve dermatological treatment together with counseling (Tampa et al., 2015). Thus, therapy for acne in teens is crucial for maintaining overall health and wellness in this high-risk group of individuals (Figure 11.6).

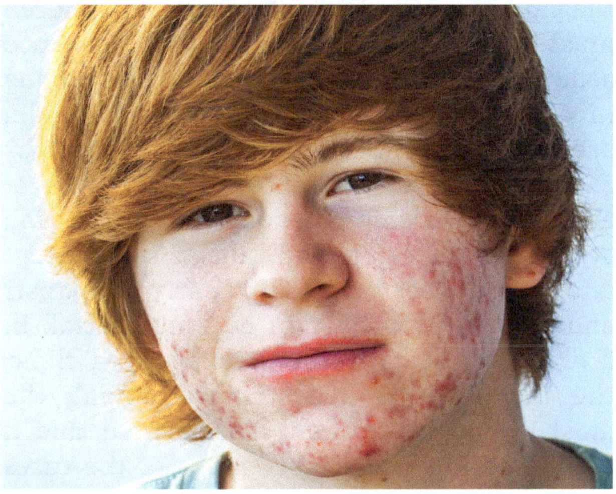

Figure 11.6. Acne in adolescents represents one of the most prevalent skin conditions encountered in pediatric dermatology, significantly impacting both physical appearance and psychological well-being.

Source: https://d148x66490prkv.cloudfront.net/c360/imported/transfer/Screen%20Shot%202014-04-04%20at%2011.46.14%20AM.png?VersionId=x.JP0XrRSHqHghFIfSo7p6nOepczL79j.

11.2.1. Definition and Types of Acne

Acne is a chronic inflammatory dermatosis by the occurrence of comedones, pustules, and nodules, predominantly in teenagers but also found in children. It results from a combination of various factors, including overactive sebaceous glands, hormonal disturbances, and proliferation of *Cutibacterium acnes*, an otherwise normal skin-dwelling bacterium. The types of acne can be collectively divided into non-inflammatory and inflammatory types. Non-inflammatory acne comprises open and closed comedones, also known as blackheads and whiteheads, respectively. Inflammatory acne, however, includes papules, pustules, and cystic lesions, which, if not treated, lead to scarring. The psychosocial impact of acne among adolescents and children is significant, tending to affect quality of life as well as self-esteem. Thus, proper identification and management of all forms of acne are crucial in pediatric dermatology to avoid potential long-term physical and psychological consequences (Burden-Teh et al., 2016; Chukwu & Mankila, 2018).

11.2.2. Causes of Acne in Adolescents

Adolescence is a foundational development period for the formation of acne, primarily due to the hormonal changes that occur during puberty.

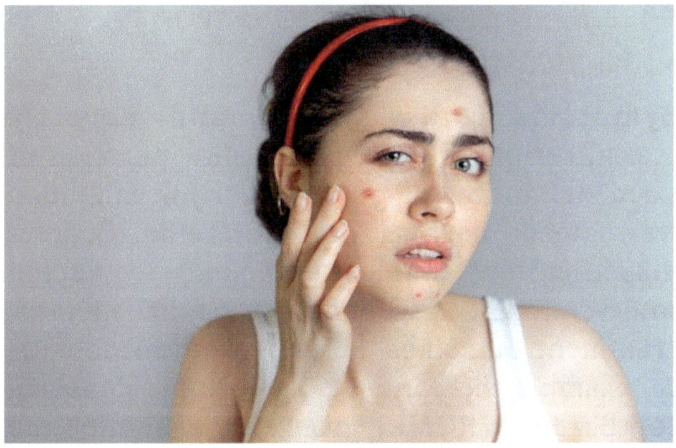

Figure 11.7. Adolescence is a critical period for the onset of acne, primarily due to the hormonal changes that occur during puberty.

Source: https://ssbhealthcare.com/wp-content/uploads/2023/06/portrait-young-woman-examines-her-face-with-pimples_1200x800.jpg.

Greater androgen release leads to heightened sebaceous gland function, resulting in an overproduction of sebum, one of the leading causes of acne formation. The effect of excess oil on skin cells can cause pores to become enlarged, paving the way for bacteria to multiply, providing a perfect environment for *Propionibacterium acnes*, the acne-causing bacteria, to grow.

Environmental factors such as poor hygiene, food influences, and stress also trigger the condition. Studies have established that in certain populations, adolescent acne prevalence is common and constitutes approximately 11.8% of dermatological conditions, emphasizing the importance of the condition in child dermatology (Oninla et al., 2016). Furthermore, socioeconomic status may also have a role to play in sustaining healthy skin, and studies have demonstrated poor living conditions and low hygiene practices to be related to a higher rate of dermatological conditions, including acne (Polat et al., 2018). There is a need to understand these intricate causes to be able to treat and manage them effectively (Figure 11.7).

11.2.3. Symptoms and Severity Classification

Symptomatic assessment and severity classification are integral to the practice of paediatric dermatology, particularly in childhood dermatoses such as atopic eczema. Correct classification enables clinicians to design interventions in a more effective way and monitor treatment outcomes. Emergent advancements, for example, the Harmonising Outcome Measures for Eczema (HOME) programme, signify the need to harmonize measuring instruments to improve comparability across studies and practices. Through the application of these harmonised approaches, clinicians are able to quantify severity in terms of objective measures, thereby refining the evaluation of efficacy and safety of treatment. Besides, the establishment of an essential dataset for the TREatment of ATopic eczema (TREAT) Registry allows not just national but international collaboration in evaluating treatment strategies to atopic eczema, given the heterogeneity of findings across different populations (Bousquet et al., 2016; Vermeulen et al., 2019). Such a systematic approach eventually enhances clinical practice and enhances research activities in pediatric dermatology.

11.2.4. Diagnosis and Assessment of Acne

Diagnosis and assessment of acne in children must be achieved with sensitivity because acne is a frequent disorder, usually beginning in adolescence. History and physical exam are generally followed by the clinician as an initial step to assess severity and type of acne lesions, from comedones to papules and cysts. As acne significantly affects self-concept and emotional well-being, early diagnosis and correct classification become crucial. In a review of pediatric dermatology in a clinic, the incidence of acne ranked among the most frequent conditions documented, and it accounted for a high percentage of the cases presented, particularly among males (Sciberras & Boffa, 2013). Furthermore, epidemiological studies reveal that acneiform eruptions are found to manifest among teenagers, and this emphasizes the importance of specialty management strategies (Ayanlowo et al., 2018). By prioritizing early diagnosis and personalized treatment, medical professionals can optimize the physical and psychological needs of afflicted children and adolescents (Figure 11.8).

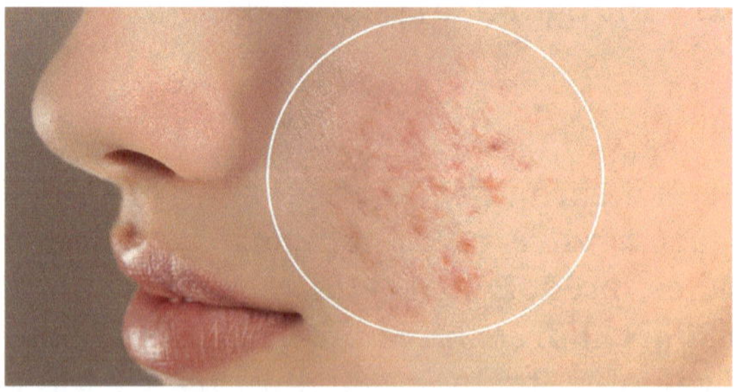

Figure 11.8. Clinicians typically begin with a thorough history and physical examination, assessing the type and severity of acne lesions, which range from comedones to inflammatory papules and cysts.

Source: https://www.apexhospitals.com/_next/image?url=https%3A%2F%2Fbed.apexhospitals.com%2Fuploads%2Facne2_83f52b7980.jpg&w=1920&q=75.

11.2.5. Treatment Options for Acne

Acne, which is one of the most frequent skin conditions in the child and adolescent population, primarily occurs in young children and teenagers and needs timely treatment options according to age-specific needs. For neonatal and infantile acne, superficial topical treatments in the form of benzoyl peroxide or topical antibiotics may be enough. Mid-childhood and prepubertal acne, however, may necessitate more intensive treatments in the form of retinoids or oral antibiotics, depending on severity. It is worth noting that the early treatment is able to prevent long-term scarring and psychological impact, thus emphasizing the importance of proper diagnosis and treatment approaches (Gencler et al., 2017). Moreover, there exists a synergy between dermatological and mental health because if the acne remains untreated, it can result in depression and anxiety in the affected children. Thus, the integration of mental health evaluation along with dermatological treatments continues to be core to the delivery of comprehensive care in pediatric dermatology clinics (Kraft, 2024). Practitioners are able to enhance the quality of life of children with this condition with a holistic approach.

11.2.6. Importance of Skincare Routines

Skincare regimens continue to be core to the treatment of the majority of childhood skin conditions and emphasize the need for preventive interventions in pediatric dermatology. Good skin care not only cures short-term symptoms of skin disease but also has a significant role in ensuring long-term skin health and quality of life. For instance, in the management of atopic dermatitis (AD), a chronic regimen with anti-inflammatory agents is key to achieving clear skin and preventing flare-ups, as highlighted by the consensus guidelines of Boguniewicz et al. (2024). Moreover, conditions like epidermolytic ichthyosis (EI) underline the great role of skincare habits, where inadequate care leads to unnecessary discomfort and compromised quality of life in children, as research assessing the burden of EI disease suggests (Frommherz et al., 2025). Thus, it is crucial to introduce individualized skincare regimens for maximizing skin health, enhancing comfort, and enhancing treatment compliance in caregivers and patients (Figure 11.9).

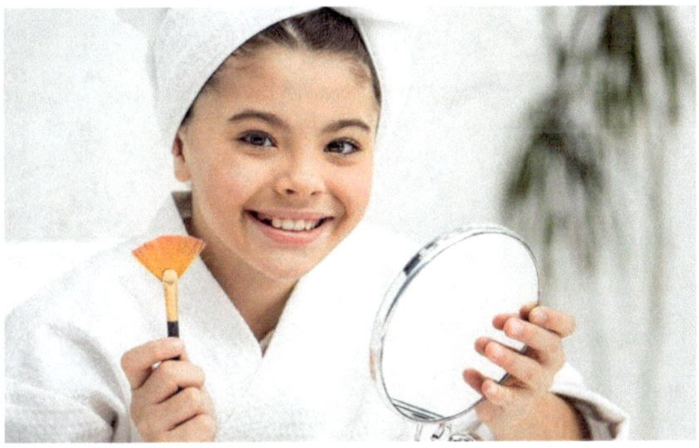

Figure 11.9. Skincare routines play a pivotal role in managing various childhood skin conditions, emphasizing the necessity for proactive measures in pediatric dermatology.

Source: https://images.onlymyhealth.com/imported/images/2024/March/15_Mar_2024/1.jpg.

11.2.7. Psychological Effects of Acne on Teenagers

Acne is a widespread skin condition in adolescents that profoundly impacts psychological well-being, in most instances encouraging high levels of concern, depression, and social withdrawal. The appearance of acne can lead to negative self-esteem and affect peer relationships, and so perpetuate feelings of loneliness and low self-esteem. Research has indicated that adolescents with skin conditions, such as acne, experience a measurable decrease in quality of life (QoL) when using the T-QoL tool developed to measure how these conditions affect adolescents emotionally and socially (Basra et al., 2018). In addition, pediatric primary care providers

(PCPs) may be challenged in the management of acne, which can delay effective treatment and compound psychological distress due to the long-term uncertainty of treatment efficacy (Char, 2024). Thus, addressing the psychological effect of acne, as well as medical treatment, is crucial in preserving the overall health of affected teenagers.

11.2.8. Myths and Misconceptions About Acne

The common myths and misconceptions surrounding acne can significantly influence the emotional health of afflicted children and their families.

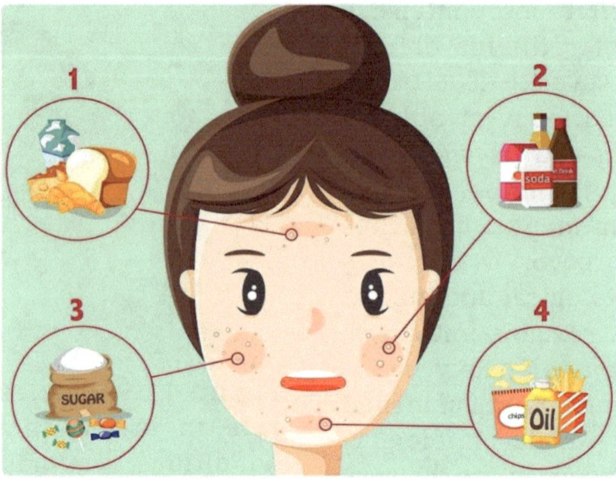

Figure 11.10. Many individuals associate the severity of acne with dietary choices, particularly the consumption of chocolate or greasy foods, although current research indicates that such dietary factors may have minimal influence on acne development.

Source: https://www.news-medical.net/image-handler/picture/2019/10/By_Wanwisspaul.jpg.

One of the most common falsehoods is the belief that acne is caused significantly by unclean skin, which can lead to over-washing and inflammation of the skin and further exacerbate the condition. Also, the majority of people attribute the intensity of acne to diet, that is, consumption of chocolate or greasy food, though contemporary research establishes that these types of dietary factors most likely will exert minimal effect on the formation of acne. The psychological influence of these myths is great; children suffering from acne will feel embarrassed or develop low self-esteem, which will adversely affect their quality of life and social relationships. Besides, the need for appropriate psychological care is also brought to light since misconceptions can prevent individuals from receiving appropriate treatment (Hughes, 2025). Hence, debunking these myths is relevant in creating awareness and acceptance of acne as a normative skin condition (Figure 11.10).

11.2.9. Role of Diet and Lifestyle in Acne Management

Recent research increasingly indicates the very significant role that diet and lifestyle play in the management of acne, particularly among children. A diet high in glycemic index, like sugars and refined carbohydrates, has been shown to exacerbate acne by increasing insulin resistance and increasing sebum production. Consumption of dairy has also been linked to higher rates of acne, which suggests that some dietary options may determine the health of the skin. Lifestyle, including stress and sleep, can also cause worsening of acne by disturbing hormonal balances as well as inflammatory responses. Though pediatric dermatologists aim to address these common skin ailments that afflict children, treatment protocols must incorporate patient education regarding healthy eating habits and lifestyle modification. Interdisciplinary modalities that address both the medical and lifestyle aspects of treatment can contribute to making the patient an active partner in managing their disease, which ultimately contributes to better compliance with treatment and ideal outcomes in the management of acne (Kandhari et al., 2022; Chukwu & Mankila, 2018).

Test Your Knowledge

1. What hormonal changes contribute to adolescent acne?
2. What is the difference between inflammatory and non-inflammatory acne?

11.3. Psoriasis in Children

Learning Outcome

1. Understand Definition and Types of Psoriasis;
2. Explain Symptoms and Clinical Presentation;
3. Focus on Causes and Risk Factors for Psoriasis;
4. Describe Diagnosis and Differential Diagnosis;
5. Learn Treatment Options for Pediatric Psoriasis;
6. Discuss Importance of Early Intervention;
7. Know Impact of Psoriasis on Children's Social Life;
8. Understand Long-term Management and Follow-up Care;
9. Explain Support Groups and Resources for Families.

Psoriasis in children is a significant childhood dermatologic condition with a characteristic abnormal skin cell proliferation, producing inflammatory lesions of varying severity. With their usual symptom of red scaling patches, this autoimmune condition has the possibility to have a significant impact on a child's quality of life, physical and emotional. A pediatric dermatology clinic clinical survey determined that psoriasis was among the most frequent conditions encountered, confirming its clinical significance (Sciberras & Boffa, 2013). Treatment approaches generally aim at topical therapy; conversely, a fixed formulation of calcipotriene plus betamethasone dipropionate has been found to be effective in adolescents, with resolution in a majority of patients without impacting safety (Eichenfield et al., 2015). Treatment for children with psoriasis requires individualized management of the physical and psychosocial consequences of the disease, with an integrated care model that addresses the individual.

11.3.1. Definition and Types of Psoriasis

Psoriasis is a chronic inflammatory disease that is mediated by the immune system and is characterized by the rapid growth of skin cells, where scaly, thick plaques develop on the surface of the skin. In children and adolescents, psoriasis can take many forms, the most frequent of which is plaque psoriasis. It usually begins on the scalp, limbs, and trunk with noteworthy incidence among schoolchildren and adolescents. Another significant characteristic of psoriasis in children is its association with heredity, in the sense that nearly half of the children who have the condition have an affected first-degree relative. Knowledge regarding the various psoriasis types, including guttate, inverse, and pustular forms, is crucial for correct diagnosis and management in children since chronicity of the condition can have a very adverse impact on physical as well as psychosocial well-being. Thus, continued research into childhood psoriasis remains essential for providing improved long-term health care and clinical practice (Burden-Teh et al., 2016; Burden-Teh, 2020) (Figure 11.11).

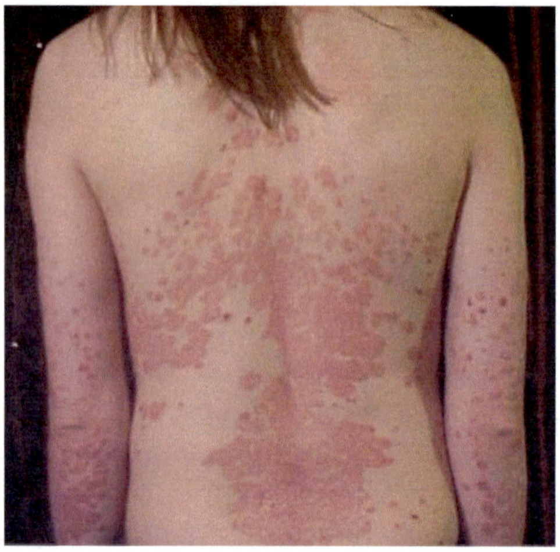

Figure 11.11. Psoriasis is an immune-mediated chronic inflammatory condition characterized by the rapid proliferation of skin cells, leading to the formation of thick, scaly plaques on the skin's surface.

Source: https://upload.wikimedia.org/wikipedia/commons/f/f5/Psoriasis_on_back1.jpg.

11.3.2. Symptoms and Clinical Presentation

The clinical presentation of cutaneous diseases in children is highly varied, reflecting the wide variety of underlying etiologies and the unique physiology of children's skin. Symptoms are highly variable and may range from benign rashes to severe states necessitating immediate treatment. For instance, the coexistence of a purpuric rash and systemic symptoms may be an indicator of underlying conditions like cardiac myxomas, in cases where presentations thereof have led to severe consequences when not properly diagnosed (Macias et al., 2018). Additionally, psoriasis also occurs predominantly in the form of plaque lesions, in locations like the scalp, limbs, and trunk, with typical high prevalence among girls and older children (Burden-Teh et al., 2016). Knowing these symptoms and their implications for treatment is important for prompt diagnosis and proper management. Therefore, knowing the heterogeneity of skin diseases among children is an integral part of pediatric dermatology that ensures improved outcomes for affected children.

11.3.3. Causes and Risk Factors for Psoriasis

Psoriasis, a chronic inflammatory skin disease, has etiologies and risk factors that are multifactorial and specifically impact children. Genetic susceptibility is also a significant factor, whereby studies have indicated that nearly 48.8% of affected children have a family history of psoriasis, which indicates strong hereditary influence (Burden-Teh et al., 2016). Additionally, environmental stimuli such as infections, stress, and skin injuries can provoke or exacerbate the condition in genetically susceptible individuals. The changing comprehension of the cutaneous microbiome has also brought into focus its possible impact on psoriasis, where it is postulated that dysbiosis of microbial communities can influence the immune system and exacerbate disease severity (Paller et al., 2019). It is crucial to continue studying, where it is important to recognize other risk factors in order to improve early diagnosis and intervention tactics in children, leading to better management outcomes for this chronic skin disease. Understanding these complex interactions is essential while designing targeted therapeutic strategies in pediatric dermatology (Figure 11.12).

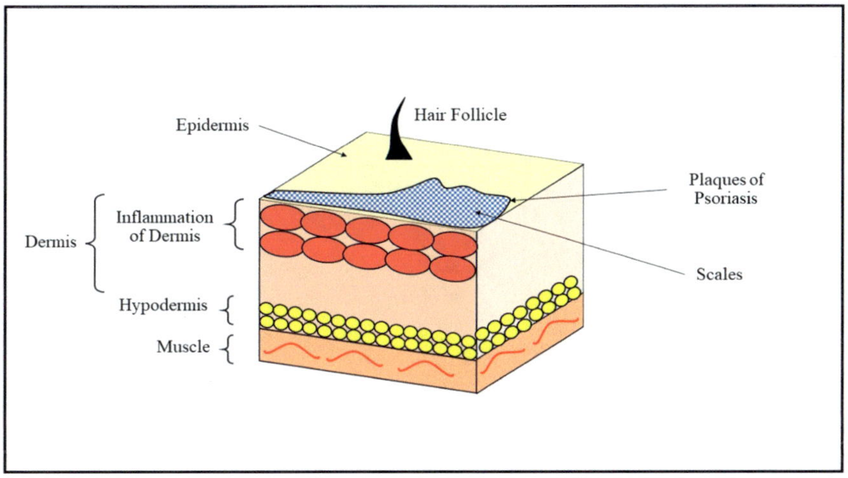

Figure 11.12. Genetic predisposition plays a significant role, with studies revealing that nearly 48.8% of affected children have a family history of psoriasis, indicating a strong hereditary component.

Source: https://pub.mdpi-res.com/biomedicines/biomedicines-11-01589/article_deploy/html/images/biomedicines-11-01589-g001.png?1685450315.

11.3.4. Diagnosis and Differential Diagnosis

The diagnosis and differential diagnosis in children's dermatology are significant due to the enormous number of skin conditions that occur in the pediatric population. Diagnosis often rests on the characteristic appearance of various rashes and lesions, which may provide significant clues to underlying systemic disease. For instance, a purpuric rash with constitutional symptoms will lead clinicians to consider cardiac myxomas since such rare tumors will behave differently in the child population. Delayed diagnosis of such conditions will result in significant morbidity, highlighting why they need to be put in the differential diagnosis early (Macias et al., 2018). In addition, illnesses like photosensitivity can be an indicator of serious systemic diseases, such as lupus erythematosus or rare genetic diseases, and thus need to be assessed properly to prevent sun-related problems (Sjerobabski-Masnec et al., 2010). Differential diagnosis should be done carefully for the treatment of cutaneous and systemic effects.

11.3.5. Treatment Options for Pediatric Psoriasis

Effective management of children with psoriasis needs an integrative understanding of the treatment modalities appropriate to the varying needs of children. Topical treatments, such as corticosteroids and vitamin D analogues, are typically the initial treatment, providing localized action and reducing inflammation with minimal systemic toxicity. However, in severe to moderate psoriasis, systemic management, including methotrexate and biologics, is justified even in children despite their side effects. Phototherapy is a promising option, as it is highly effective for treating childhood psoriasis. Evidence suggests that phototherapy has been proven to produce promising outcomes, with approximately 81.8% of patients suffering from psoriasis showing improvement after therapy sessions, indicating the effectiveness of the technique in symptom amelioration without posing systemic toxicity (Brasileiro et al., 2013). Moreover, data standardization concerning such therapies is also expected to enhance pediatric dermatology comparative effectiveness research, thus resulting in better treatment strategies for the vulnerable population (Vermeulen et al., 2019) (Figure 11.13).

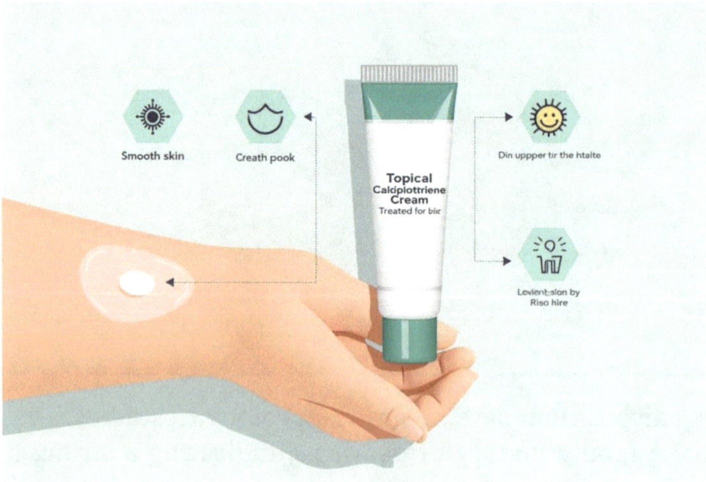

Figure 11.13. Topical therapies, such as corticosteroids and vitamin D analogs, are often the first line of treatment, providing localized relief and reducing inflammation with minimal systemic effects.

Source: https://www.kaya.in/media/mageplaza/blog/post/t/o/topical-calcipotriene.jpg.

11.3.6. Importance of Early Intervention

Early treatment of dermatological conditions in children is vital to optimize therapeutic outcomes and avoid long-term complications. Early intervention not only abates symptoms temporarily but also addresses possible psychosocial impacts associated with visible skin diseases, such as atopic eczema and psoriasis, which can have an impact on the self-perception and relationships of a child. What is evident is that children with these conditions can be significantly enhanced by early and effective management, as indicated in the elevated rate of childhood psoriasis related to familial history, suggesting the utilization of proactive interventions in susceptible groups (Burden-Teh et al., 2016). Further, while there exists considerable heterogeneity of treatment effectiveness for atopic eczema, early intervention pathways can have a positive outcome in the quality of life as reported by evidence with credible benefits from different treatment approaches (Nankervis et al., 2016). Thus, integrating early treatment and diagnosis interventions is required in pediatric dermatology to foster healthier prospects.

11.3.7. Impact of Psoriasis on Children's Social Life

The influence of psoriasis on the social life of children is profound and multifaceted, and typically casts insurmountable emotional and psychological challenges. Patients with psoriasis may develop feelings of embarrassment and isolation due to the outward lesions of the disease. This stigma might deter them from participating in normal social activities, like sports and social interactions with people of their own age group, and may even affect their self-esteem and academic performance. The unpredictable and chronic character of this inflammatory dermatosis further exacerbates these issues, as these breakouts can erupt unexpectedly and thus further increase anxiety in self-presentation in social contexts (Ujiie et al., 2022). Furthermore, inasmuch as treatment modalities have shown promising advancements, the question of accessible dermatologic care is key, particularly in its help toward children's integration into social environments as well as to their quality of life (Marasca et al., 2022). Management of the psychosocial effect of psoriasis is therefore a high priority in pediatric dermatology (Figure 11.14).

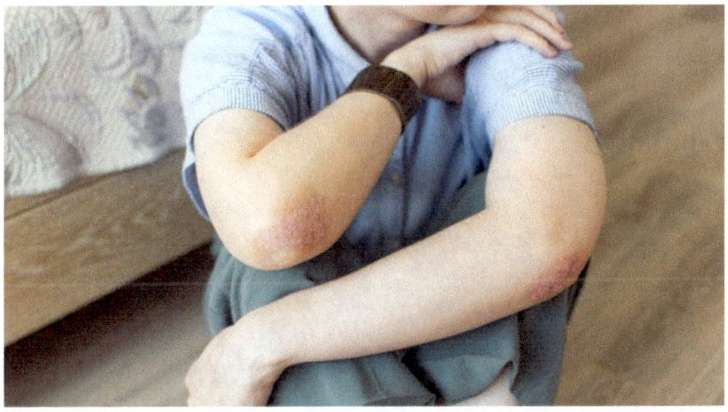

Figure 11.14. Children with psoriasis may experience feelings of embarrassment and social isolation due to the visible lesions associated with the condition.

Source: https://images.onlymyhealth.com/imported/images/2024/January/30_Jan_2024/psoriasis.jpg.

11.3.8. Long-term Management and Follow-up Care

Effective long-term management and follow-up care are essential in the management of pediatric skin conditions because they have the potential to be chronic and recurrent. For instance, after a severe asthma attack requiring intensive care, patients have a greater risk of recurrence and need ongoing follow-up for treatment improvement in accordance with the Global Initiative for Asthma guidelines, which has been statistically significant for those whose treatment adjustments were performed post-discharge (Selmanoğlu et al., 2025). Similarly, juvenile localized scleroderma is a less frequent but clinically significant condition that requires close follow-up and most often a multidisciplinary therapeutic approach over time. The recent emphasis on consensus treatment protocols has led to increased utilization of systemic therapies with improved coordination of care and effectiveness of treatment protocol (Egeli et al., 2025). This long-term management plan is detailed and helps to minimize complications and maximize the quality of life of children with such conditions, emphasizing the importance of continuous follow-up in pediatric dermatology.

11.3.9. Support Groups and Resources for Families

The knowledge of pediatric dermatology, particularly that of common skin diseases, typically places enormous pressure on families. Support groups and resources help a great deal to relieve such pressure through useful emotional and practical support. These networks would focus on creating relationships between families facing similar problems, and in this way, their quality of life can be significantly enhanced. For instance, it has been proven that chronic illness significantly impacts family life and emotional well-being, and 92% of the surveyed demonstrated extreme emotional impact, while 91% had interference with daily living (Golics et al., 2013). On top of that, educational materials and psychological interventions have proved useful, particularly in diseases like atopic eczema, in assisting families in their adoption of effective topical treatment alongside addressing their psychological needs (Ersser et al., 2014). By providing support from the community and providing essential information, materials are able to assist families in being more in charge of their children's diseases, providing a much-needed safety net during their caregiving journey (Figure 11.15).

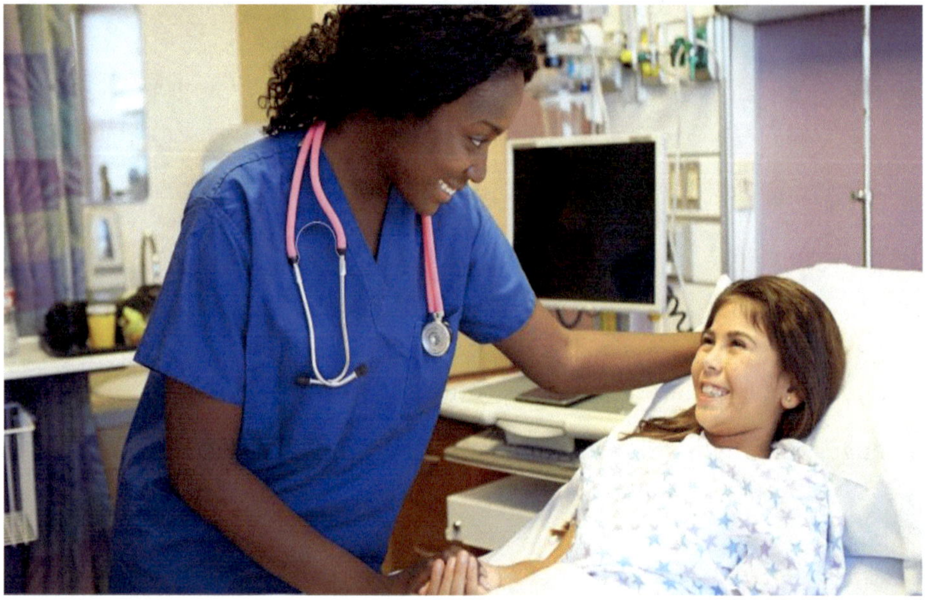

Figure 11.15. Support groups and resources play a pivotal role in alleviating this burden, providing essential emotional and practical assistance.

Source: https://theresiliencysolution.com/how-can-nurses-provide-emotional-support-for-patients/nurse-with-happy-patient.png.

Test Your Knowledge

1. How does pediatric psoriasis differ from adult-onset psoriasis?
2. What is the role of family history in childhood psoriasis?

11.4. Infectious Skin Conditions

Learning Outcome

1. Understand Overview of Common Infectious Skin Conditions;
2. Explain Impetigo: Causes, Symptoms, and Treatment;
3. Focus on Fungal Infections: Types and management;
4. Describe Viral Infections: Warts and Molluscum Contagiosum;
5. Learn Scabies: Symptoms and Treatment Options;
6. Discuss the Importance of Hygiene in Prevention;
7. Know Diagnosis Challenges in Pediatric Patients;
8. Understand Impact of Infections on School Attendance;
9. Explain Parental Guidance on Prevention and Care.

Nonsuppurative infectious skin conditions are one of the significant groups of pediatric dermatologic disorders, commonly presenting as rashes, lesions, or infections that can complicate the child's health and life. Cutaneous bacterial infections like impetigo and cellulitis arise from innocuous skin or skin condition injury with consequent serious complications if left unmanaged.

Further, viral infections like herpes simplex and varicella zoster are prevalent among children, with high morbidity and requiring careful management to prevent transmission and reduce symptoms. The interaction between psychological problems and skin conditions is prevalent, particularly that of obsessive-compulsive disorder, with the potential to cause skin disorders like eczema or dermatitis by severe washing or irritation (Tampa et al., 2015). In addition, systemic conditions such as cardiac myxomas have cutaneous manifestations, making it crucial to have an integrated approach to diagnosis and management of children who present with infectious and systemic manifestations (Macias et al., 2018).

11.4.1. Overview of Common Infectious Skin Conditions

There are a number of common infectious cutaneous diseases in pediatric dermatology, each with its unique set of problems and requiring unique management approaches. Some of the infections include impetigo, primarily due to *Staphylococcus aureus* and *Streptococcus pyogenes*, which produce highly contagious, crusted lesions that most frequently occur on and around the nose and mouth. Similarly, tinea capitis, a fungal infection of the scalp, may lead to alopecia as well as significant pain.

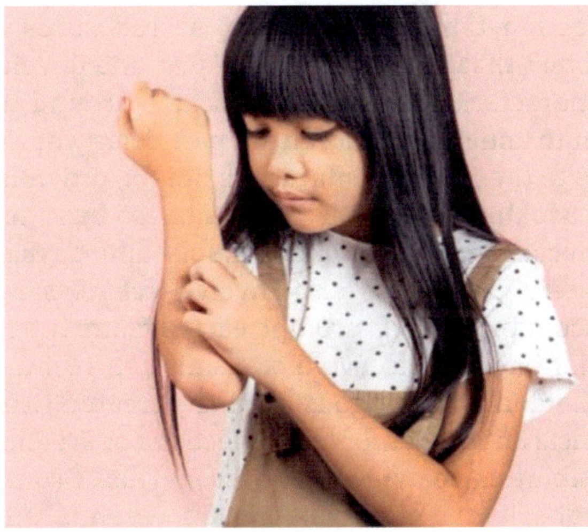

Figure 11.16. In pediatric dermatology, various infectious skin conditions are prevalent, each presenting unique challenges and requiring tailored management strategies.

Source: https://womenandchildren.avisena.com.my/wp-content/uploads/2024/06/article-skin-conditions-intro.jpg.

Additionally, viral infections such as herpes simplex and verrucae vulgaris (warts) are prevalent in children, for which treatment and watchful observation are needed to alleviate symptoms and prevent transmission. Aside from impacting the child's physical health, these also have psychosocial and emotional impacts, thus treatment becomes a holistic process. An interdisciplinary team approach among healthcare providers is required to deal with both the medical and the psychological impact of these conditions on children and their families, with a focus on holistic care in pediatric dermatology (Golics et al., 2013; Tampa et al., 2015) (Figure 11.16).

11.4.2. Impetigo: Causes, Symptoms, and Treatment

Impetigo is a highly contagious skin infection most commonly seen in children and caused most commonly by either *Streptococcus pyogenes* or *Staphylococcus aureus* bacteria. The infection typically manifests as red sores or blisters that can rupture, ooze pus, and develop a characteristic crust, often located around the mouth and nose. Children are particularly at risk due to their close contact with others, providing an avenue for easy transmission of infection, especially in places like schools and daycare centers. Symptoms also involve itchiness and discomfort, which prompt early treatment for relief and also to avoid transmission to other individuals. Impetigo is normally treated using topical antibiotics for local infections or systemic antibiotics in widespread scenarios. Prompt diagnosis and management are essential, not just to accelerate recovery but also to prevent potential complications, i.e., cellulitis or nephritis, which are life-threatening sequelae of untreated impetigo (Western University, 1957; Alqahtani et al., 2023).

11.4.3. Fungal Infections: Types and Management

Fungal infections are a significant category of skin conditions in pediatric dermatology, with most kinds creating diverse clinical presentations. Common fungal diseases among children are tinea capitis, tinea corporis, and candidiasis, each with varying symptoms and requiring separate treatment. Tinea capitis, for instance, is a scalp infection caused by fungi, which usually presents with loss of hair and lesions on the scalp and requires systemic antifungal therapy to cure it. Candidiasis that occurs frequently in wet skin areas may require topical antifungals in addition to proper hygiene measures to avoid relapse. According to a pediatric dermatology clinic review, fungal infections were among the most common presenting conditions, hence highlighting clinician suspicion during diagnosis and treatment (Sciberras & Boffa, 2013). Finally, teamwork between dermatologists and specialists is crucial, particularly in managing underlying psychological problems related to skin habits that can lead to such infections, as given by similar research (Tampa et al., 2015) (Figure 11.17).

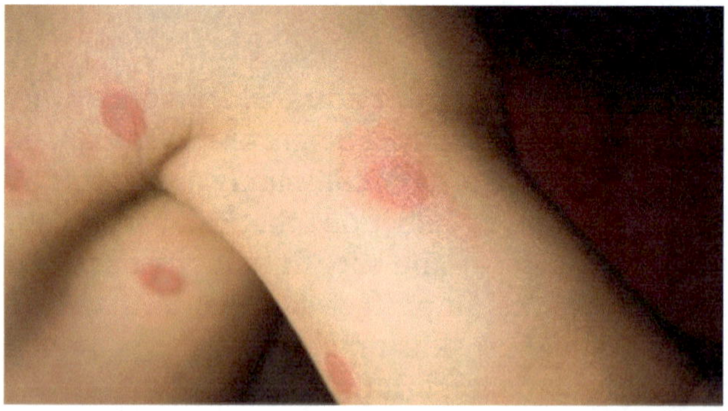

Figure 11.17. Fungal infections represent a significant category of skin conditions in pediatric dermatology, with various types causing diverse clinical presentations.

Source: https://www.dermatology.org.sg/wp-content/uploads/2019/12/fungal-infection.jpg.

11.4.4. Viral Infections: Warts and Molluscum Contagiosum

Viral infections such as warts and molluscum contagiosum are prevalent skin diseases in pediatric dermatology, with distinct clinical features and modes of transmission. Warts, secondary to human papillomavirus (HPV), typically occur as raised, hardened lesions on the skin and are generally benign, though painful and socially stigmatizing in children. Conversely, molluscum contagiosum, driven by a poxvirus, is viewed as small, pearly, dome-shaped papules that are grouped together. Both, though self-limiting, may be parent-concerning because they are contagious and impact children's self-esteem. While recent evidence has emphasized the aetiology and treatment of such infections, there remains a considerable necessity to increase awareness of their importance in diverse paediatric groups, particularly with reported variation in presentation noted in children of different skin types (Daniel et al., 2024; Karampinis et al., 2024). Hence, it is necessary to be aware of these viral infections so as to manage them properly and reassure patients presenting with such infections.

11.4.5. Scabies: Symptoms and Treatment Options

Scabies, caused by *Sarcoptes scabiei* var hominis mite, is a common skin infection that occurs in millions of individuals worldwide, particularly in children. Scabies, as manifested by rash and severe itching usually seen in burrows, can cause significant discomfort and secondary infections unless treated. Clinical suspicion combined with patient history and examinations constitutes the diagnosis, with dermoscopy having the capacity to enhance accuracy in confirmation (Thompson et al., 2021). Treatment is essentially comprised of first-line topical scabicides such as permethrin, which target the infestation itself. Treating all close intimate contacts is also crucial in a bid to prevent reinfestation risks, as highlighted by recent research supporting full management regimens involving individual as well as environmental interventions (van der Linden et al., 2018). In addition, for stubborn cases or for high-risk populations, oral ivermectin may be utilized, emphasizing the need for personalized approaches to best treat scabies in children (Figure 11.18).

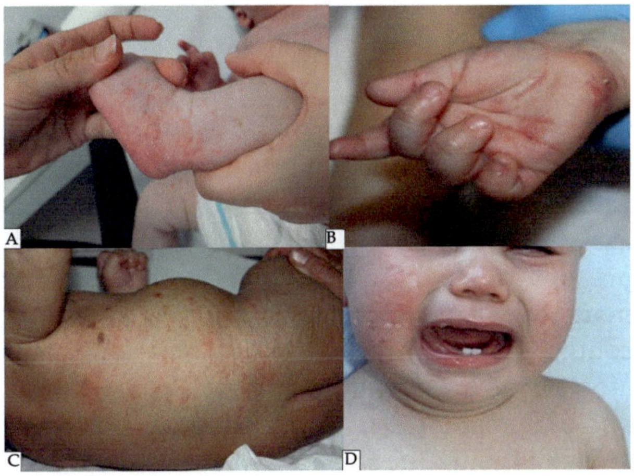

Figure 11.18. Scabies in pediatric populations.

Source: https://www.mdpi.com/children/children-11-00443/article_deploy/html/images/children-11-00443-g001.png.

11.4.6. Importance of Hygiene in Prevention

Adequate hygienic habits have a pivotal role in preventing a wide range of skin conditions in children, particularly communicable ones. Skin also serves as a primary barrier to pathogens, and the maintenance of its integrity by proper hygiene can go a long way in the prevention of skin dermatological diseases such as impetigo or cutaneous bacterial infections. Evidence indicates that a balanced microbiome is part of the defense system of the skin and that enhancing hygiene procedures can result in an improved microbial environment, ultimately warding off infections (Kamel et al., 2024). Besides, illnesses like Turner Syndrome, which may be due to a weakened immune system, present the need for rigorous hygiene practices against complications or secondary infection (Fiot et al., 2022). Generally, through the promotion of good hygiene practices in young kids, caregivers promote general wellness as well as lay a long-term dermatological health foundation, remarkably reducing cases of common skin conditions among children.

11.4.7. Diagnosis Challenges in Pediatric Patients

In pediatric dermatology, accurate diagnosis is of paramount importance, but with the availability of vast challenges due to the unusual presentation of skin conditions in children. For instance, atopic dermatitis (AD), a prevalent condition in children, often coexists with other atopic conditions, which enables its management and diagnostic clarity to be doubtful (Ginsberg & Eichenfield, 2016).

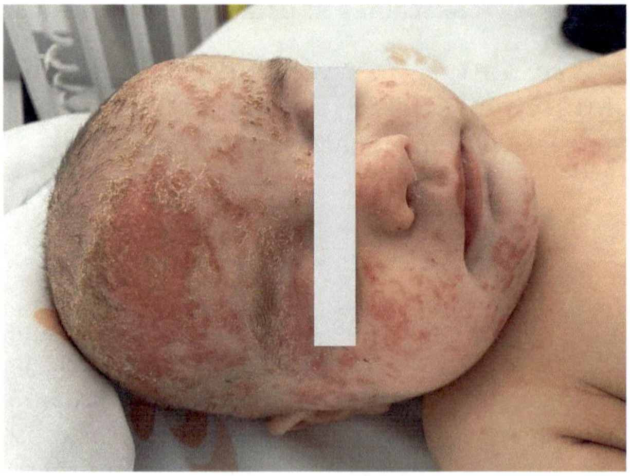

Figure 11.19. Atopic dermatitis (AD), a prevalent childhood condition, often intertwines with other atopic disorders, complicating its management and diagnostic clarity.

Source: https://assets.cureus.com/uploads/figure/file/745752/article_river_b8d666804bd511ee9038adc2e998b745-tempImagemmI8gT.png.

The instability of biomarkers like IgE then makes these issues even more complicated, with higher levels not always corresponding to disease severity or clinically relevant allergies. Moreover, certain diseases like dermatofibrosarcoma protuberans (DFSP), though rare, demonstrate diagnostic challenges when they appear as benign lesions and are most likely to be misdiagnosed (Cassalia et al., 2025). Correct differentiation from other conditions is crucial to prevent treatment delay and proper management. Enhanced awareness and advanced diagnostic methods are thus necessary in pediatric dermatology to allow early, correct diagnosis of these complex skin conditions (Figure 11.19).

11.4.8. Impact of Infections on School Attendance

Infections, particularly skin infections, have detrimental impacts on school attendance among children. Skin infections such as impetigo and other infectious skin diseases can lead to high absenteeism due to the fact that children often remain at home to prevent contracting the infection from other pupils. A study carried out at Lagos University Teaching Hospital sets up the prevalence of infections among children, where such infections are at their peak during childhood and adolescence (Ayanlowo & Okesola, 2017). The necessity of proper treatment and management of these skin infections is not only critical to the health of the infected child but also in keeping their studies uninterrupted. While infections like atopic dermatitis are not infectious, their chronic nature can be a multiplier of school absenteeism due to pain or treatment schedules prompted thereby, as reflected in the Taiwanese Dermatological Association's consensus guidelines in the management of atopic dermatitis (Chen et al., 2015). Thus, active dermatological care is necessary in aiding students' attendance as well as general welfare.

11.4.9. Parental Guidance on Prevention and Care

Effective parental counseling plays a vital role in the prevention and management of common skin conditions in children, notably atopic dermatitis.

Parents are often the first line of defense for the child's skin and may greatly influence the efficacy of treatments by proper education of skin care routines. For instance, studies have revealed that treatments such as crisaborole ointment lead to a considerable improvement in the quality of life for children and families, indicating the importance of understanding and adhering to directed therapy protocols (Simpson et al., 2018). Moreover, educational and psychological interventions supplement conventional treatments and have also been observed to enhance the effectiveness of overall treatment for child atopic eczema (Ersser et al., 2014). Through the construction of an active response encompassing ongoing communication with health care providers and acceptance of recommended preventive measures, parents empower themselves and children and therefore diminish the quality-of-life burden of skin disease significantly (Figure 11.20).

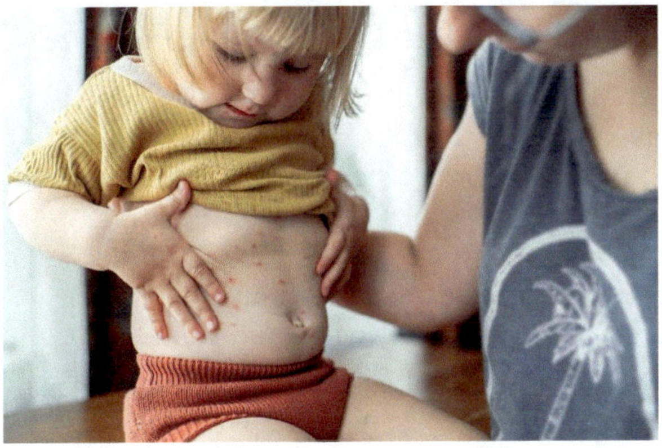

Figure 11.20. Effective parental guidance plays a crucial role in the prevention and care of common childhood skin conditions, particularly atopic dermatitis.

Source: https://epidermatology.com.sg/wp-content/uploads/2023/08/epi-blog-common-paediatric-featured.jpg.

Test Your Knowledge

1. What is molluscum contagiosum, and how does it present?
2. What are the common features of scabies in children?

SUMMARY

The literature on common skin disease in children, particularly atopic dermatitis (AD), highlights the need for an integrative treatment that takes physical as well as quality-of-life factors into account. Literature now reflects the complexity of AD, such as the comorbidity with other atopic conditions, which complicates diagnosis and treatment (Ginsberg & Eichenfield, 2016). Recent advances in therapies, such as the use of crisaborole ointment, have been very encouraging, demonstrating spectacular improvements in quality of life for these patients and their families, above that achieved with traditional therapies (Simpson et al., 2018). Moreover, further work is required to maximize therapeutic regimens and enhance our knowledge of the pathophysiology of these cutaneous diseases. As pediatric dermatology continues to evolve, an integrated approach with both medical treatment and psychological counseling may lead to enhanced health and improved quality of life in children suffering from skin disease.

In total, an integral understanding of common childhood skin diseases is imperative to good pediatric dermatology. Key issues discussed are conditions such as atopic dermatitis, psoriasis, and food allergy, which all impact the quality of life of children and must be kept under observation. For instance, food allergy is present in approximately 2–4% of children, where avoidance of recognized allergens is required, along with taking into account personalized therapeutic options such as oral immunotherapy for certain allergies (Muraro et al., 2022). Treatment of inflammatory skin diseases, as highlighted in a number of systematic reviews, is testament to the viability of new therapies such as biological agents, which have transformed treatment protocols (Marasca et al., 2022). Teledermatology has also made specialty care more accessible, notably for children who are located far from healthcare facilities, thereby enhancing outcomes in general. These are the kind of discussions that confirm the need for ongoing research and creativity in pediatric dermatology.

KEY TERMS FROM THIS CHAPTER

- Pediatric dermatology
- Lifestyle
- Eczema
- Naevi
- Asthma
- Allergic rhinitis
- Atopic dermatitis
- Dyshidrotic eczema
- Education
- Stimuli
- Health
- Benign
- Acne
- Obsessive-compulsive disorder
- Allergies
- Awareness
- Seborrheic dermatitis
- Counseling
- Detergents
- Skin biopsies

CRITICAL THINKING QUESTIONS

1. **What is the most common bacterial cause of impetigo in children?**
   a. *Streptococcus pneumoniae*
   b. *Staphylococcus aureus*
   c. *Pseudomonas aeruginosa*
   d. *Corynebacterium minutissimum*
2. **Which of the following skin conditions in children is associated with "target" or "iris" lesions?**
   a. Atopic dermatitis
   b. Erythema multiforme
   c. Psoriasis
   d. Urticaria
3. **The most common site for atopic dermatitis in infants is:**
   a. Flexural surfaces
   b. Face and extensor surfaces
   c. Palms and soles
   d. Abdomen and back
4. **A child presents with itchy papules in web spaces of fingers and flexural areas. The most likely diagnosis is:**
   a. Eczema
   b. Tinea corporis
   c. Scabies
   d. Psoriasis
5. **Which skin condition is characterized by "herald patch" followed by a Christmas tree pattern on the trunk?**
   a. Pityriasis rosea
   b. Tinea corporis
   c. Lichen planus
   d. Molluscum contagiosum

Short Answer Questions

1. What are the typical clinical features of atopic dermatitis in infants and children?
2. What is the atopic triad, and how is it related to eczema?
3. What are the types of acne lesions (comedones, papules, pustules, nodules)?
4. What is the pathophysiology of acne vulgaris?
5. What are the common types of psoriasis seen in children?
6. What are the clinical features of guttate psoriasis and its usual trigger?
7. What are the clinical features of impetigo, and what organisms cause it?
8. How is tinea corporis diagnosed and treated in children?

Answers to Critical Thinking Questions

1. (b); 2. (b); 3. (b); 4. (c); 5. (a)

REFERENCES

1. Brenninkmeijer, E. E., Legierse, C. M., Sillevis Smitt, J. H., Last, B. F., Grootenhuis, M. A., & Bos, J. D. (2009). The course of life of patients with childhood atopic dermatitis. *Pediatric dermatology*, *26*(1), 14–22. https://doi.org/10.1111/j.1525-1470.2008.00745.x(accessed on 23rd July 2025).
2. Burden-Teh, E., Thomas, K. S., Ratib, S., Grindlay, D., Adaji, E., & Murphy, R. (2016). The epidemiology of childhood psoriasis: a scoping review. *The British journal of dermatology*, *174*(6), 1242–1257. https://doi.org/10.1111/bjd.14507(accessed on 23rd July 2025).
3. Bousquet, J., Hellings, P. W., Agache, I., Bedbrook, A., Bachert, C., Bergmann, K. C., Bewick, M., Bindslev-Jensen, C., Bosnic-Anticevitch, S., Bucca, C., Caimmi, D. P., Camargos, P. A., Canonica, G. W., Casale, T., Chavannes, N. H., Cruz, A. A., De Carlo, G., Dahl, R., Demoly, P., Devillier, P., ... Zidarn, M. (2016). ARIA 2016: Care pathways implementing emerging technologies for predictive medicine in rhinitis and asthma across the life cycle. *Clinical and translational allergy*, *6*, 47. https://doi.org/10.1186/s13601-016-0137-4(accessed on 23rd July 2025).
4. van der Linden, N., van Gool, K., Gardner, K., Dickinson, H., Agostino, J., Regan, D. G., Dowden, M., & Viney, R. (2019). A systematic review of scabies transmission models and data to evaluate the cost-effectiveness of scabies interventions. *PLoS neglected tropical diseases*, *13*(3), e0007182. https://doi.org/10.1371/journal.pntd.0007182(accessed on 23rd July 2025).
5. Alqahtani, S. M., Awaji, B. H., Mahdi, A. M., Althawab, F. H., Aljohani, H. M., Rayes, R. A., Shafie, R. K., Aljohani, R. A., Alkhorayef, S., & Alghamdi, M. K. (2023). Assessment and Management of Atopic Dermatitis in Primary Care Settings: A Systematic Review. *Cureus*, *15*(9), e44560. https://doi.org/10.7759/cureus.44560(accessed on 23rd July 2025).
6. Macias, E., Nieman, E., Yomogida, K., Petrucci, O., Javidan, C., Baszis, K., & Anwar, S. (2018). Rare presentation of an atrial myxoma in an adolescent patient: a case report and literature review. *BMC pediatrics*, *18*(1), 373. https://doi.org/10.1186/s12887-018-1313-6(accessed on 23rd July 2025).
7. Brasileiro, A., Campos, S., Fidalgo, M., Correia, T., Apetato, M., et al. (2013). Phototherapy in childhood: A 17-year retrospective study regarding effectiveness and safety. https://core.ac.uk/download/71737759.pdf (accessed on 23rd July 2025).
8. Vermeulen, F. M., Gerbens, L. A. A., Bosma, A. L., Apfelbacher, C. J., Irvine, A. D., Arents, B. W. M., Barbarot, S., Deleuran, M., Eichenfield, L. F., Manca, A., Schmitt, J., Vestergaard, C., Wall, D., Weidinger, S., Middelkamp-Hup, M. A., Spuls, P. I., Flohr, C., & International TREAT Registry Taskforce (2019). TREatment of ATopic eczema (TREAT) Registry Taskforce: consensus on how and when to measure the core dataset for atopic eczema treatment research registries. *The British journal of dermatology*, *181*(3), 492–504. https://doi.org/10.1111/bjd.17715 (accessed on 23rd July 2025).
9. Kandhari, S., Girdhar, M., Kulkarni, D. S., Arsiwala, S., Sakhiya, J., Karthikeyan, K., Murthy, S., Dhawan, S., Mallela, V. B., & Rathi, S. (2022). Expert consensus on the management of acne in India. *International Journal of Research in Medical Sciences*, *10*(4), 980–990. https://doi.org/10.18203/2320-6012.ijrms20220998(accessed on 23rd July 2025).
10. Ayanlowo, O., & Okesola, O. (2017). Pattern of skin disorders across age groups. https://core.ac.uk/download/478463608.pdf (accessed on 23rd July 2025).

11. Ayanlowo, O., Puddicombe, O., & Gold-Olufadi, S. (2018). Pattern of skin diseases amongst children attending a dermatology clinic in Lagos, Nigeria. *The Pan African medical journal, 29*, 162. https://doi.org/10.11604/pamj.2018.29.162.14503(accessed on 23rd July 2025).

12. Nankervis, H., Thomas, K. S., Delamere, F. M., Barbarot, S., Smith, S., Rogers, N. K., & Williams, H. C. (2017). What is the evidence base for atopic eczema treatments? A summary of published randomized controlled trials. *The British journal of dermatology, 176*(4), 910–927. https://doi.org/10.1111/bjd.14999(accessed on 23rd July 2025).

13. Golics, C. J., Basra, M. K., Salek, M. S., & Finlay, A. Y. (2013). The impact of patients' chronic disease on family quality of life: an experience from 26 specialties. *International journal of general medicine, 6*, 787–798. https://doi.org/10.2147/IJGM.S45156(accessed on 23rd July 2025).

14. Cassalia, F., Danese, A., Cocchi, E., Vaienti, S., Bolzon, A., Franceschin, L., Mazzetto, R., Caroppo, F., Melandri, D., & Belloni Fortina, A. (2025). Congenital Dermatofibrosarcoma Protuberans-An Update on the Ongoing Diagnostic Challenges. *Cancers, 17*(1), 158. https://doi.org/10.3390/cancers17010158(accessed on 23rd July 2025).

15. Tampa, M., Sarbu, M. I., Matei, C., Benea, V., & Georgescu, S. R. (2015). Common Dermatoses in Patients with Obsessive Compulsive Disorders. *Journal of Mind and Medical Sciences, 2*(2), 150-158. https://doi.org/10.22543/2392-7674.1022(accessed on 23rd July 2025).

16. Sciberras, C., & Boffa, M. J. (2013). A review of a pediatric dermatology clinic in Malta. https://core.ac.uk/download/46602353.pdf (accessed on 23rd July 2025).

17. Simpson, E. L., Paller, A. S., Boguniewicz, M., Eichenfield, L. F., Feldman, S. R., Silverberg, J. I., Chamlin, S. L., & Zane, L. T. (2018). Crisaborole Ointment Improves Quality of Life of Patients with Mild to Moderate Atopic Dermatitis and Their Families. *Dermatology and therapy, 8*(4), 605–619. https://doi.org/10.1007/s13555-018-0263-0(accessed on 23rd July 2025).

18. Boguniewicz, M., Levy, M. L., Eichenfield, L. F., Lauren, C. T., Leung, D. Y. M., Schneider, L. C., Siegfried, E. C., Tom, W. L., & Paller, A. S. (2024). Managing Childhood and Adolescent Atopic Dermatitis in Primary Care: A US Expert Group Consensus. *Journal of pediatrics. Clinical practice, 14*, 200121. https://doi.org/10.1016/j.jpedcp.2024.200121(accessed on 23rd July 2025).

19. Burden-Teh, E. (2020). Improving our understanding of childhood psoriasis: Identifying opportunities for early intervention for the prevention of long-term harm. https://core.ac.uk/download/552443070.pdf (accessed on 23rd July 2025).

20. Char, C. (2024). Empowering primary care providers to transform pediatric acne care: A quality improvement project. https://core.ac.uk/download/643773271.pdf (accessed on 23rd July 2025).

21. Chen, H. C., Chen, Y. J., Chu, C. Y., Dai, Y. S., Hsieh, C. W., et al. (2015). Taiwanese Dermatological Association consensus for the management of atopic dermatitis. https://core.ac.uk/download/pdf/82420700.pdf (accessed on 23rd July 2025).

22. Chukwu, R., & Mankila, J. (2018). Dermatology nurses' job description: Literature review. https://core.ac.uk/download/161432240.pdf (accessed on 23rd July 2025).

23. Ersser, S. J., Cowdell, F., Latter, S., Gardiner, E., Flohr, C., Thompson, A. R., Jackson, K., Farasat, H., Ware, F., & Drury, A. (2014). Psychological and educational interventions for atopic eczema

in children. *The Cochrane database of systematic reviews, 2014*(1), CD004054. https://doi.org/10.1002/14651858.CD004054.pub3(accessed on 23rd July 2025).

24. Daniel, S. S., Peterman, C., & Awasthi, S. (2024). Updates on postinfectious skin rashes in pediatric dermatology. *Current Opinion in Pediatrics, 36*, 431–435. https://www.semanticscholar.org/paper/eb4289f2d33761ead99444bdd3c6f3f8b0030891 (accessed on 23rd July 2025).
25. Basra, M. K. A., Salek, M. S., Fenech, D., & Finlay, A. Y. (2018). Conceptualization, development and validation of T-QoL© (Teenagers› Quality of Life): a patient-focused measure to assess quality of life of adolescents with skin diseases. *The British journal of dermatology*, *178*(1), 161–175. https://doi.org/10.1111/bjd.15853(accessed on 23rd July 2025).
26. Egeli, B., Dallas, J., Reusch, D. B., Shaw, K. S., Gellis, S., Sundel, R., Son, M., et al. (2025). Juvenile localized scleroderma: A large retrospective cohort study from a tertiary care center. *Pediatric Rheumatology, 23.* https://www.semanticscholar.org/paper/6dfb07f30f10a74dc340aecee4f264e8b9578b8d (accessed on 23rd July 2025).
27. Ginsberg, D. N., & Eichenfield, L. F. (2016). Debates in allergy medicine: Specific immunotherapy in children with atopic dermatitis, the "con" view. *The World Allergy Organization journal*, *9*, 16. https://doi.org/10.1186/s40413-016-0107-2(accessed on 23rd July 2025).
28. Eichenfield, L. F., Ganslandt, C., Kurvits, M., & Schlessinger, J. (2015). Safety and efficacy of calcipotriene plus betamethasone dipropionate topical suspension in the treatment of extensive scalp psoriasis in adolescents ages 12 to 17 years. *Pediatric dermatology*, *32*(1), 28–35. https://doi.org/10.1111/pde.12429(accessed on 23rd July 2025).
29. Fiot, E., Alauze, B., Donadille, B., Samara-Boustani, D., Houang, M., De Filippo, G., Bachelot, A., et al. (2022). Turner syndrome: French National Diagnosis and Care Protocol (NDCP). *Orphanet Journal of Rare Diseases, 17.* https://doi.org/10.1186/s13023-022-02423-5 (accessed on 23rd July 2025).
30. Giua C, Floris NP, Schlich M, Keber E, Gelmetti C (2021) Dermatitis in community pharmacies: a survey on italian pharmacists' management and implications on corticophobia. Pharmacia 68(3): 671-677. https://doi.org/10.3897/pharmacia.68.e70452(accessed on 23rd July 2025).
31. Paller, A. S., Kong, H. H., Seed, P., Naik, S., Scharschmidt, T. C., Gallo, R. L., Luger, T., & Irvine, A. D. (2019). The microbiome in patients with atopic dermatitis. *The Journal of allergy and clinical immunology*, *143*(1), 26–35. https://doi.org/10.1016/j.jaci.2018.11.015(accessed on 23rd July 2025).
32. Gencler, B., Keseroglu, O., Kartal, S. P., & Gonul, M. (2017). Pediatric Acne. InTech. doi: 10.5772/66141(accessed on 23rd July 2025).
33. Hughes, O. (2025). *Mindfulness-Based Online Support for Children and Families Affected by Skin Conditions.* https://core.ac.uk/download/595951183.pdf (accessed on 23rd July 2025).
34. Jones, A. (2024). Developing thick skin: Pediatric eczema in vulnerable communities and FDA regulation of cosmetic products. https://core.ac.uk/download/624158048.pdf (accessed on 23rd July 2025).
35. Kamel, M., Aleya, S., Alsubih, M., & Aleya, L. (2024). Microbiome dynamics: A paradigm shift in combatting infectious diseases. *Journal of Personalized Medicine, 14*, 217–217. https://doi.org/10.3390/jpm14020217 (accessed on 23rd July 2025).
36. Karampinis, E., Toli, O., Georgopoulou, K., Papadopoulou, M. M., Vardiampasi, A., Zafiriou,

E., Lazaridou, E., et al. (2024). Exploring pediatric dermatology in skin of color: Focus on dermoscopy. *Life, 14*. https://www.semanticscholar.org/paper/9cb574b228f1cf530983be030b4ef874e6e80f7b (accessed on 23rd July 2025).

37. Kraft, E. (2024). *It's More Than Skin Deep: Evaluating Mental Health Care in Dermatology Settings*. https://core.ac.uk/download/624274604.pdf (accessed on 23rd July 2025).

38. Marasca, C., Annunziata, M. C., Camela, E., Di Guida, A., Fornaro, L., Megna, M., Napolitano, M., et al. (2022). Tele dermatology and inflammatory skin conditions during COVID-19 era: New perspectives and applications. *Journal of Clinical Medicine, 11*, 1511–1511. https://doi.org/10.3390/jcm11061511 (accessed on 23rd July 2025).

39. Mohod M., Thakare S. Critical Review on Various Skin Disorders and Ayurvedic Management: A Holistic Approach. AYUSCRIPT 2025;4(1):32-37 DOI: http://doi.org/10.55552/AYUSCRIPT.2025.4107(accessed on 23rd July 2025).

40. Muraro, A., de Silva, D., Halken, S., Worm, M., Khaleva, E., Arasi, S., DunnGalvin, A., et al. (2022). Managing food allergy: GA2LEN guideline 2022. *World Allergy Organization Journal, 15*, 100687–100687. https://doi.org/10.1016/j.waojou.2022.100687 (accessed on 23rd July 2025).

41. Oninla, O., Oninla, S., Onayemi, O., & Olasode, O. (2016). Pattern of pediatric dermatoses at dermatology clinics in Ile-Ife and Ilesha, Nigeria. *Pediatrics and International Child Health*. https://www.semanticscholar.org/paper/13678bf0f869761a64e8b0dfdc2cb5059d005c9e (accessed on 23rd July 2025).

42. Polat, A. K., Yesilova, Y., Alataş, E., Belli, A., Dogan, G., & Picakciefe, M. (2018). Prevalence of skin diseases of the pediatric population in the Southeastern Anatolia, Turkey. *Medicine Science | International Medical Journal, 7*, 664. https://www.semanticscholar.org/paper/141d1756e2986e78e1acdb0bff353cd838401190 (accessed on 23rd July 2025).

43. Selmanoğlu, A., Çelik, H. I., Genis, C., Koçkuzu, E., Emeksiz, Z., & Mısırlıoğlu, E. (2025). Evaluation of asthma course in patients hospitalized in pediatric intensive care unit due to severe asthma exacerbation. *Medicina, 61*. https://www.semanticscholar.org/paper/990e7253760ad5b87817923952a5d061e51a9db9 (accessed on 23rd July 2025).

44. Sena, T. (2019). Managing childhood atopic dermatitis: Utilizing a written eczema action plan to improve caregiver self-efficacy. https://core.ac.uk/download/214384237.pdf (accessed on 23rd July 2025).

45. Sjerobabski-Masnec, I., Kotrulja, L., Šitum, M., Poduje, S., & Ožanić-Bulić, S. (2010). Photosensitivity skin disorders in childhood. https://core.ac.uk/download/14422812.pdf (accessed on 23rd July 2025).

46. Thompson R, Westbury S, Slape D. Paediatrics: how to manage scabies. *Drugs Context*. 2021;10:2020-12-3. Published 2021 Mar 26. doi:10.7573/dic.2020-12-3(accessed on 23rd July 2025).

47. Suliman, O., Abd Elmagid, A., Abd Elmagid, R., & Abd Elmagid, R. (2025). Colostomy-related morbidity in children following stoma formation and closure: Systemic review. *Journal of Advances in Medicine and Medical Research*. https://www.semanticscholar.org/paper/352c427f177b096025079178764bb7e691cf2772 (accessed on 23rd July 2025).

48. Ujiie, H., Rosmarin, D., Schön, M. P., Ständer, S., Boch, K., Metz, M., Maurer, M., et al. (2022). Unmet medical needs in chronic, non-communicable inflammatory skin diseases. *Frontiers in Medicine, 9*. https://doi.org/10.3389/fmed.2022.875492 (accessed on 23rd July 2025).
49. Western University. (1957). *UWOMJ, 27*(1), January 1957. https://core.ac.uk/download/61657207.pdf (accessed on 23rd July 2025).

NEONATAL DERMATOLOGY AND BIRTHMARKS

12

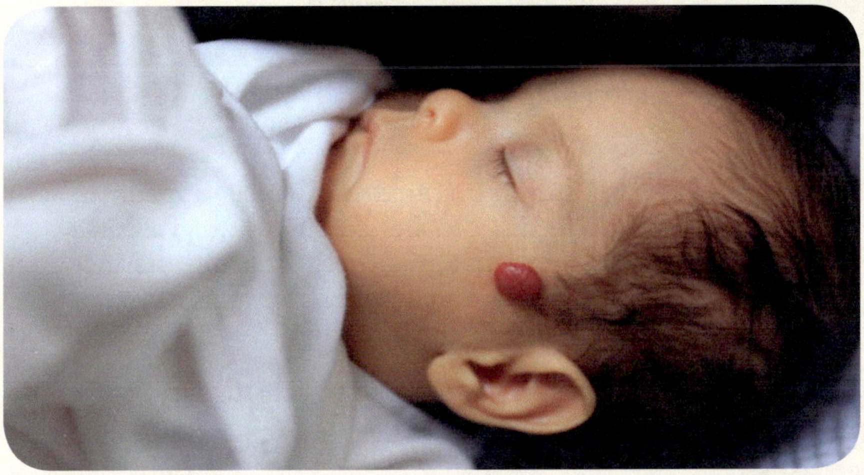

LEARNING OBJECTIVES

After studying this chapter, you will be able to:

1. Understand Types of Birthmarks;
2. Explain Diagnosis and Assessment;
3. Describe Treatment Options;
4. Focus on Prevention and Care.

Introduction

Neonatal dermatology is an important field of study in understanding the various skin illnesses that occur in neonates, particularly focusing on birthmarks and other dermatoses. The cutaneous lesions can range from benign pigmented macules to vascular hamartomas, and there has to be a refined way of their treatment and diagnosis. Recent studies reveal that vascular hamartomas, which are usually in the form of lesions, may be linked to certain perinatal risk factors like preterm birth and maternal factors, as revealed by the significant variations in occurrence by race and maternal health (Conn, 2025). Such common transient cutaneous disorders as Mongolian spots and erythema toxicum are also prevalent, showing the variability of neonatal dermatoses (Marwah et al., 2018). Identification of these conditions does more than add to clinical practice; it also raises parental awareness and reassurance and emphasizes the pivotal role dermatological examinations have in neonatal examination.

12.1. Types of Birthmarks

Learning Outcome

1. Understand Vascular Birthmarks: Definition and Examples;
2. Explain Pigmented Birthmarks: Definition and Examples;
3. Focus on Differences between Congenital and Acquired Birthmarks;
4. Describe Common Types of Vascular Birthmarks;
5. Learn Common Types of Pigmented Birthmarks;
6. Discuss Rare Birthmarks and their Implications;
7. Know Genetic Factors Influencing Birthmark Development;
8. Understand Environmental Factors Affecting Birthmarks;
9. Explain Psychological Impact of Visible Birthmarks on Infants.

Birthmarks, found in countless variations, can be classified into vascular and pigmented birthmarks, both with distinctive characteristics and implications on neonatal health. Vascular birthmarks, such as infantile hemangiomas and port-wine stains, are brought about by blood vessel anomalies. Infantile hemangiomas are also common in the newborn and typically follow a proliferation phase and involution, with strict follow-up as they tend to resolve spontaneously without intervention.

In large cases or where there is suspicion of complications, laser therapy has proved to be an effective option, with more favorable outcomes when applied early in the hemangioma development (Kendrick, 2025). On the other hand, pigmented birthmarks include nevi, which may be manifested as congenital melanocytic nevi or café-au-lait macules. These lesions need to be continuously monitored to rule out malignant evolution, particularly in larger or atypical presentations. Lymphatic malformations, although less frequent, can also impact the patient's quality of life due to complications such as compression of vital structures (Ghaffarpour, 2018) (Figure 12.1).

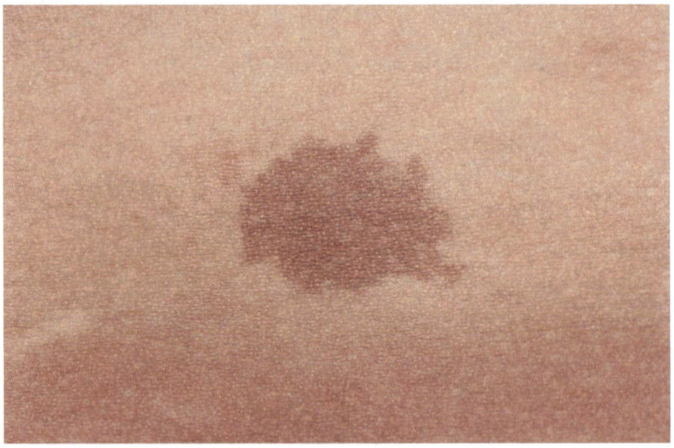

Figure 12.1. Birthmarks, which appear in various forms, can be classified into vascular and pigmented types, each bearing distinct characteristics and implications for neonatal health.

Source: https://www.mymed.com/image/2625/medicalarticle/800.

12.1.1. Vascular Birthmarks: Definition and Examples

Vascular birthmarks, typically segregated into vascular malformations and hemangiomas, are a focal point of study in neonatal dermatology. Hemangiomas, or strawberry marks, are proliferating tumors of endothelial cells and, in the case of most types, typically appear in infancy with a growth phase followed by involution. They most commonly appear on the face, neck, and scalp and illustrate the vascular nature of their development. This is unlike vascular malformations, such as port-wine stains and arteriovenous malformations, that are present at birth and never involuted. Their management is often a multidisciplinary approach due to potential complications like psychological impact and the need for interventions like sclerotherapy for symptom relief. Furthermore, preterm birth and maternal conditions like gestational diabetes have been found to be linked with the presence of these anomalies and hence warrant complete awareness of their etiology and management modalities (Kerr, 2014) (Figure 12.2).

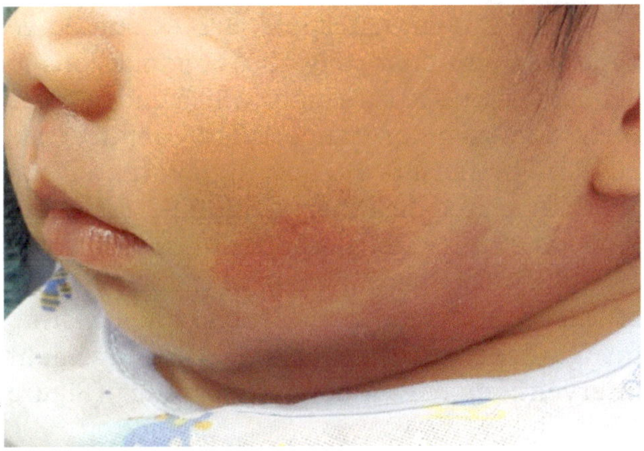

Figure 12.2. Vascular birthmarks.

Source: https://www.dermatologyinc.com/wp-content/uploads/Vascular-birthmark-symptoms.jpg.

12.1.2. Pigmented Birthmarks: Definition and Examples

Pigmented nevi or pigmented birthmarks are a benign type of cutaneous marking present at birth or shortly after. Areas of raised melanin that occur in localized patches, such as birthmarks, are pretty diverse in nature, and appear as café-au-lait spots, congenital nevi, or melanocytic nevi, among others. For instance, café-au-lait macules are light brown macules that signal soon-to-happen genetic disorders when they are present in great numbers, while congenital nevi are larger in size and have a predisposition to become malignant melanoma over time. It is essential to understand these distinctions within the branch of neonatal dermatology because early detection and intervention can prevent complications. The effectiveness and safety of treatment of pigmented birthmarks, e.g., observation and potential excision, must be evaluated in terms of psychological impact and quality of life in the patient because it is along this intersection that these two are equally valued: patient safety and appropriate care (de Leeuw, 2009; Díaz et al, 2019).

12.1.3. Differences between Congenital and Acquired Birthmarks

It is important to recognize the distinctions between acquired and congenital birthmarks in neonatal dermatologic practice.

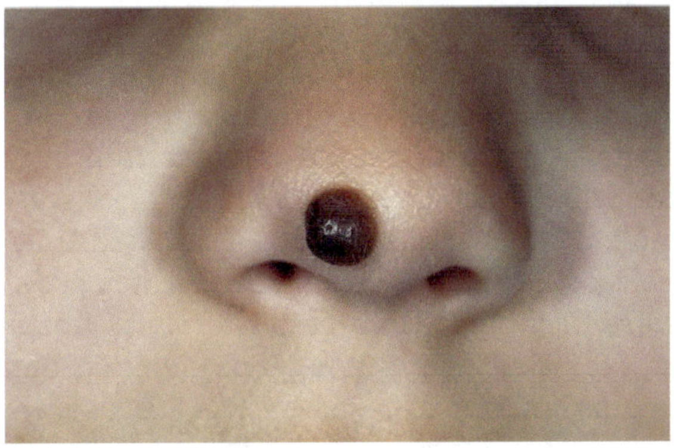

Figure 12.3. Congenital birthmarks.

Source: https://upload.wikimedia.org/wikipedia/commons/4/4c/Congenital_melanocytic_nevus_01.jpg.

Congenital birthmarks, which occur at birth or shortly thereafter, are a result of some of the following: genetic predispositions, as well as developmental abnormalities that arise during pregnancy. Classic examples include nevus simplex and Mongolian spots, which can typically be followed up but are typically benign (Vemu et al., 2024). On the other hand, acquired birthmarks present after birth, often as a result of environmental influences from the external world or body physiological changes. These may include conditions such as café-au-lait spots and post-inflammatory hyperpigmentation, arising due to trauma or irritation. Differentiation between these two categories is necessary to enable appropriate diagnosis, management, and allaying parents' fears, as most congenital marks are benign, but some acquired marks might indicate associated medical conditions. Thus, both neonatologists and pediatric dermatologists need to have a deep understanding of their etiology and outcomes (Figure 12.3).

12.1.4. Common Types of Vascular Birthmarks (e.g., Hemangiomas)

Vascular birthmarks, and hemangiomas in particular, are the most frequent among all conditions encountered in neonatal dermatology. These are benign tumors characterized by localized vascular proliferation that may manifest as red or purple discoloration of the skin, which may resemble a bruise or blistered lesion. Hemangiomas typically occur in the initial weeks of life and may exhibit accelerated growth before they begin to regress afterward. Despite the fact that the etiology of hemangiomas remains unknown, research has discovered a potential correlation with preterm delivery and maternal conditions, suggesting that population knowledge may be employed to establish clinical management (Conn, 2025). Treatment for hemangiomas is variable, with observation as one approach, as well as, in certain patients, laser therapy, which has proven highly effective in reducing their size and cosmesis if begun early in their development (Kendrick, 2025). Hence, early education and assessment of parents are crucial in the management of issues with these vascular lesions.

12.1.5. Common Types of Pigmented Birthmarks (e.g., Café-au-lait Spots)

Among the many pigmented birthmarks encountered in neonatal dermatology, café-au-lait spots stand out due to their significance as markers for inherent genetic diseases. The light brown, coffee-colored pigmented macules can be of varied size and may or may not be present at birth, but may also appear in early childhood. The existence of over one café-au-lait mark, particularly in association with other clinical findings, may indicate conditions such as neurofibromatosis type 1, as these marks are classically associated with this genetic disorder. In fact, congenital anomalies and pigmented nevi, including café-au-lait spots, are estimated to appear on approximately 10% of admissions to neonatal intensive care units, which underscores their clinical importance (Vlădăreanu et al., 2017). Furthermore, such pigmentation can also be related to other syndromic disorders with other cutaneous manifestations (Mitri et al., 2021). The identification of the importance of these birthmarks is crucial in assisting the guidance of diagnosis and management interventions within neonatal practice (Figure 12.4).

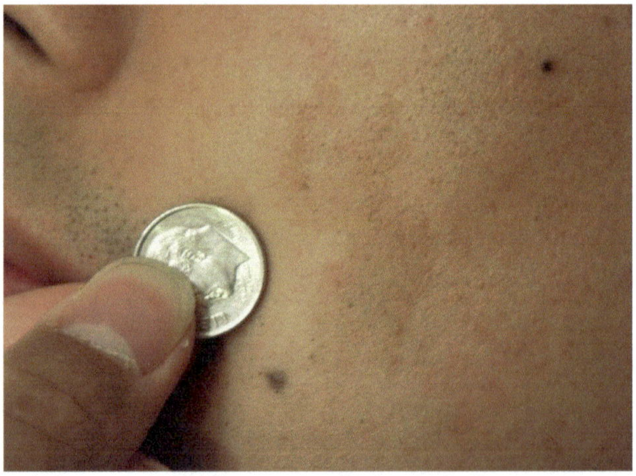

Figure 12.4. Café-au-lait spots.

Source: https://upload.wikimedia.org/wikipedia/commons/thumb/f/f3/CALSpot.jpg/1200px-CALSpot.jpg.

12.1.6. Rare Birthmarks and Their Implications

Rare birthmarks, even infrequently encountered in clinical practice, are highly diagnostic and management-demanding within neonatal dermatology. Fibrosarcoma, dermatofibrosarcoma protuberans and rare congenital vascular malformations may initially mimic benign lesions, and thus there may be a lag in management and misguidance in therapeutic strategies. For instance, the congenital form of DFSP can simulate hemangiomas of the common type, and hence an impromptu understanding of differential diagnoses is imperative not to miss management (Cassalia et al., 2025). Also, the prevalence of some birthmarks, such as Mongolian spots, demonstrates the importance of geographic and cultural variation in recognition and implications. In a study of Mongolian newborns, the incidence of Mongolian spots was strongly predominant at 91.3%, indicating their frequency, but introducing potential diagnostic confusion with other skin conditions (Batbaatar et al., 2017). Together with the knowledge of these rare birthmarks and their implications, it is essential to advance clinical practice and appropriately treat the affected neonates.

12.1.7. Genetic Factors Influencing Birthmark Development

The intricate interaction between genetic factors and the development of birthmarks is a topic of growing interest in neonatal dermatology. The evidence indicates that a high percentage of congenital anomalies, some of them other birthmarks, may have a genetic etiology; it has been mentioned in the literature that one-third of them are due to genetic causes (Vlădăreanu et al., 2017). This suggests a potential hereditary component in such conditions as congenital pigmented nevi and vascular malformations. Genetic aberrations and chromosomal mutations could initiate the formation of such skin markings even at the embryonic stage, both in the type and the body distribution. To this complicated picture, the majority of birthmarks would not be accompanied by severe malformations but could also occur within the generalized malformation syndromes, tracing the complexity of the genetic influences in neonatal cutaneous manifestations (Vlădăreanu et al., 2017). Awareness of such genetic predispositions is valuable for the planning of proper management and for facilitating correct diagnosis in clinical settings (Figure 12.5).

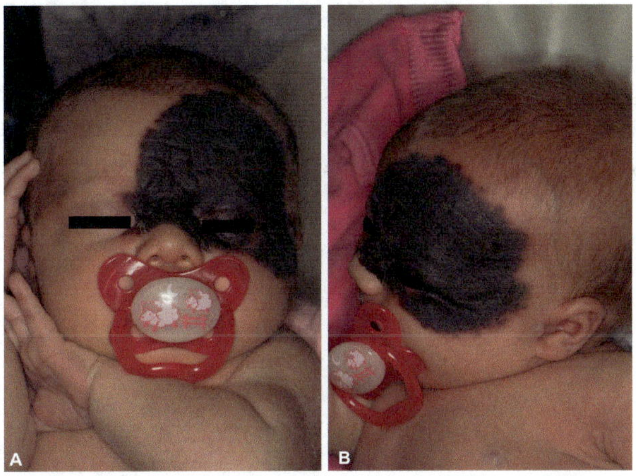

Figure 12.5. Congenital pigmented nevi.

Source: https://www.jaadcasereports.org/cms/10.1016/j.jdcr.2023.02.011/asset/76e3718e-3ae2-47a0-b22a-7e598d92c002/main.assets/gr1_lrg.jpg.

12.1.8. Environmental Factors Affecting Birthmarks

Environmental factors greatly affect the occurrence of birthmarks in neonates, with several maternal and neonatal parameters influencing their occurrence. For instance, between May 2008 and November 2009, a study documented a strong association between mode of delivery, gestational age, and the occurrence of dermatological conditions like birthmarks in 1,000 children. Importantly, it made it clear that 72% of the children showed signs of birthmarks, suggesting that obstetric variables could be an influencing factor in their development. Further, certain lifestyle traits, such as maternal smoking and drug use in pregnancy, had correlations with the presence of certain birthmarks, further attesting to the importance of environmental factors in neonatal skin diseases. Accordingly, it is useful to know these factors, considering that congenital abnormalities, including skin diseases, have multifactorial causes, and environmental factors may be interacting with genetic determinants (Vlădăreanu et al., 2017).

12.1.9. Psychological Impact of Visible Birthmarks on Infants

The psychological impact of visible birthmarks in infants is a multifaceted process that carries profound implications for their emotional adaptation and psychological development. Infants with visible birthmarks, such as hemangiomas or other congenital vascular malformations, may face challenges in forming secure attachment and social connections as they grow up.

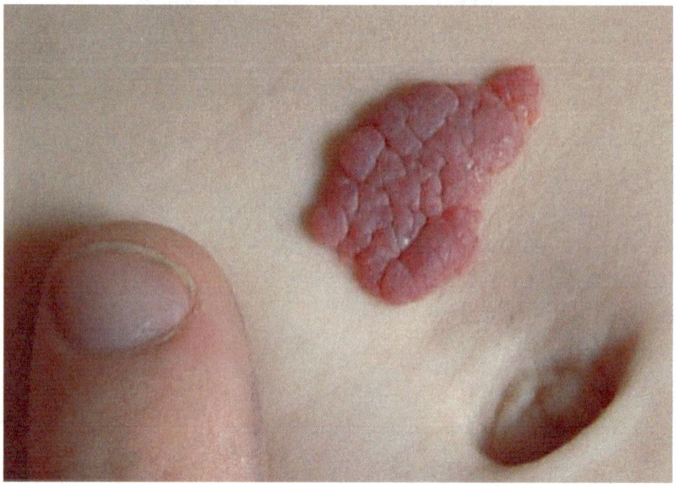

Figure 12.6. Infants with noticeable birthmarks, such as hemangiomas or other vascular malformations, may face challenges in forming secure attachments and social relationships as they grow.

Source: https://birthmark.org/wp-content/uploads/2018/06/Capillary_haemangioma.jpg.

The visibility of the birthmarks may also elicit reactions of rejection by caregivers and peers, thereby bringing feelings of stigma or isolation. Research has revealed that congenital abnormalities occur in at least 10% of newborns, the majority of whom have explanations which are not straightforward, contributing to parental concern during diagnosis and care (Vlădăreanu et al., 2017). Secondly, treatment and classification of vascular malformations should consider both physical appearances as well as psychological effects, as these birthmarks can prove to be a source of long-term distress for the infant (Lakshmi, 2010). So, addressing psychological factors is critical for the comprehensive care of infants with birthmarks (Figure 12.6).

Test Your Knowledge

1. What is the clinical significance of a port-wine stain (nevus flammeus)?
2. How can salmon patches be differentiated from port-wine stains?

12.2. Diagnosis and Assessment

Learning Outcome

1. Understand Clinical Examination Techniques for Neonatal Skin;
2. Explain the Importance of Patient History in Diagnosis;
3. Focus on Use of Imaging Techniques in Assessment;
4. Describe Differentiating Between Benign and Concerning Birthmarks;
5. Learn Role of Pediatric Dermatologists in Diagnosis;
6. Discuss Common Diagnostic Tools and Methods;
7. Know Challenges in Diagnosing Skin Conditions in Neonates;
8. Understand the Importance of Early Diagnosis for Treatment Outcomes.

In neonatal dermatology, accurate diagnosis and assessment of skin lesions are critical to establishing the correct approaches to management. Conditions such as dermatofibrosarcoma protuberans (DFSP) and epidermal choristoma are examples of the challenges of clinical examination. DFSP may be clinically indistinguishable from benign lesions externally, and hence differential diagnosis by means of advanced molecular techniques, including identification of the COL1A1-PDGFB fusion gene using FISH and RT-PCR. These techniques enhance diagnostic precision, especially in treatment planning like Mohs micrographic surgery to ensure oncologic safety without compromising aesthetic integrity (Cassalia et al., 2025). Epidermal choristoma is a rare congenital anomaly that usually occurs as pigmented oral lesions and is benign (Cassalia et al., 2025). In such instances, observation is preferred to invasive excision and highlights the importance of good clinical evaluation and a customized response to each individual case (Hughes et al., 2021).

12.2.1. Clinical Examination Techniques for Neonatal Skin

Systematic clinical examination of neonatal skin is important to enable proper diagnosis and management of different dermatological conditions, such as birthmarks. These findings involve a systematic assessment of skin color, texture, and the presence of lesions, which are measurable indicators for potential underlying pathological processes.

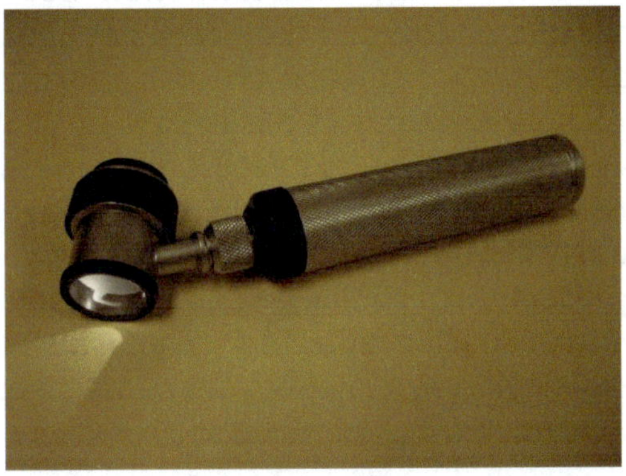

Figure 12.7. Pediatric practitioners should engage in meticulous observation, utilizing dermatoscopes for enhanced visualization of superficial skin structures, thereby facilitating better differentiation of benign from potentially malignant lesions.

Source: https://upload.wikimedia.org/wikipedia/commons/e/e6/Dermatoscope1.JPG.

Pediatricians should be observant, employing dermatoscopes to better visualize superficial skin architecture, thereby being able to differentiate better between benign and potentially malignant lesions. In neonates, congenital anomalies may occur as skin manifestations; for example, birthmarks such as port-wine stains or hemangiomas should be closely observed to determine if any need for intervention (Cassalia et al., 2025). Moreover, a sharp inspection can ascertain mild dysmorphic features, which could be linked to genetic syndromes warranting immediate medical management. Because roughly 50%–60% of congenital anomalies are of indeterminate etiology, the use of a detailed clinical examination is important in guiding future diagnostic steps for optimal management (Vlădăreanu et al., 2017) (Figure 12.7).

12.2.2. Importance of Patient History in Diagnosis

The importance of patient history in the diagnosis of neonatal dermatoses cannot be overstated, particularly in the discrimination between various birthmarks and their relevance. A good patient history provides critical information regarding the timing of onset, rate of growth, and associated symptoms necessary for accurate diagnosis. For instance, dermatofibrosarcoma protuberans (DFSP) and infantile hemangiomas can present with similar visual manifestations but with radically differing prognostic hopes and treatment requirements. Examination of the family history, the gestational age sequence, and exogenous influences also facilitates increased diagnostic specificity, allowing for proper interventions and management programs. As elucidated in recent publications, misdiagnosis of such conditions can result in serious delays in treatment, and therefore, an integrated approach with a convergence of the histopathology and molecular testing on one hand and the patient story on the other is inevitable (Cassalia et al., 2025; Kendrick, 2025). Finally, a detailed history of the patient acts as a pillar in guaranteeing successful outcomes in neonatal dermatology, highlighting the pivotal relationship between clinical evaluation and patient-oriented care.

12.2.3. Use of Imaging Techniques in Assessment

Imaging methods are at the forefront of the evaluation of skin diseases in neonates, particularly in the accurate diagnosis of congenital birthmarks and associated anomalies. Ultrasound, magnetic resonance imaging (MRI), and optical coherence tomography are non-invasive methods that provide critical anatomical information and help to distinguish between benign and malignant disease. For instance, a link between vascular birthmarks and underlying structures can be made evident through advanced imaging, increasing the precision of clinical evaluation. Moreover, as discussed in the discussion regarding rare conditions like dermatofibrosarcoma protuberans, imaging can be utilized to aid in distinguishing these from benign lesions and thus guide management (Cassalia et al., 2025). Besides, in congenital anomalies with unknown etiology, imaging can assist in effective assessments that can aid in the identification of the underlying genetic conditions, as approximately 50–60% of such anomalies are of an unknown etiology (Vlădăreanu et al., 2017). Such supplementation of imaging in dermatological assessments for its role in neonatal care validates its significance (Figure 12.8).

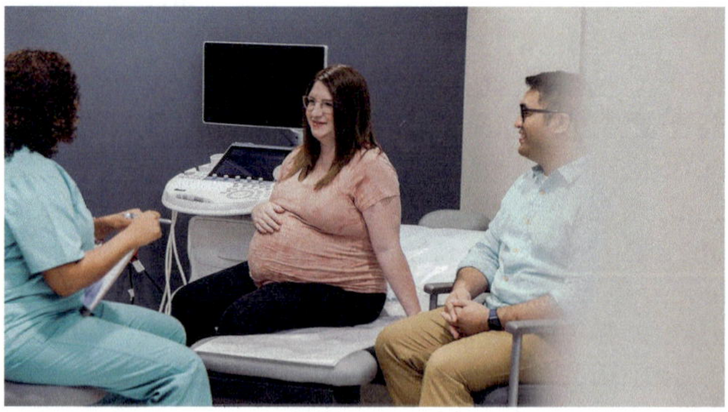

Figure 12.8. Imaging techniques play a pivotal role in the assessment of neonatal dermatological conditions, particularly concerning the accurate diagnosis of congenital birthmarks and associated anomalies.

Source: https://post.healthline.com/wp-content/uploads/2023/08/nurse-talking-to-pregnant-mother-couple-1296x728-header.jpg.

12.2.4. Differentiating Between Benign and Concerning Birthmarks

Benign vs. concerning birthmarks differentiation is important in neonatal dermatologic practice for correct management, as well as reassuring parents.

The most common tumors in infancy are benign birthmarks, such as hemangiomas. Benign birthmarks have a predictable involution pattern, which tends to alleviate parental anxiety as they disappear over time (Tom, 2011). Conversely, more significant lesions, including epidermal choristomas, while histologically benign, can be problematic to diagnose since they can cause misdiagnosis with other diseases, thereby implying the need for accurate observation rather than excision (Hughes et al., 2021).

Practitioners need to ensure that they employ a systematic approach when evaluating birthmarks, taking into consideration factors like appearance, location, and growth patterns. In the process, practitioners can provide families with specialist advice and effective intervention where necessary, thus enhancing the overall care of neonates with various skin lesions.

12.2.5. Role of Pediatric Dermatologists in Diagnosis

Pediatric dermatologists play an important role in diagnosing and treating various skin conditions, particularly birthmarks, some of which can appear as diagnostic challenges in neonatal dermatology. Their high level of skill enables them to differentiate between benign lesions and harmful conditions, with timely and proper interventions. For instance, a proper analysis of skin lesions is important because the majority of common presentations like erythema toxicum and mongolian spots are benign, while others may reflect hidden dermatological disorders that need to be scrutinized and monitored, as in a study with 50.8% of hospitalized neonates presenting with cutaneous lesions (Eftekhari et al., 2023). Further, higher forms of diagnostic techniques, including molecular diagnostics and imaging technology, are valuable assets to pediatric dermatologists, which increase the degree through which they can identify complex conditions such as dermatofibrosarcoma protuberans (Cassalia et al., 2025). Such proficiency brings maximum outcomes for infants, illustrating the crucial role of their professional contribution toward primary diagnosis and effective management of neonatal dermatological disorders (Figure 12.9).

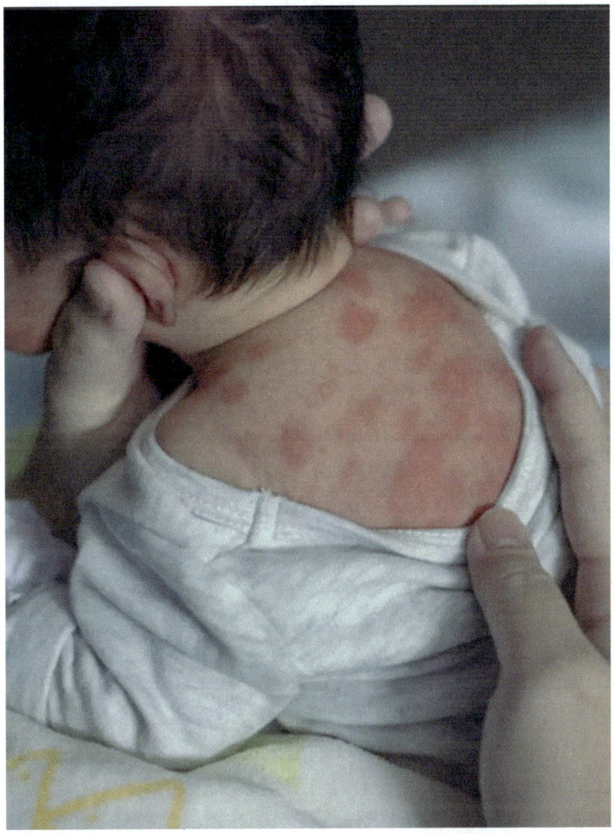

Figure 12.9. Diligent evaluation of skin lesions is vital, as many common manifestations like erythema toxicum and Mongolian spots are often benign.

Source: https://cdn2.momjunction.com/wp-content/uploads/2021/06/Erythema-Toxicum-In-Newborns-Causes-Symptoms-And-Treatment-1.jpg.webp.

12.2.6. Common Diagnostic Tools and Methods

An accurate diagnosis of birthmarks and related conditions is imperative for appropriate management and treatment in neonatal dermatology. Professionals tend to employ a combination of clinical observation and advanced diagnostic tools to differentiate among various dermatoses. For instance, differentiation of rare tumors such as dermatofibrosarcoma protuberans (DFSP) from common benign lesions such as hemangiomas largely relies on histopathological examination and molecular techniques, i.e., fluorescence *in situ* hybridization (FISH) to identify specific genetic markers (Cassalia et al., 2025). Similarly, while deciding the cutaneous manifestations of moyamoya angiopathy, doctors should examine skin manifestations such as café-au-lait spots and hypomelanosis cautiously with careful observation supplemented by imaging modalities as appropriate (Mitri et al., 2021). This kind of a multidisciplinary diagnostic approach not only enhances the precision in detection but also guides the following therapeutic interventions, which is the reason for incorporating a variety of techniques in neonatal dermatology.

12.2.7. Challenges in Diagnosing Skin Conditions in Neonates

Diagnosis of neonatal skin diseases presents a unique challenge, and this makes clinical evaluation difficult. Neonatal skin is soft in texture and shows dynamic changes during the first few weeks of life, with no clear delineation between benign and pathological states. For instance, entities such as dermatofibrosarcoma protuberans (DFSP) can mimic other benign lesions and be late misdiagnosed and treated; novel sophisticated molecular techniques have been proposed to assist in the accurate identification (Cassalia et al., 2025). In the same way, infantile hemangiomas, the most common vascular anomaly of infancy, can present with complicated inheritance patterns and varied presentations among themselves, further complicating diagnosis. These nuances underscore the necessity for a comprehensive and interdisciplinary assessment of neonatal skin as timely and precise diagnoses take top priority in effective treatment and best outcomes for this vulnerable population (Figure 12.10).

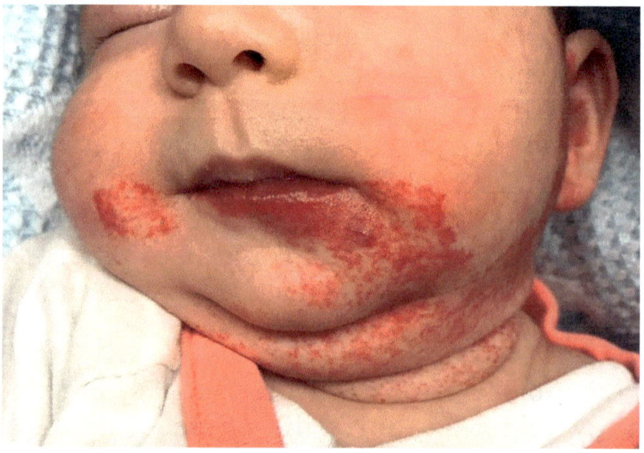

Figure 12.10. Infantile hemangiomas, the most common vascular anomaly of infancy, can exhibit complex inheritance patterns and varying presentations that further obscure diagnosis.

Source: https://www.derm.theclinics.com/cms/10.1016/j.det.2022.06.004/asset/2521628b-7667-4e57-8b08-707f705174cc/main.assets/gr3_lrg.jpg.

12.2.8. Importance of Early Diagnosis for Treatment Outcomes

Early diagnosis is also of great importance in the treatment outcome of neonatal skin diseases, particularly of birthmarks such as lymphatic malformations (LMs). The possibility of early detection of such conditions facilitates performing procedures that significantly minimize the complications of airway compression and chronic infection (Ghaffarpour, 2018). In addition, it provides parents with an opportunity to engage in a multidisciplinary treatment plan, eliminating their uncertainty and enhancing their decision-making efficiency towards treatments (Kerr, 2014). Because LMs can lead to both aesthetic and psychological effects, an early diagnostic intervention is necessary not only to gain the best clinical outcomes but also to ensure the child's general well-being. Early resolution of such complications supports the development of an effective management plan, which ultimately leads to improved long-term quality of life in affected infants and families. Early diagnosis as a priority thus remains important in the achievement of favorable therapeutic results in neonatal dermatology.

Test Your Knowledge

1. How is the diagnosis of neurocutaneous syndromes made in the presence of pigmented birthmarks?
2. What is the role of dermoscopy in assessing birthmarks?

12.3. Treatment Options

Learning Outcome

1. Understand Observation and Monitoring of Benign Birthmarks;
2. Explain Medical Treatments for Problematic Birthmarks;
3. Focus on Surgical Interventions for Severe Cases;
4. Describe Laser Therapy for Vascular Birthmarks;
5. Learn Topical Treatments for Pigmented Birthmarks;
6. Discuss Role of Pediatricians in Treatment Planning;
7. Know Parental Education on Treatment Options;
8. Understand Ethical Considerations in Treating Birthmarks;
9. Explain Long-term Outcomes of Various Treatment Approaches.

Neonatal skin disorders, particularly birthmarks, necessitate an advanced understanding of the etiology as well as the variations in treatment modalities available because these can significantly impact outcomes for affected infants. The treatment decision would generally be based on the nature and magnitude of the birthmark; vascular hamartomas, for instance, would require close monitoring or treatment depending on their growth pattern as well as comorbidities with it, as shown by the research on an association with preterm deliveries (Conn, 2025). Also, benign neonatal skin findings such as erythema toxicum and milia typically resolve on their own and are managed with nontraumatic skin care practices, highlighted by the importance of reassurance for parents. In more persistent cases, therapeutic interventions may include laser therapy or surgery in later infancy. Most of all, the promotion of an effective working relationship between caregivers, dermatologists, and healthcare providers provides the optimal treatment modalities that are appropriate to each individual newborn's unique needs.

12.3.1. Observation and Monitoring of Benign Birthmarks

Monitoring and observation of benign birthmarks are critical in neonatal dermatology to facilitate optimal management and intervention. Most benign birthmarks, such as café-au-lait macules and nevus simplex, are benign and not the subject of any required immediate treatment. Follow-up will allow monitoring of size change, color change, and change in texture, which will require further evaluation or interventions. For instance, while others occur spontaneously, some, such as enlarging hemangiomas, may need to be followed more closely since they may be problematic if not managed correctly. Research highlights the importance of conservative management and the encouragement of simple observation rather than radical removal for particular congenital lesions, such as in the suggested management of epidermal choristoma (Hughes et al., 2021). Besides, advances in laser therapy have been promising in the treatment of some birthmarks while emphasizing the need for constant observation, particularly for infantile hemangiomas (Shi et al., 2024) (Figure 12.11).

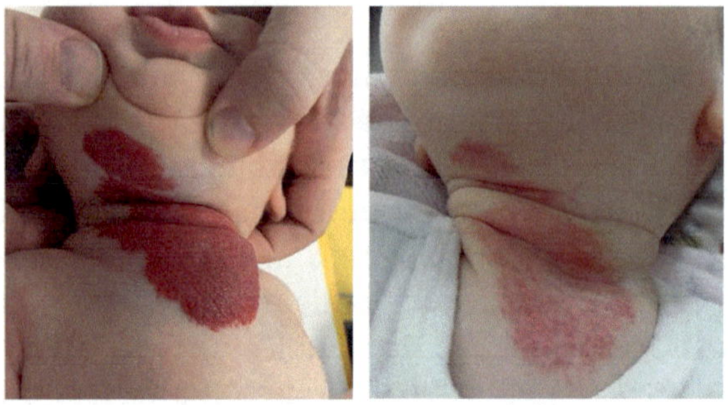

(a) (b)

Figure 12.11. Routine examinations allow for the assessment of changes in size, color, and texture, which can indicate the necessity for further evaluation or interventions.

Source: https://pub.mdpi-res.com/children/children-11-01397/article_deploy/html/images/children-11-01397-g001.png?1731947377.

12.3.2. Medical Treatments for Problematic Birthmarks

The management of problematic birthmarks in the newborn requires sufficient knowledge of their types and the variety of medical interventions. Some birthmarks, such as hemangiomas, may have to be treated due to their complex nature and cosmetic concerns. Therapies may vary from observation in small, non-troublesome lesions to drug treatment, with the use of drugs such as beta-blockers, such as propranolol, which have been proven to be very effective in reducing the size of hemangiomas. In more serious instances, surgical treatment might be necessary, especially in cases of vascular birthmarks that prove resistant to medication. It is essential that healthcare professionals, such as childbirth educators, provide information regarding the monitoring of these conditions, since early treatment is often more successful. Education and reassurance of caregivers are also essential in managing the psychological impact of these skin diseases on the neonate and caregivers alike.

12.3.3. Surgical Interventions for Severe Cases

Severe cases of neonatal dermatological disease are often treated using surgical treatments, particularly if non-surgical methods fail.

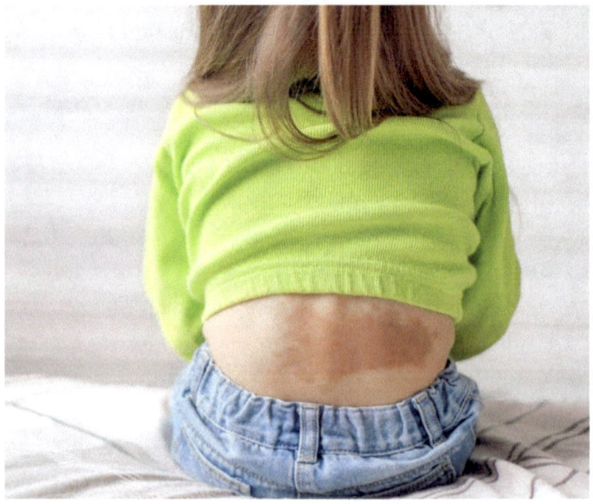

Figure 12.12. Surgical procedures may be employed for a range of birthmarks and vascular anomalies, including hemangiomas and other malformations that could lead to complications, such as ulceration or functional impairment.

Source: https://ysm-res.cloudinary.com/image/upload/c_fill,f_auto,g_faces:auto,h_960,q_auto,w_1280/v1/yms/prod/8f5f046d-7c04-4091-a712-a828d0462fe1.

Surgical treatment can be used for a range of birthmarks and vascular lesions, including hemangiomas and other malformations that can progress to complications, like ulceration or functional deficit. In fact, approximately 1 in 40 newborns are born with some form of major malformation, including complex syndromes requiring urgent medical intervention in an effort to offer the optimum possibilities for the infant (Vlădăreanu et al., 2017). In the treatment of infantile hemangiomas, considerable precaution is taken in balancing the risk and benefit of surgical excision, especially in those cases for which histories of complications of sclerotherapy are available. An interdisciplinary team environment is therefore essential to provide conjoint care and guarded decision-making inasmuch as surgical procedures are involved and are performed in the best interest of the neonate (Figure 12.12).

12.3.4. Laser Therapy for Vascular Birthmarks

Laser therapy has emerged as a key intervention in the treatment of vascular birthmarks, port-wine stains, and infantile hemangiomas in neonatal dermatology. Such conditions, normally a source of worry to new mothers and fathers, must be well taken care of to avoid occurrence and the consequent psychological effect. Pulsed dye laser therapy, now since 1999 widely available in most health centers, has been specifically emphasized for its capability to remove vascular lesions, as it specifically targets the hemoglobin of these abnormal vessels for destruction with minimal destruction of surrounding tissue (Boffa, 2001). Moreover, systematic reviews indicate that laser treatment in the early stages is shown to significantly enhance the effects of infantile hemangiomas by reducing their redness and surface area effectively in all skin types (Kendrick, 2025). Therefore, laser therapy is a significant advancement in the therapeutic management of vascular birthmarks, having clinical efficacy in addition to positive psychosocial properties for worried families.

12.3.5. Topical Treatments for Pigmented Birthmarks

Topical drugs for pigmented birthmarks represent a precious advancement in therapy for these common skin lesions of the newborn.

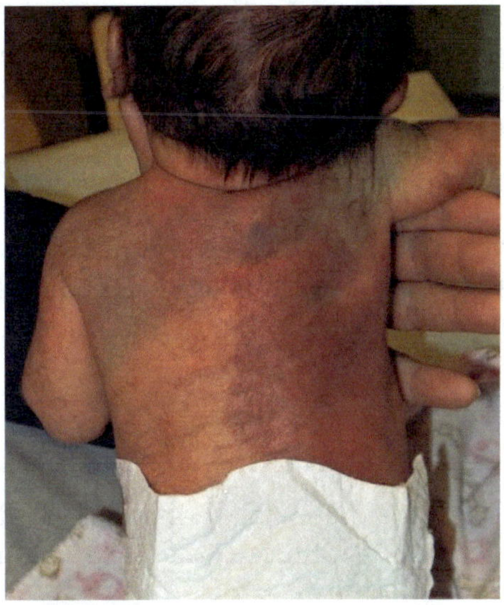

Figure 12.13. Topical treatments for pigmented birthmarks represent a significant advancement in the management of these common dermatological conditions in neonates.

Source: https://media.springernature.com/lw685/springer-static/image/chp%3A10.1007%2F978-3-319-45134-3_25-1/MediaObjects/393492_0_En_25-1_Fig90_HTML.jpg.

Hydroquinone and retinoids are two of the medications utilized to whiten the pigmented lesions through inhibition of melanin production and stimulation of the turnover of skin cells. Although these medications might have positive results, their administration must be approached cautiously since neonatal skin is very fragile and susceptible to complications and irritation. New modalities are also brought in, such as laser therapies, which have been proposed for the use in more resistant birthmarks, with the pulsed dye laser being of benefit for treating vascular lesions like port-wine stains, with the same clinical challenges (Boffa, 2001). Generally, treatment selection should be informed primarily by concerns about safety and efficacy, such that the intervention undertaken is commensurate with the individual needs of the neonate and addresses parental anxiety regarding skin irregularities (Figure 12.13).

12.3.6. Role of Pediatricians in Treatment Planning

Pediatricians will have an essential role to fulfill in neonatal dermatology with regard to skin treatment planning, particularly when it involves multiple birthmarks and related skin conditions. They are not limited to merely diagnosing the lesions; they are engaged in creating integrated management plans that weigh both the developmental and medical interests of the infant. In congenital vascular malformations, early diagnosis and characterization by imaging and clinical evaluation allow the pediatrician to separate lesions that are not needed from lesions that require treatment, generally taking on a multidisciplinary approach for the best outcome (Fiore et al., 2024). Furthermore, in cases like dermatofibrosarcoma protuberans, pediatricians' capacity to detect minimal clinical signs is crucial since misdiagnosis has the potential to cause significant treatment delay (Cassalia et al., 2025). Pediatricians are thus not just early caregivers but also central care coordinators, delivering timely and effective treatment planning for newborns with dermatological conditions.

12.3.7. Parental Education on Treatment Options

In the context of neonatal dermatology and more generally birthmarks such as infantile hemangiomas, it is important to educate the parents on treatment options.

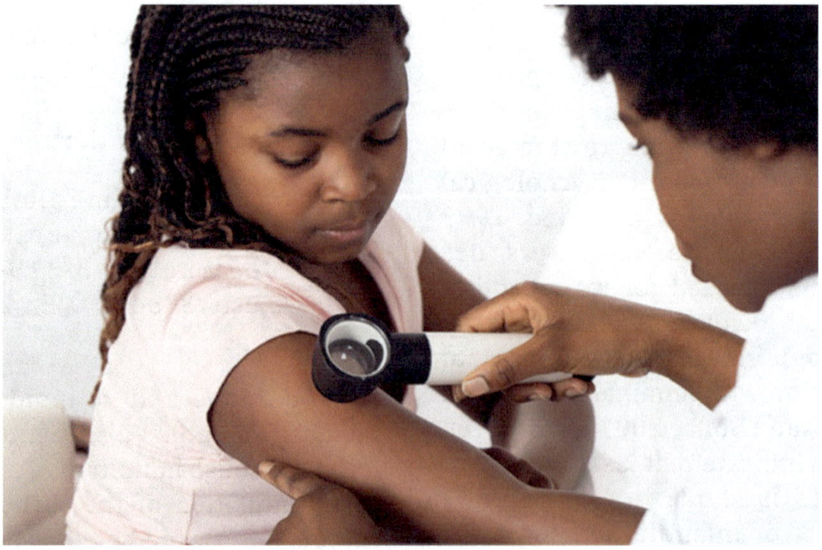

Figure 12.14. Parents frequently experience anxiety upon learning about these benign tumors, necessitating clear and comprehensive communication from clinicians.

Source: https://www.thedermspecs.com/wp-content/uploads/2013/04/pediatric-derm.png.

Parents become anxious upon learning about these benign neoplasms, and therefore, clear and comprehensive communication from doctors is required. Parent education includes not only the demarcation of the nature and pattern of development of hemangiomas but also the explanation of treatment possibilities, such as laser treatment, with proof of positive outcomes in eradicating superficial hemangiomas (Kendrick, 2025). The processing of ambiguity is also very important; parents tend to weigh all the information and are left having to make informed decisions amidst the complexity of their child. Engaging parents in treatment planning not only empowers them to take care of these problems but also fosters a culture of support that avoids the sensation of being overwhelmed (Kerr, 2014). Therefore, brilliant parental education ends up enhancing decision-making ability and building confidence in managing their child's dermatological problems (Figure 12.14).

12.3.8. Ethical Considerations in Treating Birthmarks

Birthmark treatment in the newborn is a significant ethical problem that must be resolved to bring about well-being in concerned infants and their families. Therefore, the primary issue for healthcare providers is how to treat surgically or in a less invasive fashion, i.e., by sclerotherapy, especially in lymphatic malformations, and which may lead to both physical as well as psychological complications in the child and family (Ghaffarpour, 2018). The ethical standard of beneficence requires that interventions be designed to serve the child's best interests, while minimizing risks for treatment-complication-related harm. Secondarily, parents' autonomy must be upheld in decision-making, although treatment options and the visibility of some birthmarks make it difficult for them to make informed decisions. Hence, an overall ethical guideline is essential in guiding practitioners when handling the diverse implications of neonatal birthmark treatment.

12.3.9. Long-term Outcomes of Various Treatment Approaches

Treatment of neonatal dermatoses, particularly birthmarks, calls for careful consideration regarding the long-term consequences of various treatment modalities.

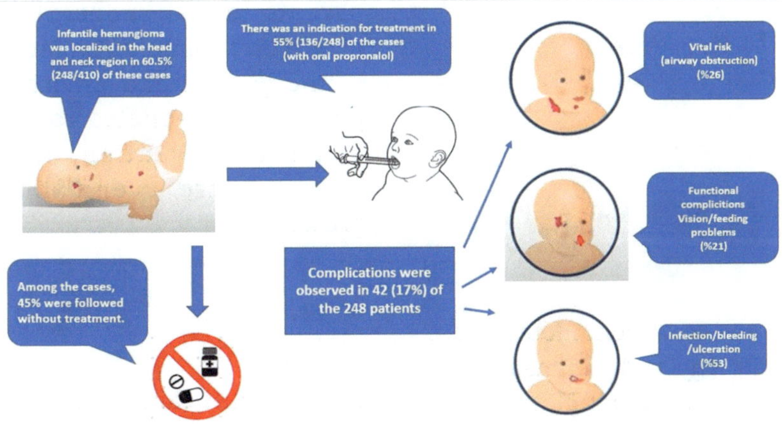

Figure 12.15. Infantile hemangiomas, prevalent among neonates, often undergo spontaneous regression, leading many clinicians to opt for a watchful waiting strategy.

Source: https://pub.mdpi-res.com/children/children-11-00311/article_deploy/html/images/children-11-00311-ag.png?1709712513.

For instance, infantile hemangiomas are prevalent among neonates and are likely to spontaneously regress, such that many clinicians opt to use a watchful waiting strategy. But in cases where intervention is warranted, modalities such as laser therapy have been reported to have promising results. Studies have indicated that early laser treatment was able to significantly reduce the size and pigmentation of superficial hemangiomas, resulting in better cosmetic outcomes in patients (Kendrick et al. 2025). However, surgical treatment is critical in the management of tumors like dermatofibrosarcoma protuberans, for which extensive resection should be carried out to decrease the rate of recurrence and achieve satisfactory functional and aesthetic results in the long run (Cassalia et al., 2025). Evaluating the efficacy of such treatments is also crucial since their long-term consequences have a substantial effect on the social and psychological well-being of children as they develop (Figure 12.15).

Test Your Knowledge

1. What are the indications for laser therapy in port-wine stains?
2. How does oral propranolol work in the treatment of infantile hemangiomas?

12.4. Prevention and Care

Learning Outcome

1. Understand Importance of Skin Care in Newborns;
2. Explain Preventive Measures for Skin Conditions;
3. Focus on the Role of Nutrition in Skin Health;
4. Describe Educating Parents on Skin Monitoring;
5. Learn Recognizing Signs of Skin Infections;
6. Discuss the Importance of Regular Pediatric Check-ups;
7. Know Cultural Perceptions of Birthmarks and Skin Care;
8. Understand Community Resources for Skin Health Education.

Successful prevention and treatment methods are key in neonatal dermatology to the management of skin conditions such as hemangiomas, the most common benign infantile tumors. The understanding of their pathophysiology reveals that excessive overexpression of angiogenesis drives them, and thus, therapeutic interventions targeting this process would significantly improve outcomes. Therapeutic interventions presently available, from observation to medical therapy, demand careful handling due to side effects, pointing towards the need for individualized care plans in such affected babies (Mabeta & Pepper, 2011). Given the usual phases of hemangiomas—proliferative, quiescent, and involuting—it is crucial for health professionals to observe these lesions carefully and alert parents to the spontaneous fading normally observed (Tom, 2011). Moreover, the discovery of the genetic and environmental factors that predispose neonates to such birthmarks will enhance prevention and facilitate overall neonatal care, eventually leading to healthy growth.

12.4.1. Importance of Skin Care in Newborns

Correct skin care in newborns is important in ensuring both their immediate comfort and long-term health, especially when viewed in the context of neonatal dermatology. Newborns possess sensitive and delicate skin that still remains highly predisposed to a range of dermatoses, including illnesses like erythema toxicum and milia, that can frequently arise during the first weeks of life. It has been proven through research that nearly 87.3% of neonates demonstrate some form of skin condition at this stage, which indicates the necessity of proper skin care practices (Eftekhari et al., 2023). Proper skin care not only avoids common conditions like diaper dermatitis and cutis marmorata but also contributes significantly towards early identification of more serious skin diseases that may develop (Eftekhari et al., 2023). With the high incidence of such benign yet alarming changes, caregivers need to be instructed on optimum skin care methods to ensure healthy skin and prevent possible complications in their newborns (Figure 12.16).

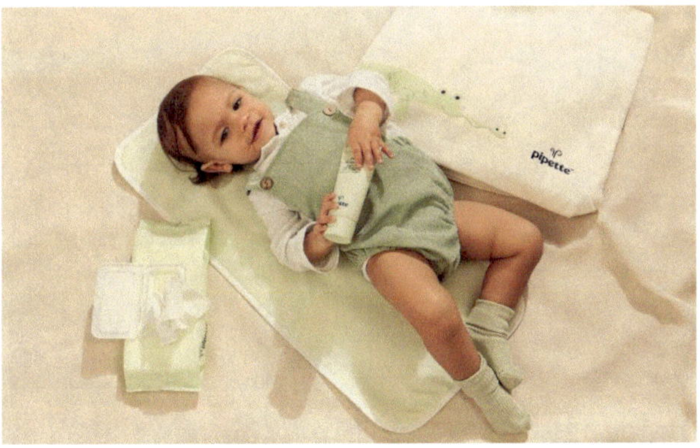

Figure 12.16. Effective skin care in newborns is paramount for ensuring both their immediate comfort and long-term health, specifically within the context of neonatal dermatology.

Source: https://www.pipettebaby.com/cdn/shop/articles/The_Complete_Guide_to_Baby_Skin_Care_27de2b27-c7ab-4fd6-8f5d-ce7c7384669e.jpg?v=1739984506.

12.4.2. Preventive Measures for Skin Conditions

Preventive treatment for neonatal skin diseases is essential in maintaining healthy skin growth and avoiding long-term dermatological complications. Early diagnosis and treatment are imperative, most particularly in addressing common skin conditions such as neonatal jaundice, whose lack of treatment can have fatal repercussions. Interventions such as the application of low-cost mHealth solutions, for example, smartphone applications for screening jaundice, have proven to effectively improve early detection and monitoring and thus provide support in various healthcare settings (Díaz, 2019). Additionally, parent education on frequent dermatological manifestations, combined with proper skincare practices, is able to substantially lower the frequency of environmental factor- and infection-induced skin lesions (Mahajan, 2019). Through targeted preventive measures and increased diagnostic access, healthcare providers can better meet newborns' dermatological needs, ultimately improving overall well-being and quality of life for these vulnerable populations.

12.4.3. Role of Nutrition in Skin Health

Skin, the largest organ of the body, plays a vital role in protecting against environmental stressors, and nutrition plays an enormous role in its health. Good nutrition is what supplies the necessary vitamins and minerals important in sustaining skin integrity and function. For neonates, good maternal nutrition during pregnancy is essential since a deficiency can cause different manifestations of the skin in newborns, such as birthmarks and dermatoses. Specifically, studies identify that maternal smoking may be associated with an increased incidence of certain neonatal skin conditions, such as salmon patches and neonatal erythema, which have been linked to nutrition deficiencies. Moreover, the immunological bases of skin health, particularly in diseases like lymphatic malformations and lymphangiomas, may be aggravated by improper nutrition, paving the way for infections and inflammation (Ghaffarpour, 2018). Thus, nutritional optimization is essential to ensuring healthy neonatal skin development and the prevention of dermatological complications (Figure 12.17).

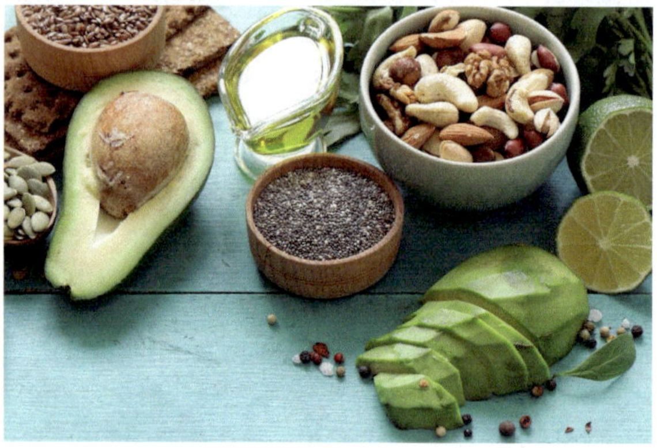

Figure 12.17. Proper nutrition provides essential vitamins and minerals, which are critical for maintaining skin integrity and function.

Source: https://i0.wp.com/cdn-prod.medicalnewstoday.com/content/images/articles/322/322986/high-fat-plant-foods-containing-omega-3-fatty-acids-including-olive-oil-avocado-nuts-and-seeds.jpg?w=1155&h=1558.

12.4.4. Educating Parents on Skin Monitoring

Excellent parent education on skin monitoring is essential within the context of neonatal dermatology, including the identification of birthmarks and other skin conditions. Well-informed parents regarding the appearance and growth of their child's skin can also be beneficial in early identification of potential problems, and hence improving outcomes. The education needs to include information about normal variability in skin and symptomatic signs that require professional evaluation. Research identifies that long-term conditions predominantly come about as a result of events during the perinatal period, thereby highlighting the significance of meticulous monitoring from birth (Simpson et al., 2018). Further, awareness of skin monitoring contributes to the minimization of parental anxiety regarding dermatological disorders and facilitates an increased proactive approach in seeking medical consultation when the same is needed (van Zuuren et al., 2017). By educating parents, health workers can facilitate the overall pattern of growth in children and improve the quality of life and health.

12.4.5. Recognizing Signs of Skin Infections

Identification of skin infections in the context of neonatal dermatology is crucial because infants have especially vulnerable immune systems.

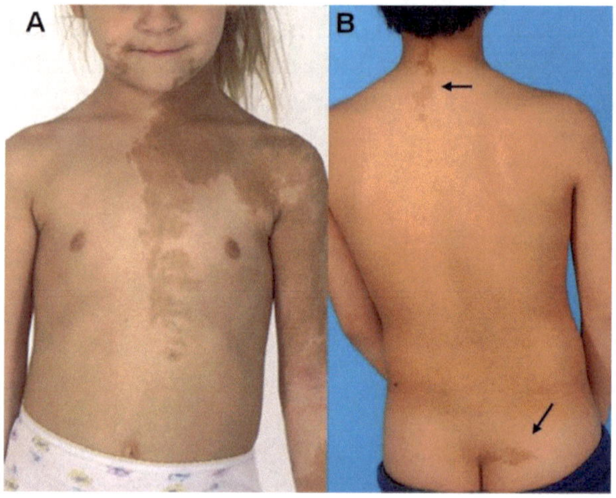

Figure 12.18. Care providers and parents must understand that certain dermatological manifestations, such as café-au-lait spots or hypomelanosis of Ito.

Source: https://media.springernature.com/lw1200/springer-static/image/art%3A10.1186%2F1750-1172-3-12/MediaObjects/13023_2007_Article_112_Fig1_HTML.jpg.

Early presentations often consist of abnormal redness, swelling, and warmth over localized areas, which may signal inflammation. Also, the presence of vesicles or pustules may suggest infection of greater severity, such as herpes simplex virus or impetigo. Along with these classic signs, the systemic manifestations of fever or lethargy may accompany skin manifestations and mandate immediate medical referral. Parents and caregivers should be aware that certain dermatological presentations, such as café-au-lait spots or hypomelanosis of Ito, may also present alongside systemic illness, thus complicating diagnosis and management (Mitri et al., 2021). Thus, a clear understanding of such manifestations can significantly enhance early treatment and diagnosis and subsequently neonatal outcome in high-risk populations (Díaz, 2019) (Figure 12.18).

12.4.6. Importance of Regular Pediatric Check-ups

Regular pediatric check-ups are essential for monitoring the overall well-being and development status of children and infants, especially during the pivotal early years when most dermatologic conditions, including birthmarks, will occur. Such routine checks enable medical doctors to diagnose issues at an early stage, which further facilitates timely intervention and improved future results. For instance, the identification of congenital skin conditions through such checks can prevent issues associated with certain birthmarks that should be further examined or treated. Also, there needs to be an understanding of the prevalence of chronic disorders and skin diseases in children to plan health services; this is exemplified by programs such as the one explained here, whereby data on chronic conditions are applied in informing health policies and practices tailored to the needs of children (Simpson et al., 2018). In this context, regular visits in pediatrics not only guarantee coverage for direct health but also enable a universal notion of childhood wellness (van Zuuren et al., 2017).

12.4.7. Cultural Perceptions of Birthmarks and Skin Care

Cultural attitudes towards skin care and birthmarks greatly influence how individuals treat skin, particularly in neonatal dermatology, where these flaws are treated with a response that varies between societies. In other societies, birthmarks can be of beauty or even symbols of uniqueness, but in others, they might be stigmatized and assigned negative connotations.

The difference in perception is what will dictate the parental attitude towards birthmarks during infancy, and have an emotional impact on both the caregiver and the child. For instance, as parents navigate the complexities of caring for a child with marks evidence, they might experience uncertainty and worry related to societal expectations and opinions (Kerr, 2014). Moreover, perceptions of neonatal skin trauma, as explained by mixed methods studies, illustrate that such perceptions could prevent best care, justifying culturally sensitive practices in pediatric dermatology (August, 2022). Lastly, an aware understanding of cultural contexts surrounding birthmarks is essential for effective skin care management and parental nurturing.

12.4.8. Community Resources for Skin Health Education

Community resources used for skin health education are significant in enabling parents and caregivers to learn about neonatal dermatology, which includes birthmarks and skin conditions. Such resources can be in the form of workshops, internet forums, and community health interventions that provide important information on identification and care for newborn common skin ailments.

For instance, training sessions can call attention to early disease identification, such as neonatal jaundice, which, if left without care, can have severe consequences like bilirubin encephalopathy (Díaz, 2019). Similarly, comprehensive programs of awareness can ensure that parents can identify and control resultant skin damage disproportionately affecting neonates based on research detailing their unique risks (August, 2022). Through these community efforts, caregivers can be enabled to maximize health surveillance and upkeep of healthy skin in the infant, thereby leading to improved outcomes among the vulnerable population (Figure 12.19).

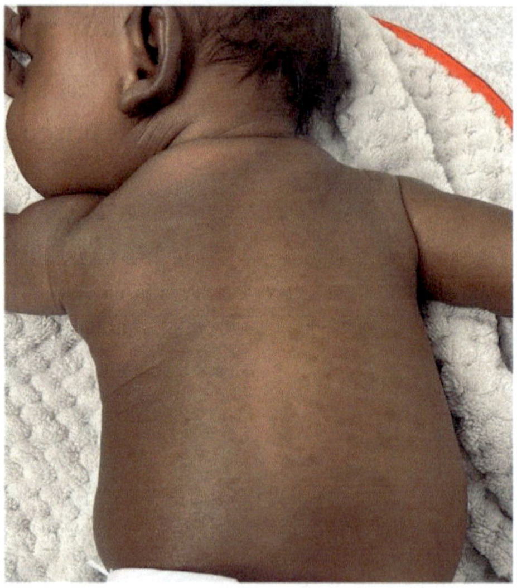

Figure 12.19. Community resources for skin health education play a critical role in assisting parents and caregivers in understanding neonatal dermatology, particularly in relation to birthmarks and skin conditions.

Source: https://www.derm.theclinics.com/cms/10.1016/j.det.2023.02.014/asset/dcef375e-441d-489e-9abf-5c85f940c6cd/main.assets/gr1_lrg.jpg.

Test Your Knowledge

1. What education is important for families regarding the natural history of hemangiomas?
2. What role do support groups or counseling play in the care of visible birthmarks?

SUMMARY

The study of neonatal dermatology and birthmarks shows valuable data regarding the presentation of the skin that is typical in neonates, with particular emphasis on how to differentiate transient from pathological skin conditions. Research indicates that muco-cutaneous manifestations such as Mongolian spots are very common, being found in a large percentage of infants, for example, 91.3% of Mongolian children based on new studies (Batbaatar et al., 2017). The majority of such skin lesions are benign and require no medical care, their recognition at an early stage and understanding among healthcare providers as well as parents is extremely important (Kurian et al., 2025). Not only does it enable proper management, but it also assuages the fears of parents regarding potential skin problems in their neonates. Overall, research progress in this field is necessary as it only goes to enhance awareness and practice in the management of neonatal dermatology and, by extension, improve outcomes for babies all over the world.

Overall, research into neonatal dermatology and birthmarks yields precious information on the nature, prevalence, and management of skin lesions in infants. Most significant results indicate that congenital vascular malformations (CVMs) are more common, with simple venous malformations as their characteristic, which present in a high number of cases and are often accompanied by anomalies and findings like pain and soft tissue hypertrophy (Tuleja et al., 2023). Additionally, variability of dermatological conditions in children contributes to the need for extensive epidemiological studies, as illustrated by variations in the incidence of skin disorders depending on socio-economic and environmental determinants (Mahajan, 2019). Their tendency to resolve spontaneously without intervention is the leading consequence of emphasizing physiological and developmental skin disorders, which, without treatment, tend to resolve easily, thus emphasizing the importance of accurate diagnosis and monitoring. These points together emphasize the complexity of neonatal dermatology and the necessity for personalized interventions in the treatment of birthmarks and related skin issues.

KEY TERMS FROM THIS CHAPTER

- Birthmarks
- Cutaneous lesions
- Preterm birth
- Maternal health
- Erythema toxicum
- Port-wine stains
- Hemangiomas
- Strawberry marks
- Infancy
- Involution
- Dermatoses
- Vascular hamartomas
- Race
- Mongolian spots
- Neonatal examination
- Lymphatic malformations
- Neonatal dermatology
- Endothelial cells
- Growth phase
- Sclerotherapy

CRITICAL THINKING QUESTIONS

1. **Which of the following is a common, benign, self-limited pustular eruption seen in newborns?**
   a. Erythema toxicum neonatorum
   b. Seborrheic dermatitis
   c. Neonatal acne
   d. Impetigo
2. **A "salmon patch" or "stork bite" is most commonly seen on which area of a neonate's body?**
   a. Cheeks
   b. Nape of neck
   c. Abdomen
   d. Lower back
3. **Which of the following birthmarks typically fades with time and is considered benign?**
   a. Port-wine stain
   b. Mongolian spot
   c. Infantile hemangioma
   d. Café-au-lait macule
4. **Which vascular lesion is most likely to grow rapidly after birth and then involute over years?**
   a. Capillary malformation
   b. Port-wine stain
   c. Infantile hemangioma
   d. Congenital hemangioma
5. **Which of the following is associated with Sturge-Weber syndrome?**
   a. Mongolian spot
   b. Café-au-lait macules
   c. Port-wine stain involving the trigeminal area
   d. Salmon patch

Short Answer Questions

1. What are the two main categories of birthmarks?
2. What are the differences between vascular and pigmented birthmarks?
3. What clinical tools are used to assess and monitor birthmarks in infants?
4. How do you differentiate between hemangioma and vascular malformation?
5. What is the first-line treatment for proliferating infantile hemangiomas?
6. How are large congenital melanocytic nevi managed?
7. Can birthmarks be prevented?
8. What guidance should be given to parents about sun protection in children with pigmented lesions?

Answers to Critical Thinking Questions

1. (a); 2. (b); 3. (b); 4. (c); 5. (c)

REFERENCES

1. Simpson, J., Duncanson, M., Oben, G., Adams, J., Wicken, A., Morris, S., & Gallagher, S. (2018). The Health of Children and Young People with Chronic Conditions and Disabilities in New Zealand 2016 (, Ill.). New Zealand Child and Youth Epidemiology Service. https://ourarchive.otago.ac.nz/esploro/outputs/report/The-Health-of-Children-and-Young/9926479990401891#file-0(accessed on 23rd July 2025).
2. Tuleja, A., Bernhard, S., Hamvas, G., Andreoti, T. A., Rössler, J., Boon, L., Vikkula, M., Kammer, R., Haupt, F., Döring, Y., & Baumgartner, I. (2023). Clinical phenotype of adolescent and adult patients with extracranial vascular malformation. *Journal of vascular surgery. Venous and lymphatic disorders*, *11*(5), 1034–1044.e3. https://doi.org/10.1016/j.jvsv.2023.03.012(accessed on 23rd July 2025).
3. van Zuuren, E. J., Fedorowicz, Z., Christensen, R., Lavrijsen, A., & Arents, B. W. M. (2017). Emollients and moisturisers for eczema. *The Cochrane database of systematic reviews*, *2*(2), CD012119. https://doi.org/10.1002/14651858.CD012119.pub2(accessed on 23rd July 2025).
4. August, D. L. (2022). *Neonatal Skin Injuries from Mechanical Forces: A Multicenter, Mixed Methods Study*. https://core.ac.uk/download/542341107.pdf (accessed on 23rd July 2025).
5. Batbaatar, S., Sharkhuu, M., Badrakh, B., Sonom, D., Altangerel, G., et al. (2017). Prevalence of Blue Spot among Mongolian Newborn Infants. Central Asian Journal of Medical Sciences. https://doi.org/10.24079/CAJMS.2017.11.007(accessed on 23rd July 2025).
6. Cassalia, F., Danese, A., Cocchi, E., Vaienti, S., Bolzon, A., Franceschin, L., Mazzetto, R., Caroppo, F., Melandri, D., & Belloni Fortina, A. (2025). Congenital Dermatofibrosarcoma Protuberans-An Update on the Ongoing Diagnostic Challenges. *Cancers*, *17*(1), 158. https://doi.org/10.3390/cancers17010158(accessed on 23rd July 2025).
7. Vlădăreanu, S., Boț, M., Berceanu, C., Mehedințu, C., & Popescu, S. (2018). The Neonate with Minor Dysmorphisms. InTech. doi: 10.5772/intechopen.71902 (accessed on 23rd July 2025).
8. Mitri, F., Bersano, A., Hervé, D., & Kraemer, M. (2021). Cutaneous manifestations in Moyamoya angiopathy: A review. *European journal of neurology*, *28*(5), 1784–1793. https://doi.org/10.1111/ene.14754(accessed on 23rd July 2025).
9. Boffa, M. J. (2001). Laser treatment of Port-wine stains. https://core.ac.uk/download/93183910.pdf (accessed on 23rd July 2025).
10. Fiore, M., Bortoli, M., Sambri, A., Lotrecchiano, L., Lovato, L., Mirelli, M., Neri, I., De Paolis, M., Piraccini, B. M., & Gargiulo, M. (2024). Soft Tissue Vascular Anomalies of the Extremities: A Proposed Diagnostic Approach. *Life (Basel, Switzerland)*, *14*(6), 670. https://doi.org/10.3390/life14060670(accessed on 23rd July 2025).
11. Conn, M. (2025). Identification of demographics and comorbidities associated with vascular hamartomas. https://core.ac.uk/download/62785131.pdf (accessed on 23rd July 2025).
12. de Leeuw, J. (J.). (2009). *Innovative Use of Pulsed Dye Laser and Liposomes in Dermatology*. https://core.ac.uk/download/18511518.pdf (accessed on 23rd July 2025).
13. Hughes, C., Ferro, A., Dubb, S., Gass, J., Hook, L., Santhanam, V., Kinsler, V., & Polubothu, S. (2021). Epidermal choristoma: a case series and review of the literature. *Pediatric dermatology*, *38*(5), 1243–1246. https://doi.org/10.1111/pde.14589(accessed on 23rd July 2025).

14. Eftekhari, H., Mahdipour, S., Masoudi, H., Poorsaravani, M., Gharibzadeh, S., et al. (2023). Investigating the frequency of skin manifestation in newborns admitted to a children's hospital in the north of Iran. https://core.ac.uk/download/568483289.pdf (accessed on 23rd July 2025).

15. Shi, W., Jin, L., Xu, A., Gao, Y., & Zhang, N. (2024). Timing and Efficacy Evaluation of 755-nm Long Pulse Alexandrite Laser and 2% Carteolol Hydrochloride Eye Drops Co-Treatment for Thicker Superficial Infantile Hemangioma. *Clinical, cosmetic and investigational dermatology*, *17*, 2009–2019. https://doi.org/10.2147/CCID.S483141(accessed on 23rd July 2025).

16. Ghaffarpour, N. (2018). *Treatment Aspects, Prognostic Factors and Outcome Measures of Lymphatic Malformations*. https://core.ac.uk/download/154171838.pdf (accessed on 23rd July 2025).

17. Jiménez Díaz, G. (2019). Validation of a new smartphone app to assess neonatal jaundice in a Mexican population. https://core.ac.uk/download/646155275.pdf (accessed on 23rd July 2025).

18. Kendrick, R. P. (2025). Effectiveness of pulse dye laser versus no treatment in the treatment of infantile hemangiomas. https://core.ac.uk/download/pdf/48843945.pdf (accessed on 23rd July 2025).

19. Kerr, A. M. (2014). Communication during first-time multidisciplinary clinic visits: Navigating parental decision making and uncertainty management in pediatric chronic illness. https://core.ac.uk/download/232563066.pdf (accessed on 23rd July 2025).

20. Kurian, A., Patidar, R., Kumar, G. V., & Narendra, G. (2018). A clinical study to assess the patterns of muco-cutaneous changes in newborns during the first five days after birth. Indian Journal of Child Health, 5(4), 294-297. https://doi.org/10.32677/IJCH.2018.v05.i04.015(accessed on 23rd July 2025).

21. Marwah, P., Marwah, A., Kumar, S., & Kumar, R. (2018). Profile of neonatal dermatoses in a tertiary care teaching hospital of Haryana. *International Journal of Research in Medical Sciences*, *6*(3), 955–958. https://doi.org/10.18203/2320-6012.ijrms20180622(accessed on 23rd July 2025).

22. Lakshmi, S. V. (2010). A clinical study of hemangiomas and vascular malformations. https://core.ac.uk/download/235653886.pdf (accessed on 23rd July 2025).

23. Mabeta, P., & Pepper, M. S. (2011). Hemangiomas - current therapeutic strategies. *The International journal of developmental biology*, *55*(4-5), 431–437. https://doi.org/10.1387/ijdb.103221pm(accessed on 23rd July 2025).

24. Mahajan, S. S. (2019). Clinic-epidemiological profile of dermatological manifestations in preschool-going children in a tertiary health care center. https://core.ac.uk/download/235670531.pdf (accessed on 23rd July 2025).

25. Passas, M. A., & Teixeira, M. (2016). *Infantile Haemangioma*. https://core.ac.uk/download/71743534.pdf (accessed on 23rd July 2025).

26. Tom, L. (2011). Pericyte, neural crest and adipocyte differentiation markers: Support for a novel hypothesis for the origin of hemangiomas. https://core.ac.uk/download/232770130.pdf (accessed on 23rd July 2025).

INDEX

A

aberrant distribution 74, 92
acne 233, 237, 238, 239, 240, 241, 242, 243, 254, 255, 256, 257
adaptability 2, 5
aetiology 98, 111
age 2, 3, 10, 11, 21
airway obstruction 118
albinism 97, 98, 99, 100, 101, 102, 103, 104, 105, 106, 107, 108, 109, 110, 111, 112, 114
allergic rhinitis 234, 254
allergies 234, 252, 254
anticancer chemotherapy 4
antifungal activity 5, 24
antimicrobials 4, 5
antiparasitic drugs 28, 38
aorta 162, 164, 165, 176
appendages 3
arthralgia 142, 152
aspiration pneumonia 143, 144, 145, 151, 152
asthma 234, 247, 254, 256, 259
athlete's foot 2
atopic dermatitis 234, 235, 236, 237, 238, 241, 252, 253, 254, 255, 256, 257, 258, 259
autoantibodies 118, 119, 120, 123, 124, 125, 126, 128, 129, 130, 132, 135, 136, 142, 147, 148, 149, 150, 152, 153, 156, 159
autoimmune 97, 98, 99, 110, 111, 113
autoimmune diseases 117, 130, 134, 135
autoimmune hypothesis 98, 111
autoimmune illnesses 98, 111
autoimmune rheumatic diseases 141, 151, 156, 159
awareness 234, 242, 251, 252, 254
Ayurveda 98

B

bacillus Calmette-Guérin (BCG) vaccine 49, 68
bacterium 48, 53, 55, 69
BCG vaccination 48
benign 233, 244, 251, 252, 254
biofilm production 2
biomarkers 142, 148
birthmarks 261, 262, 263, 264, 265, 266, 267, 268, 269, 270, 271, 272, 273, 274, 275, 276, 277, 278, 279, 280, 281, 282
bisphosphonates 5
blindness 118
blistering 213, 218, 219, 221, 227
blisters 117, 118, 119, 120, 122, 123, 124, 128, 134, 135
blood vessels 161, 162, 165, 166, 167, 168, 170, 180
bullae 117, 119, 120, 126, 127, 135
bullous pemphigoid 117, 119, 120, 121, 122, 123, 124, 125, 126, 127, 128, 129, 130, 131, 132, 133, 134, 135, 136, 137

C

café-au-lait spots 263, 264, 270, 278, 279
Candida albicans 7, 13, 15, 18, 21
Candida auris 4
Candida species 2, 7, 15, 16
cell adhesion 118, 119, 123, 135
cell density 2, 16
cellular integrity 118
chemicals 143
chronic cough 188, 193, 207
clinicians 1, 3
coinfection 48, 50, 68
colossal 74, 92
complications 161, 162, 163, 164, 165, 170, 174, 175, 176, 177, 178, 179, 180
concomitant disorders 187, 207
congenital nevi 263
connective tissue diseases 141, 142, 143, 144, 145, 146, 147, 148, 149, 150, 152, 153, 154, 155, 156, 158, 159, 160
cosmetic problem 74, 92
counseling 235, 238, 252, 254
COVID-19 pandemic 161, 180
crisaborole ointment 236, 253, 254
Crohn's disease 187, 190, 196, 197, 207, 211
cryoglobulinaemia 163, 172, 177
Cryptococcus neoformans 7
culture 4, 8, 17, 19
cutaneous lesions 261, 269, 281
cutaneous microbes 48
cutaneous tuberculosis 47, 48, 50, 51, 54, 55, 56, 57, 58, 59, 60, 61, 62, 63, 64, 65, 66, 68, 69, 72
cyclophosphamide 162, 177, 178, 180

D

deep mycoses 1, 2, 4, 6, 7, 8, 9, 10, 12, 13, 15, 16, 17, 18, 20, 25
depigmentation 97, 98, 99, 100, 101, 103, 104, 105, 106, 108, 109, 110, 111, 113
depigmented skin 97, 103, 111
dermatological disorders 75
dermatology 73, 74, 76, 78, 91, 92, 94, 95
dermatomyositis 141, 143, 144, 145, 146, 147, 148, 149, 150, 151, 152, 153, 154, 155, 156, 157, 158, 159
dermatophytes 2, 3, 4, 5, 9, 10, 11, 19, 24
dermatoses 261, 268, 270, 275, 277, 281, 284
desmogleins 118, 135
desmosomes 118
detergents 235, 254
diabetes mellitus 4
diagnosis 2, 3, 4, 6, 7, 8, 14, 18, 19, 20, 22, 23
direct microscopy 4
disease 1, 6, 7, 8, 9, 10, 15, 16, 19, 20, 21, 24
distress 142
drug reactions 161, 172, 180
drug resistance 5, 6, 22
dysphagia 142, 143, 144, 145, 151, 152, 153, 156
dysregulation 75, 79

E

ecological determinants 1
eczema 233, 234, 235, 236, 237, 238, 240, 246, 248, 249, 253, 254, 255, 256, 257, 258, 259
endogenous 74, 92
endothelial cells 262, 281
environmental exposure 2
environmental niches 47, 68
epidemiological factors 2
epidemiology 47, 68, 70
epidermal adhesion 117, 135
epidermis 118, 119, 120, 123, 135
epidermolysis bullosa 213, 215, 216, 217, 219, 220, 221, 222, 223, 224, 225, 226, 227, 228
epidermolysis bullosa (EB) 213, 219, 220, 221, 224, 227
erythema nodosum 188, 191, 192, 193, 196, 197, 200, 202, 207
erythema toxicum 261, 269, 271, 277, 281
etiology 2
eumycetoma 1, 9
exacerbation 97, 111
exhumation 151
exogenous pigments 74, 92
extrinsic factors 73, 92
eye issues 97, 111

F

fatigue 142, 144, 146, 154
fever 4, 8
fluconazole 6, 8, 21, 22, 25
fungal growth 4, 10, 11
fungal infections 2, 4, 5, 6, 7, 8, 10, 11, 12, 13, 14, 17, 18, 19, 20
fungi 1, 2, 4, 5, 7, 8, 12, 14, 16, 17, 18, 19, 22, 24

G

gene mutations 213, 219, 227
genetic 97, 99, 100, 102, 103, 104, 105, 109, 111, 113, 114
genetic correction 214, 227
genetic disorder 97, 111
genetic model 189
genetic mutations 213, 214, 215, 218, 219, 221, 227
gestational diabetes 263
glomeruli 162, 180
glomerulonephritis 162, 163, 165, 168, 169, 170, 174, 175, 177, 178, 180, 183, 184
glucocorticoids 162, 169, 173, 180
granulomas 187, 188, 189, 190, 191, 198, 199, 200, 203, 207, 208
granulomatous lesions 49, 50, 72
granulomatous skin illnesses 187, 207
growth phase 262, 281

H

hair 2, 4, 6
health 233, 238, 239, 241, 242, 243, 244, 249, 250, 252, 253, 254
health authorities 28, 32, 42
healthcare 28, 29, 30, 32, 36, 40
health issues 1
hemangiomas 262, 264, 265, 266, 267, 268, 269, 270, 271, 272, 273, 274, 275, 276, 280, 281, 282, 284
Henoch-Schönlein purpura (HSP) 163, 167, 172, 173, 176, 185
hepatitis C 162, 163, 164, 165, 173, 175, 177, 182
heterogeneous group 117, 135
human health 27
human immunodeficiency virus (HIV) 4
hypercalcemia 188, 203, 207, 209
hyperpigmentation 73, 74, 75, 76, 77, 78, 79, 80, 81, 82, 83, 84, 85, 86, 87, 88, 89, 90, 91, 92, 93, 94
hypopigmentation disorders 97, 98, 100, 104, 106, 107, 109, 111

I

ichthyosis 213, 214, 215, 216, 217, 219, 220, 221, 222, 223, 224, 225, 226, 227, 228, 229, 230
Identify-Isolate-Inform (3I) Tool 28, 42
immune cells 188, 189, 190, 207
immune checkpoint inhibitors (ICPi) 161, 180
immunity 3, 7
immunocompromised hosts 189, 193, 201
immunosuppression 48, 49, 68
infancy 262, 269, 270, 271, 279, 281
infecting agents 1
infections 1, 2, 3, 4, 5, 6, 7, 8, 9, 10, 11, 12, 13, 14, 15, 16, 17, 18, 19, 20, 22, 23, 24, 25
inflammation 74, 75, 76, 78, 81, 83, 84, 91, 92
inflammatory 48, 49, 54, 55, 56, 72
innate immune system 47, 68
in situ 3
interleukin-6 (IL-6) 190
interstitial lung disease (ILD) 141, 144, 149, 153, 155, 156
intravenous (IV) fluconazole 7
involution 262, 269, 281
itching 4
ivermectin 27, 28, 30, 32, 34, 35, 38, 39, 40, 42, 44

K

keratinocyte differentiation 214, 227
kidney 162, 163, 168, 178, 180, 184
knowledge 1, 14, 16

L

Large vessel vasculitis (LVV) 162
leishmaniasis 27, 29, 30, 31, 34, 35, 36, 37, 38, 39, 40, 41, 42, 43
leprosy 47, 48, 49, 50, 51, 53, 54, 55, 56, 57, 58, 59, 60, 61, 62, 63, 64, 65, 66, 67, 68, 69, 70, 72

lesions 29, 30, 34, 38, 43
levamisole-adulterated cocaine 163, 172, 183, 185
lice 27, 29, 30, 31, 33, 34, 35, 36, 38, 39, 40, 42, 43
lifestyle 233, 237, 242, 254
lungs 188, 191, 192, 193, 200, 207
lupus 141, 142, 143, 144, 145, 146, 147, 148, 149, 150, 152, 153, 154, 155, 156, 157, 160
Lymphatic malformations 262, 281
lymphatic system 188, 207

M

macrophages 48, 50, 54, 68
Madurella mycetomatis 1, 7, 17
malaise 4
malnutrition 48, 68
maternal health 261, 281
medication 27, 37, 42
melanin 73, 74, 75, 76, 77, 79, 80, 83, 84, 85, 89, 90, 91, 92, 93
melanin synthesis 74, 85, 92
melanocyte density 74, 92
melanocytic nevi 262, 263, 282
melasma 73, 74, 75, 76, 77, 78, 79, 80, 81, 82, 84, 85, 86, 87, 88, 89, 90, 91, 92, 93, 95
microbial virulence 48, 53
Microsporum canis 3
mixed connective tissue disease (MCTD) 141, 156
molecular diagnostics 4
Mongolian spots 261, 263, 265, 269, 281
morbidity 7, 12, 13, 14, 17, 20
mortality 6, 7, 8, 12, 13, 14, 18, 20
mucosal lesions 118, 124, 134, 137
mucous membranes 1
mutualism 48
mycobacterial species 47, 68
Mycobacterium leprae 47, 53, 54, 55, 57, 58, 59, 60, 68, 69
Mycobacterium tuberculosis 47, 48, 49, 50, 51, 54, 57, 60, 68, 69

N

naevi 233, 254
nails 2, 3, 4, 6
neonatal dermatology 262, 263, 264, 265, 267, 268, 269, 270, 271, 273, 274, 276, 277, 278, 279, 280, 281
neonatal examination 261, 281
nephritis 142
nervous system 142
neurological impairment 142, 156
niche 4
nodules 50, 56, 61, 69
nomenclature 117, 135
non-dermatophytic molds 2
nonspecific symptoms 162
nutrient deprivation 2
nutritional status 142, 156

O

obsessive-compulsive disorder 233, 249, 254
onychomycosis 2, 4, 12, 17, 19, 21
organ ischemia 162
organisms 48, 54, 68
organ system 142, 145, 156

P

parasites 27, 28, 30, 33, 34, 35, 37, 38, 39, 40, 42, 43, 45
parasitic infections 28, 30, 34, 35, 36, 38, 44
parasitic infestations 27, 29, 30, 31, 33, 34, 35, 36, 38, 39, 40, 42
parasitic skin infections 27, 42
pathogenetics 98
pathogenicity 1, 4
pathogens 2, 3, 4, 5, 6, 7, 8, 10, 12, 13, 14, 15, 16, 18, 19, 20, 23, 25
patient history 4
patient management 97, 111
pediatric dermatology 233, 236, 238, 239, 240, 241, 243, 244, 246, 247, 249, 250, 252, 254, 257, 258, 259
pemphigus 117, 118, 119, 120, 121, 122, 123, 124, 125, 126, 127, 128, 129, 130, 131, 132, 133, 134, 135, 136, 137, 138, 139
pemphigus foliaceous 117, 118, 135
personal hygiene 4
pet ownership 2
phagocyte activation 47, 68
phenotype 213, 227, 229

phenotypic heterogeneity 213, 227
physical examination 4
plant 4
plaques 50
port-wine stains 262, 266, 267, 273, 274, 276, 281
post-inflammatory hyperpigmentation (PIH) 73, 74, 75, 76, 77, 78, 79, 80, 81, 82, 84, 85, 86, 87, 88, 89, 90, 91, 92
post-transplantation 7
potential renal failure 162, 180
predispose patients 1
predisposition 263
preterm birth 261, 262, 281
prevention 28, 29, 30, 35, 36, 38, 42
Propionibacterium acnes 188, 189, 210
pruritus 28, 29, 30, 31, 34, 38
psychological health 97, 103, 111
psychosocial impact 73, 75, 83, 84, 92
public health 2, 5, 7, 10, 11, 12, 13, 14, 16, 18, 19, 20
pulmonary hypertension 188, 207
purpuric vasculitic pattern 161, 180

Q

quality of life 73, 74, 75, 77, 78, 79, 81, 82, 83, 84, 85, 86, 88, 89, 90, 91, 92, 94

R

race 261, 281
rash 142, 146, 147, 157
recognition 1
redness 4
reflectance confocal microscopy (RCM) 2, 8
renal dysfunction 142, 156
respiratory impairment 4
respiratory tract 47, 68
revertant mosaicism (RM) 215, 218, 227
ringworm 2

S

sarcoidosis 187, 188, 189, 190, 191, 192, 193, 194, 195, 196, 197, 198, 199, 200, 201, 202, 203, 204, 205, 206, 207, 208, 209, 210
Sarcoptes scabiei 28, 29, 31, 38, 39, 40, 41, 42, 43
sarcoptic mange 27, 42
scabicides 28, 42
scabies 27, 28, 29, 30, 31, 32, 34, 35, 36, 38, 39, 40, 42, 43
scaling 4, 21
scalp 3
scleroderma 141, 143, 144, 145, 146, 148, 149, 150, 151, 152, 153, 154, 155, 156, 157
sclerodermatomyositis 142, 148, 151, 152, 156
sclerotherapy 262, 273, 275, 281
Seborrheic dermatitis 234, 254
self-esteem 73, 74, 77, 81, 82, 83, 86, 92
Shwitra 98
skin 1, 2, 3, 4, 5, 6, 8, 9, 10, 22, 23, 25, 26
skin architecture 213, 227
skin biopsies 236, 254
skin folds 29
skin lesions 188, 196, 200, 203, 207
skin parasites 1
Small vessel vasculitis 163
social embarrassment 97, 99, 111
soft tissues 47, 68
soil 4, 7
stimuli 117, 123, 135, 235, 244, 254
stratum corneum 4
strawberry marks 262, 281
stroke 162, 170
subepidermal splitting 117, 135
sun exposure 74, 76, 81, 83, 92
sun sensitivity 97, 111
superficial mycoses 1, 2, 3, 4, 11, 12, 17
susceptibility 2, 7, 8, 18, 29
symptomatology 187, 192, 207
symptoms 28, 29, 30, 34, 39, 42
systemic infections 2
Systemic Lupus Erythematosus (SLE) 141, 142, 156

T

targeted therapy 188, 207
T-cell proliferation 188
therapeutic drugs 2
therapeutic protocols 141, 156

therapy 236, 237, 238, 243, 245, 250, 253, 257
thyroid diseases 98, 111
tinea corporis 3
tinea pedis 2, 3, 4, 12
tinea versicolor 3
tissue ischemia 162, 170
T-lymphocytes 48, 68
toxicity 161, 166, 180
treatment 2, 3, 4, 5, 6, 8, 11, 13, 14, 15, 16, 17, 18, 19, 20, 21, 24
treatment modalities 27, 30, 42
Trichophyton mentagrophytes 3
Trichophyton rubrum 2, 3, 21
tumor necrosis factor-alpha (TNF-α) 190

U

ulcers 50
ultraviolet (UV) radiation 75, 78, 79, 80, 81, 84, 89

V

vascular hamartomas 261, 271, 281, 283
vasculitis 161, 162, 163, 164, 165, 166, 167, 168, 169, 170, 171, 172, 173, 174, 175, 176, 177, 178, 179, 180, 181, 182, 183, 184, 185
vesiculobullous diseases 117, 118, 120, 121, 122, 123, 125, 126, 127, 128, 129, 130, 131, 132, 133, 134, 135, 136, 137
veterinary medicine 27, 36, 42
viral infections 161, 180
vitamin D metabolism abnormalities 188, 207
vitiligo 97, 98, 99, 100, 101, 103, 104, 105, 106, 107, 108, 109, 110, 111, 112, 113, 114, 115
vulnerable populations 27, 31, 42

W

water 4

Y

yeasts 2, 4

Z

zoonotic disease 27, 42